Michael Strobel Jürgen Eichhorn
Wilfried Schießler

Basic Principles of Knee Arthroscopy

Normal and Pathological Findings
Tips and Tricks

With a Foreword by Wilhelm Klein

Translation by Terry C. Telger

With 235 Figures (Mostly in Color)
Containing 410 Separate Illustrations
and 23 Tables

Springer-Verlag
Berlin Heidelberg New York
London Paris Tokyo
Hong Kong Barcelona
Budapest

Dr. Michael Strobel
Klinik und Poliklinik für Unfall- und Handchirurgie
Westfälische Wilhelms-Universität, Jungeblodtplatz 1
D-4400 Münster

Dr. Jürgen Eichhorn
Belegabteilung für Orthopädie und Arthroskopische Chirurgie
Elisabeth-Krankenhaus
D-8440 Straubing

Dr. Wilfried Schießler
Zentrum für Chirurgie, Fachabteilung Unfallchirurgie
Klinikum der Stadt Nürnberg, Flurstr. 17
D-8500 Nürnberg 91

Translator
Terry C. Telger
6112 Waco Way, Ft. Worth, TX 76133, USA

Title of the German Edition
Arthroskopische Untersuchung des Kniegelenkes
ISBN 3-7691-0185-5; © by Deutscher Ärzte-Verlag GmbH, Köln 1989

ISBN-13:978-3-642-76331-1 e-ISBN-13:978-3-642-76329-8
DOI: 10.1007/978-3-642-76329-8

Library of Congress Cataloging-in-Publication Data
Strobel, Michael. [Arthroskopische Untersuchung des Kniegelenkes. English] Basic principles of knee arthroscopy : norma and pathological findings : tips and tricks / Michael Strobel, Jürgen Eichhorn, Wilfried Schiessler ; with a foreword by Wilhelm Klein ; translation by Terry C. Telger. p. cm.
Translation of: Arthroskopische Untersuchung des Kniegelenkes. Includes bibliographical references and index.
ISBN-13:978-3-642-76331-1
1. Knee-Examination. 2. Arthroscopy. I. Eichhorn, Jürgen, Dr. med. II. Schiessler, Wilfried. III. Title.
[DNLM: 1. Arthroscopy. 2. Knee Injuries-diagnosis. 3. Knee Injuries-surgery. 4. Knee Joint-physiology. 5. Knee Joint-surgery. WE 870 S919a]
RD561.S7613 1992 617.5'82-dc20 DNLM/DLC
for Library of Congress

Softcover reprint of the hardcover 1st edition 1992

Illustrations: Wilfried Schroeder, Münster

24/3145-543210 – Printed on acid-free paper

Foreword

No one suspected in the mid-1970s that endoscopic visualization of the joints would develop so swiftly into the class of operative procedures known as arthroscopic surgery. In the German-speaking countries arthroscopy was limited in the 1970s to a few operators who underwent a "natural" learning process involving arthroscopic inspection, confirmation by arthrotomy, and use of the arthroscope to verify clinical diagnoses. Video technology was not available, so an assistant wanting to view the joint interior had to peer through an accessory eyepiece.

The learning process in diagnostic arthroscopy was greatly enhanced by the advent of video technology. Everyone present in the operating room can witness the procedure on the video monitor as it takes place. Also, videotape recordings make the procedure accessible to persons who were not present during the operation.

The journey from diagnostic to operative arthroscopy has been a halting one. The first tentative steps taken by German physicians toward arthroscopic surgery were for the most part prompted by their North American colleagues. The first arthroscopic procedures were limited to tissue biopsies, the division of adhesions, and the resection of meniscal tags using hand-operated instruments.

The advent of motorized suction cutters from the United States has contributed much to arthroscopic surgery, laying essential groundwork for modern techniques of arthroscopic joint debridement and cruciate ligament reconstruction. The latest generation of arthroscopists now receive expert training at specialized centers.

Just as youngsters have no trouble mastering a computer, a young resident has an easier time mastering video arthroscopy. The older generation must overcome the problems of working abstractly "off the screen" without looking directly at the joint itself.

Particular difficulties are encountered by colleagues who are faced with the need to perform arthroscopic surgery but are not familiar with diagnostic arthroscopy. Unlike their predecessors, they can no longer follow the natural process of "learning by doing." They cannot contemplate the joint pathology displayed on the monitor and then check their arthroscopic findings in an open arthrotomy. Patients do not approve of this learning method. As a result, physicians not familiar with arthroscopic surgery are under considerable pressure, and increasingly they will lose their patients. It is therefore encumbent upon the still relatively small group of skilled arthroscopic surgeons to make their knowledge available to interested colleagues.

The ideal teaching process would convey both theoretical and practical knowledge within a relatively short period so that the busy surgeon could learn diagnostic arthroscopy and arthroscopic surgery at the same time. The reality, of course, is that both diagnostic and operative arthroscopy each require a long learning process. Yet this process has been made easier for the inexperienced physician by the evolution of standard, reproducible arthroscopic techniques. Newcomers have been spared the process of basic development with all its problems and frustrations.

On the other hand, the younger generation often lack the ability to find imaginative "makeshift" solutions to unexpected technical complications such as the failure of the video camera or a motorized instrument. Also, too little attention is given to the classic open joint dissection in modern arthroscopic practice.

Younger colleagues, who receive lengthy training in key points at specialized centers, have it easier today. They enjoy the additional advantage that "abstract operating" is easier for the young, although hand-to-eye coordination is not a gift possessed by all.

Books still represent the primary medium for the learner of arthroscopy. The problem is that the written word does not always match the reality of the operating room. "You don't find that in books!" is a comment frequently heard in training courses and in the operating suite. Yet it is the many unanticipated problems that can make the life of the arthroscopist an ordeal. This prompted the authors Michael Strobel, Jürgen Eichhorn, and Wilfried Schießler to publish a detailed account of their own practical arthroscopic experience. The present book is designed with the user in mind. The text is easy to understand. The many drawings aid comprehension and make the book a pleasure to read. The arthroscopic illustrations are superb. The reader will find the answers to any and all problems that confront him during the everyday practice of arthroscopy.

In short, the present book is an unqualified success, and I congratulate the authors on their remarkable achievement.

Düsseldorf

WILHELM KLEIN

Preface

In recent years arthroscopy of the knee joint has established itself as a routine procedure for diagnostic and, increasingly, therapeutic applications. Indeed, arthroscopy now belongs in the repertoire of every orthopedic, traumatologic, and surgical department, and many colleagues are now seeking to master the arthroscopic technique, due in large part to the significant benefits of arthroscopic surgery for the patient.

Because nearly all disorders of the knee joint can be treated arthroscopically, the efforts of the interested novice are too often focused on arthroscopic operations. The diagnostic role of arthroscopy is acknowledged, of course, but it is more intriguing to talk about special arthroscopic surgical techniques and new instrumentation. Sometimes it is even embarrassing to talk about diagnostic arthroscopy and the problems one has with it. In courses on arthroscopy it is common to find participants who are fully conversant with all available types of punches and shavers but do not know how to visualize the posterior horn of the meniscus.

Frequently there is too wide a gap between an individual's self-assessment and his arthroscopic proficiency.

Every beginner in arthroscopy, whether he is self-taught or guided by an experienced teacher, must struggle initially with numerous adversities, problems, and confusing situations. With this in mind, we offer a reference work in which the arthroscopic surgery-oriented procedures that have long proven effective in our practice are described in detail so that they can be reproduced by any operator. We do not consider it reasonable to demand that an operator complete 100 (or 200 or 300) diagnostic arthroscopies before he is entitled to perform arthroscopic surgery. It is far more sensible to attempt to convey the "philosophy of arthroscopy." This includes the inculcation of core principles, especially an understanding of the physical properties of oblique-viewing optical systems. The mastery of palpation with the probing hook, the accurate differentiation of normal and abnormal findings, and the assessment of their pathologic significance are key elements of arthroscopic surgery. Particular attention should be given to locating the portals for the arthroscope and instrument insertion. Optimum placement of the instrument portal is essential for a successful arthroscopic operation. A portal that gives clear access for the probing of a particular joint area can serve equally well for inserting a grasping forceps to take a synovial biopsy or extract a loose body. It is equally important to explore the many problem situations and complications that can arise during arthroscopy. After all, arthroscopy is not a simple, problem-free procedure that can be learned on a Saturday morning.

The period from the first arthroscopic examination to the first removal of a loose body is always much longer than the interval between the first arthroscopic operation and a difficult arthroscopic resection of the posterior horn of a meniscus.

The essential goal of this book is to smooth and shorten the path from the first arthroscopic examination to the first arthroscopic operation.

We are grateful to Mr. J. Kolditz, one of the fathers of arthroscopic surgery in Germany, for his many tips and suggestions. We thank our artist, Mr. W. Schroeder, for his excellent diagrams and drawings. We are indebted to

Dr. J. Grünert, Mr. A. Halder, Mr. T. Lutze, Dr. H. Neumann, Dr. H.-W. Stedtfeld, and Mrs. U. Strobel for reviewing our manuscript and offering several suggestions that were implemented in the book.

We express very sincere thanks to the staff of Springer-Verlag for their cheerful cooperation and for their outstanding production work on this book. We give special recognition and our sincere thanks to Mr. Terry C. Telger (Fort Worth, Texas) for undertaking the English translation.

Münster, Straubing, Nuremberg
August 1991

MICHAEL STROBEL, JÜRGEN EICHHORN,
WILFRIED SCHIESSLER

Contents

1 Historical Background

1.1 Early Instruments for Endoscopic Examinations

For centuries man has been intrigued by the prospect of rendering visible that which ordinarily cannot be seen. As early as 1806 the German physician Philipp Bozzini, driven by the emergent quest for knowledge during the Enlightenment, designed an instrument for illuminating the interior of human body cavities. The desire to study the inner functions of the human body was the driving force behind this development.

Bozzini's *Lichtleiter* (light conductor) consisted of a leather-sheathed metal tube containing an internal brass plate which spanned half its length. A concave mirror reflected the light from a wax candle through the tube into the body cavity. The brass partition created separate channels for illumination and reflection, allowing the examiner a glare-free view. Immersed in warm water and coated with oil, the instrument could theoretically be used to inspect the nasopharynx, rectum, vagina, bladder, and urethra. Bozzini envisioned major applications for his device in physiology, pathology, surgery, obstetrics, and even in pharmacology for testing the efficacy of medications. He foresaw the possibility of operative procedures and even designed an apparatus for performing hysterectomies that incorporated his *Lichtleiter* (Bozzini 1807).

While his discoveries were initially received with enthusiasm and stimulated spirited discussions in medical journals, interest soon dwindled. The derisive pronouncement of the Viennese Medical Society dealt a fatal blow to Bozzini's invention.

John Fisher, while still a medical student, developed an "instrument for the illumination of dark spaces." To increase the light intensity, he proposed to equip his device with an electrochemical power source in the form of galvanic cells. However, he does not appear to have applied his experimental efforts to living subjects. In 1826 Segalas independently designed his "speculum urethrocysticum" for examining the urethra and bladder.

Stimulated by the urethrocystic speculum of Segalas and building on the ideas of Bozzini, Antonin Desormeaux developed a device which he called the endoscope. First presented at the Academie de Medicine in Paris in November of 1853, this instrument became widely used in Europe and America following design improvements and refinements in the examination technique. The light source was a gazogene lamp, which burned a mixture of alcohol and turpentine, and the light was directed into the bladder by a concave mirror at the back of the instrument. The observer viewed the dimly lit interior of the bladder through an opening in the mirror.

Once it had been shown that body cavities could be examined through hollow tubes, attention focused on ways to develop simpler instruments and better light sources. The heat generated by the use of gazogene, petroleum, or burning magnesium filament often caused burns to the thigh. Moreover, the smoke produced by these lamps evoked an involuntary voiding response in anxious patients, frequently extinguishing the light source.

In 1867 the Dresden physician Max Nitze tried to solve the problem of low light intensity by developing a modification of the bladder diaphanoscope designed by Julius Bruck the same year. The light source consisted of a battery-powered incandescent platinum loop, the heat from which was dissipated by a continuous flow of water around the instrument. Nitze commissioned the Berlin optician Beneche to design a new type of lens system for expanding the field of view. The instrument maker Leiter succeeded in combining a light source, optical system, and water cooling system in one instrument only 7 mm in diameter.

Nitze, who came to examinations equipped with batteries and buckets of water, often elicted only a contemptuous smile from his colleagues with his "light and water show." Indeed, his experience is similar to that of many present-day arthroscopists who find the operating room flooded by their "waterworks" when they perform their first arthroscopic operations in a fluid medium.

The discovery of the carbon-filament incandescent light bulb by Thomas Edison in 1879 provided a compact, relatively low-temperature light source of high intensity that could be mounted at the tip of an endscope without the need for a cooling system. This invention greatly enhanced the usefulness of the Nitze urethroscope. In 1886 Leiter developed a cystoscope that was used by physicians all over the world (Fig. 1-1).

Just before the turn of the century, this new type of illumination made it possible for the first time to photograph the interior of the bladder and stomach using a special camera. In subsequent years the Leiter cystoscope underwent several modifications so that it could be sterilized to meet the requirements of aseptic technique.

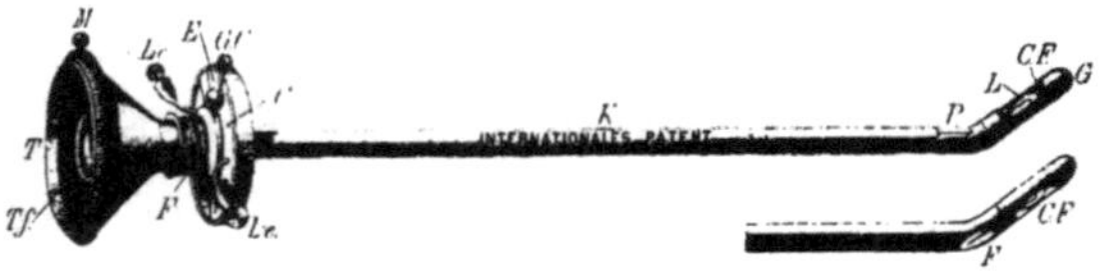

Fig. 1-1. The Leiter cystoscope (1886) (from Donner 1979)

1.2 Eugen Bircher

The difficulty of diagnosing many joint disorders, even by a very thorough clinical examination, prompted the Swiss surgeon Eugen Bircher (Fig. 1-2) in 1913 to look for improved ways to diagnose injuries of the menisci in the knee. After his father, Heinrich Bircher, director of the district hospital at Aarau, acquired the hospital's first cystoscope in 1909, Eugen Bircher began to perform endoscopic examinations of the knee joint at the same facility. He used the Jacobaeus laparoscope, which he considered to be safer and better suited for use in the knee than in the peritoneal cavity. Initially he examined cadaveric knee joints inflated with oxygen or nitrogen to facilitate insertion of the scope and illumination of the intraarticular compartments.

In 1921 Bircher published his classic paper "Die Arthro-Endoskopie" detailing the results of knee arthroscopies in 18 patients. In

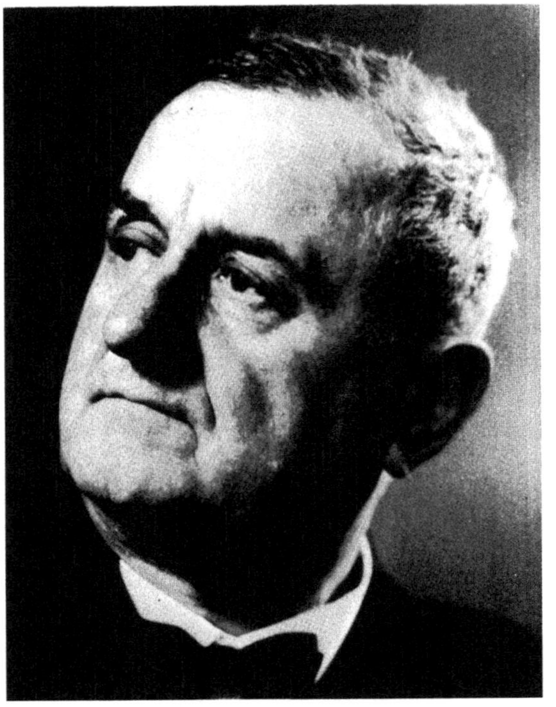

Fig. 1-2. Eugen Bircher (1882–1956)

13 cases he was able to make a correct diagnosis which was subsequently confirmed by arthrotomy. In 3 cases arthroscopic findings were equivocal, and in 2 tuberculous joints he was unable to perform a successful examination. The following year Bircher announced that he had already examined 35 patients endoscopically.

Besides being the first physician to successfully use arthroscopy clinically, Eugen Bircher gave an accurate prediction of its future development: "Arthroscopy permits us to visualize the interior of the joint and evaluate pathologic changes, and thus to establish a diagnosis by visual observation. In this respect it is superior to all other methods of examination and, like endoscopy of the bladder, can be used to define certain indications for surgery. Also like cystoscopy, it will meet with resistance but undoubtedly will gain in popularity and develop until it becomes as indispensable as cystoscopy itself" (Bircher 1922).

Today, many aspects of Bircher's arthroscopic technique remain as valid as his predictions. For example, he believed that strict surgical asepsis like that practiced in arthrotomy was the first and foremost requirement for successful arthroscopy. He exsanguinated the limb with an Esmarch bandage to obtain a bloodless field. He performed arthroscopy in a darkened room, and he distended the joint with oxygen or nitrogen using an artificial pneumothorax apparatus. Bircher also employed the basic insertion technique that is used today: a sheath and sharp trocar are introduced into the joint, the trocar is replaced by a blunt trocar, and finally the trocar is replaced by the viewing scope.

Bircher additionally offered important suggestions for orientation within the joint: "An extremely useful landmark is the patellar border, from which the examiner may track upward or downward. The wide, sharp, black line of the patellar border contrasts sharply with the glistening white surface of the patella, separating it from the bright pink inner capsule of the joint. The scope may be swept upward along the patellar border to the center of the distal femur and downward to demonstrate the cruciate ligaments" (Bircher 1922).

Bircher was also a pioneer of ambulatory arthroscopy, describing the case of one female patient who could be discharged home immediately after the examination (Bircher 1922).

Interestingly, experiments in cadavers led Bircher to conclude that arthroscopic examination was not feasible in the shoulder, elbow, hip, or ankle joints.

Besides being the father of arthroscopy, Bircher also developed arthrography and pneumoarthrography of the knee joint. He was additionally interested in surgery of the stomach and esophagus and the surgical treatment of goiter. Beyond this, Bircher was a prominent Swiss military officer and parlementarian. The excellent biography *Eugen Bircher: Doctor, Soldier, Politician*, written by Daniel Heller in 1988, highlights the controversial personality of its subject. Characterized as impulsive and high-spirited, Bircher had a coarse and even vulgar side to his nature that contrasted markedly with his meticulous work as a surgeon. He rarely minced words and spoke out vehemently against any kind of medical chicanery (Heller 1988).

1.3 Kenji Takagi

The Tokyo surgeon Kenji Takagi reported in 1939 that he had attempted to examine the interior of cadaveric knee joints with a cystoscope as early as 1918, although these initial attempts were unsuccessful (Fig. 1-3). In 1920 he developed a simple arthroscope whose large size made it impractical for routine use. His primary goal was the early detection of tuberculosis of the knee, which at that time was widespread in Japan. Through prompt diagnosis, Takagi hoped to refer his patients for early treatment and forestall the crippling effects of the disease. Takagi wrote: "There was only one case, that of an elderly woman with draining tuberculous arthritis of the knee, in which this simple arthroscope was successfully inserted from the external orifice of the fistula. We tried to visualize the interior of the

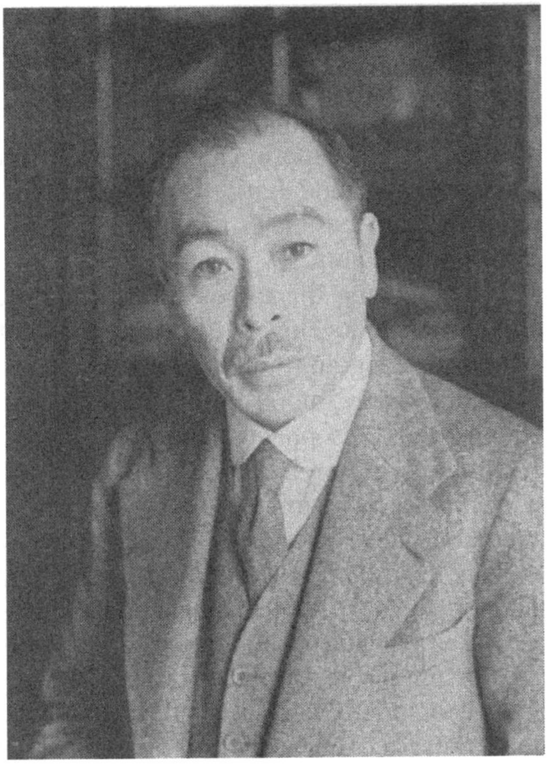

Fig. 1-3. Kenji Takagi (1888–1963) (from Watanabe 1969)

joint, but fluid leakage through the fistula prevented our ballooning the lumen."

Takagi's arthroscope did not have a lens system, and its tiny field of vision forced him to use a large-caliber instrument (7.3 mm) that was quite difficult to handle. His first concern, therefore, was to reduce the instrument diameter. This made it necessary to incorporate a lens system. Takagi designed a series of arthroscopes in subsequent years, and by 1931 he had succeeded in reducing the diameter to 3.5 mm. His thinnest model, the No. 11 arthroscope, was only 2.7 mm in diameter. His No. 12 model, 4.4 mm in diameter, was suitable for obtaining biopsies. In collaboration with Jino, Takagi was the first to photograph and film the interior of the knee joint. The first black-and-white arthroscopic photographs of the knee joint were published in 1932, and the first color photographs were taken 4 years later. In 1938 Takagi presented his results and experiences at the annual meeting of the Japanese Orthopedic Society.

1.4 Development of Diagnostic Arthroscopy

Today it seems difficult to understand the tepid response to the early reports of Bircher and Takagi. Yet skepticism prevailed, as illustrated by the Dutch physician Hustinx (1937) who claimed that the very anatomy of the knee joint made arthroscopy worthless: "How can one dare to introduce a bulky object into the knee joint to look between articular surfaces that cannot be pushed apart. Even in an arthrotomy, the posterior horn of the meniscus cannot be seen. So how can one expect to view that structure in a closed knee? It is simply impossible" (Hustinx 1937). He also considered arthroscopy to be a far more dangerous procedure than exploratory arthrotomy.

Philipp Kreuscher became the first American surgeon to advocate this new procedure for the diagnosis of meniscus lesions. He presented his study to the Illinois Medical Society in 1925, but we have no detailed information on the type of arthroscope that he used.

In 1926 the American surgeon Geist first described the potential use of an arthroscope for taking small biopsy specimens from the knee joint for microscopic examination, analogous to the procedure used by urologists. Technical problems delayed the practical application of this procedure until Harry Mayer and Leo Finkelstein of the Hospital for Joint Diseases in New York developed an arthroscope 8 mm in diameter for punch biopsies. In 1931 Michael S. Burman, today recognized as the pioneer of arthroscopy in the U.S., worked with the instrument maker Wappler to design an arthroscope that embodied some important basic features of present-day instruments. Burman, working in collaboration with Finkelstein and Mayer, performed numerous cadaver experiments which laid the groundwork for the clinical application of arthroscopy. Following the insertion of a trocar 4 mm in diameter, the joint was irrigated and distended with Ringer's solution and then inspected with a 3–mm direct-viewing arthroscope. Burman described various approaches to the knee joint and researched the potential applications of arthroscopy in the hip, ankle, shoulder, and elbow. However, technical deficiencies aroused the skepticism of many colleagues, and the *Atlas of Arthroscopy* compiled by Burman remained unpublished.

In 1937 the German physician Rene Sommer continued research on knee joint arthroscopy at the Brüder Hospital in Dortmund. He used the Graf thoracoscope manufactured by the C. G. Heynemann company of Leipzig. This instrument, which was equipped with a sharp trocar, provided easy access to the joint interior, especially when intraarticular effusion was present. In knees without effusion, Sommer initially recommended distention of the joint with O_2. He inserted the scope from the lateral side through the suprapatellar pouch with the knee extended. From there he could inspect the anterior portions of the menisci, the intercondylar fossa, and the anterior cruciate ligament. He believed that the ability to inspect the infrapatellar fat pad was a major advantage of arthroscopy. At that time inflammatory, hypertrophic, and synovial proliferative changes in the infrapatellar fat pad were frequently held responsible for functional derangements of the knee.

In 1938 the rheumatologist Vaubel performed arthroscopic examinations in patients with chronic joint disease. He hoped that serial examinations would provide a means of studying the progression of rheumatoid arthritis.

Wilke conducted systematic arthroscopic examinations of 56 cadaveric knees in 1938. He examined them with a 6–mm Kalk thoracoscope after first distending the joint with 180 ml of water. The meniscus could be plainly seen, but as time passed an emulsion formed in the joint which hampered further inspection, prompting him to change to air as an arthroscopic medium. While Wilke regarded endoscopy as a technique that enriched diagnosis, he did not recommend it as a routine procedure in live patients.

Development of this promising procedure ceased in Europe during the Second World War, and it was not until 1955 and 1956 that Hurter and Imbert reported on further arthroscopic experience in Germany.

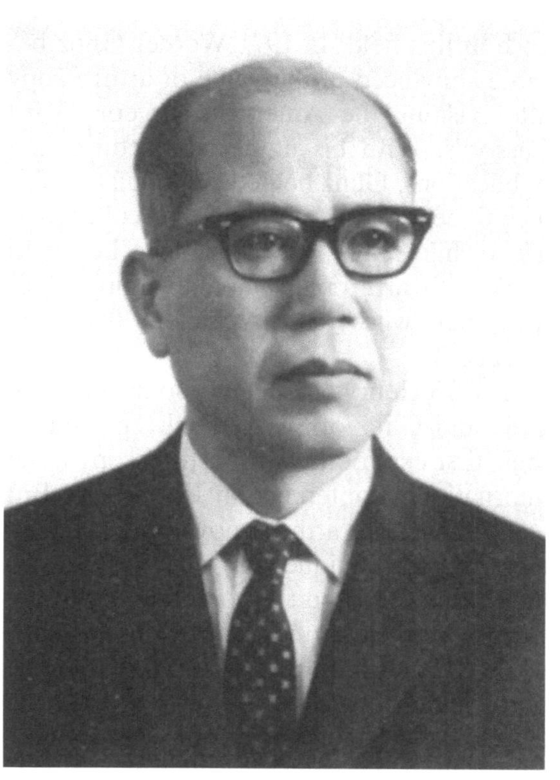

Fig. 1-4. Masaki Watanabe

Success and ongoing refinements of arthroscopic technique enabled Takagi's most outstanding pupil, Masaki Watanabe, to make arthroscopy known outside the borders of Japan (Fig. 1-4). The first edition of the *Atlas of Arthroscopy,* which Watanabe authored in collaboration with S. Takeda and H. Ikeuchi, was published in 1957. This atlas stimulated world-wide interest in arthroscopy of the knee joint and formed an important basis for its further evolution.

The great breakthrough in arthroscopy did not come, however, until the early 1970s. Watanabe developed a number of new arthroscopes, including the famous No. 21 arthroscope, which enjoyed great popularity in the United States.

The Viennese surgeon Wruhs, a colonel in the medical corps, has performed arthroscopies since the early 1970s. Since 1972 Christoph

Kieser of Zurich has also reported on experience in this field. In 1971 Werner Glinz became convinced of the value of arthroscopy after visiting the American surgeon Ward Casscells. With his numerous lectures and publications, Glinz helped to popularize this technique among many of his colleagues. Meanwhile Hans Rudolf Henche began to work with arthroscopy at the urging of E. Morscher, who was his chief at that time (Henche).

In 1973 Henry of England, Johnson of the U.S., and Glinz of Switzerland reported on their first experience with arthroscopy at an international conference in Rotterdam. But even at that time, arthroscopy was far from an established technique. As related by Glinz, the president closed the conference with the words: "Mr. Henry hospitalizes his patients, while Mr. Johnson and Mr. Glinz perform outpatient arthroscopies. I watch my patients closely for 15 minutes in my office, and I know what's wrong with their knee!" (Glinz 1985).

1.5 Development of Arthroscopic Surgery

Arthroscopic surgery traces much of its development to Watanabe, who on March 9, 1955, removed a xanthomatous giant cell tumor from the suprapatellar pouch under arthroscopic vision. On May 4, 1962, Watanabe performed the first arthroscopic meniscectomy by resecting a small meniscal flap.

Impressed by Watanabe's results, O'Connor of the U.S. visited Watanabe in 1970 to learn his arthroscopic technique. O'Connor has performed arthroscopic meniscectomies since 1974 and has developed many special operating instruments, including an arthroscope that enabled him to perform meniscectomies through a single portal. In 1976 Jackson and Dandy published the first English-language textbook on arthroscopy. Later O'Connor conducted numerous practical courses which broadened the use of the arthroscopic technique. Hans-Rudolf Henche published the first German-language textbook on arthroscopy in 1978. Capturing the intraarticular image with a video camera and transmitting it to a television screen, first described by McGinty, has contributed fundamentally to the further development of diagnostic and operative arthroscopy.

In the ensuing years, arthroscopic surgical options have expanded at an explosive pace. Lanny L. Johnson, who introduced motorized operative instruments (shaver systems) and worked extensively with arthroscopic procedures on the cartilage, is still considered one of the most influential promotors of arthroscopic surgery. In the third edition of his now two-volume work *Arthroscopic Surgery-Principles and Practice*, he devotes more than 1500 pages to describing the possibilities and principles of arthroscopic surgery.

1.6 Outlook

Today arthroscopy is still expanding, and there is no end in sight. New arthroscopic instruments and operating techniques are constantly being described.

Research is currently being done on the capabilities of arthroscopic laser surgery. Increasing attention is being focused on arthroscopic reconstruction of the anterior cruciate ligament and on meniscal repair. Moreover, arthroscopy is being applied to other joints such as the shoulder, elbow, wrist, hip, and ankle. Even very small joints like the interphalangeal and temporomandibular articulations are "not safe" from arthroscopic scrutiny. Watanabe published a book on the arthroscopy of small joints in 1985.

The scope of developments is illustrated by soft-tissue endoscopy, used for the examination and treatment of subcutaneous soft tissues (muscles, nerves, blood vessels). Through this technique, soft structures can be visually inspected and selectively biopsied. Endoscopic division of the carpal roof also has been reported.

The significance of soft-tissue endoscopy as a diagnostic and therapeutic modality will become more clear with passage of time (Watanabe 1985).

The evolutionary history of arthroscopy is best summarized by the words of Bozzini: "Every invention owes its existence to a fortuitous combination of diverse circumstances. It is always born a child and, like a child, matures and progresses in stages, becoming ever more complete" (Bozzini 1807).

2
Indications for Arthroscopy of the Knee Joint

Even an exhaustive noninvasive diagnostic workup, including clinical, radiographic (tomography, CT), sonographic, and radioisotopic studies and even magnetic resonance imaging, may not furnish a conclusive diagnosis. These cases require evaluation by more invasive procedures like arthroscopy. However, the indications for these procedures must be clearly defined.

The main danger of such a relatively complication-free procedure as arthroscopy lies in its too-frequent, uncritical application. The arthroscopic examination can supplement but cannot replace a careful history and a systematic clinical examination. Arthroscopy, then, should serve to clarify or establish a diagnosis only after all clinical methods of examination have been exhausted. Arthroscopy is too often regarded as "the" examination technique for the knee joint in general.

The options made available by arthroscopic surgery have greatly expanded the scope of indications for arthroscopy. Thus, there are many situations in which an examiner with sufficient experience in arthroscopy will gladly opt for a procedure with which he can both evaluate the knee joint and perform various therapeutic interventions.

2.1 Diagnostic Indications

Diagnostic arthroscopy is indicated in cases where:

- a definitive diagnosis is not supplied by the history, clinical examination, or radiology (e.g., hemarthrosis, locking, unexplained pain or effusion, meniscus injury, cartilage lesions);
- it is necessary to evaluate for associated injuries after trauma (e.g., after patallar dislocation);
- it is necessary to evaluate the condition of the joint prior to operation.

2.1.1 Hemarthrosis

Posttraumatic hemarthrosis most commonly results from a severe intraarticular injury, often with involvement of the anterior cruciate ligament. In patients with no evidence of bony injury, the clinical examination focuses on the exclusion or confirmation of patellar dislocation or a capsuloligamentous injury.

The specific diagnostic test for patellar dislocation is *Fairbank's apprehension test,* in which the examiner recreates the mechanism of the luxation by pressing the patella laterally while the knee is extended. The patient is then told to flex his knee. With a recent patellar dislocation, the patient experiences such pain and fear of recurrence, especially on moving the knee from extension to flexion, that he will often attempt to avoid the maneuver or will complain of severe pain.

In the absence of any other cause, such as a fracture, that might account for the posttraumatic hemarthrosis, it should be assumed that the anterior cruciate ligament is ruptured until it has been proven otherwise.

Far too often the integrity of the anterior cruciate ligament is assessed only by performing the anterior drawer test in 90° flexion. This laxity test is usually negative in the acutely traumatized knee, because intraarticular effusion either prevents knee flexion to 90° or makes such a movement extremely painful. Also, the raised intraarticular pressure in that joint position intensifies the pain, which in turn evokes a reflex contraction of the muscles of the thigh. With the knee thus flexed, a positive drawer sign cannot be elicited. The anterior drawer test is better tolerated when it is performed with the knee almost extended, and thus in a painless or relatively painless position. Known as the *Lachman test*, this maneuver represents the most important laxity test in the acutely injured knee. Isolated ruptures of the anterior cruciate ligament can be diagnosed with the Lachman test even when there is coexisting intraarticular effusion. As in all laxity tests, the examiner should assess the end-point resilience. A *firm end point* signifies that the anterior cruciate ligament may be intact (e.g., but very lax), elongated, or partially torn, whereas a *soft end point* implies a complete rupture of the ligament. It can be determined through selective questioning whether the rupture is recent or old. The pivot-shift tests are often false-negative immediately after a trauma. The subluxating forces applied in the tests (internal rotation of the upper tibia, valgus pressure) stretch the medial ligaments, which frequently are involved by the injury, and the resulting pain again incites reflex muscular guarding. Acutely injured patients rarely show a positive pivot-shift test unless examined under anesthesia (see Chap. 5).

Hemarthrosis can have causes other than a torn anterior cruciate ligament or dislocated patella (Table 2-1). If hemarthrosis develops after a trivial injury or without apparent cause, coagulation studies should be done to rule out a hematologic disorder, as before any arthroscopic procedure. In 4%–10% of cases arthroscopy reveals no identifiable morphologic cause for the intraarticular hemorrhage.

In knees with a positive Lachman test and a soft end point, arthroscopy is not indicated for the purpose of demonstrating a torn anterior cruciate ligament; this has already been satisfactorily established by the clinical examination. In terms of treatment planning, however, it is important to know whether the rupture is recent or old, whether it involves the proximal, distal or midportion of the ligament, and whether there are associated meniscal injuries. A number of pathologic conditions should be considered in the differential diagnosis of hemarthrosis (Table 2-1). Some of these are difficult or impossible to differentiate by clinical means. Thus, arthroscopy should be used to investigate hemarthrosis in all cases where a definitive diagnosis is not provided by a comprehensive noninvasive workup.

Table 2-1. Differential diagnosis of hemarthrosis

- Rupture of anterior cruciate ligament
- Patellar dislocation
- Meniscal tear
- Synovial tear
- Osteochondral fracture
- Tear of mediopatellar or infrapatellar plica
- Fissure fracture of the upper tibia or femoral condyle
- Epiphyseal plate injury
- Intraarticular tumor (e.g., hemangioma)
- Sequela of intraarticular needle insertion
- Anticoagulant medication
- Hemophilia
- Nondiscernible cause

2.1.2 Locking

Locking of the knee may occur spontaneously in the absence of trauma, or it may develop in the immediate posttraumatic period. It is manifested by an inability to flex or extend the knee completely. Various diseases and injuries can produce this condition (Table 2-2). If a diagnosis is not established by clinical and radiologic studies, diagnostic arthroscopy is indicated.

No other diagnostic procedure is as accurate as arthroscopy in identifying the cause of acute locking in the knee. Common causes are meniscal injuries as well as partial and complete ruptures of the anterior cruciate ligament.

Table 2-2. Differential diagnosis of acute locking

- Meniscal tear
- Partial rupture of the anterior cruciate ligament
- Complete rupture of the anterior cruciate ligament
- Partial rupture of the posterior cruciate ligament
- Injury of the medial collateral ligament
- Entrapment of a loose body
- Intraarticular effusion
- Chondromalacia
- False locking due to pain
- Intraarticular tumor
- Psychogenic
- No pathologic findings

Table 2-3. Differential diagnosis of intermittent locking

- Meniscal tear (bucket handle, flap tear)
- Loose body (cartilage, osteochondral fragment)
- Hypertrophic villus on infrapatellar fat pad (behaves like meniscal flap)
- Exophyte (rare)
- Ruptured cruciate ligament fibers (behaves like a meniscal flap)
- Patellar subluxation
- Plica syndrome (hypertrophic mediopatellar plica)
- Chondromatosis
- Anomaly of the lateral or medial meniscus (discoid meniscus)
- Intraarticular foreign body (glass fragment, needle)

Intermittent locking can be difficult to interpret clinically (Table 2-3), but arthroscopy is extremely helpful in identifying and perhaps eliminating the cause.

2.1.3 Recurrent Effusion

Effusion is usually secondary to degenerative conditions of the cartilage and menisci, but various other diseases may also be causative (Table 2-4).

If a mechanical cause is not found for recurrent effusion in the knee, a synovial biopsy for microscopic evaluation should be obtained routinely during arthroscopy.

Table 2-4. Causes of recurrent effusion in the knee joint

- Degenerative cartilage changes
- Meniscal lesions
- Chronic ligament instabilities
- Loose bodies
- Chronic rheumatoid arthritis
- Ankylosing spondylitis (Bekhterev's disease)
- Chondrocalcinosis
- Gout
- Collagen disease
- Enteritis
- Hemophilia
- Yersinia infection
- Sympathetic effusion due to extraarticular disease

Diagnostic arthroscopy is rarely indicated for chronic effusions, because the diagnosis is satisfactorily established by clinical and radiographic methods and by a biochemical analysis of aspirated fluid.

2.1.4 Cartilage Injuries

Clinical and radiographic studies are of limited value for the diagnostic evaluation of cartilage injuries and other cartilage disorders. Even arthrography gives only a limited view of the cartilage surface. Magnetic resonance imaging (MRI) is much better for evaluating the thickness and condition of the cartilage (see Fig. 9-1), but it is a costly study, and further experience is needed in order to assess the value of MRI of the joints.

Arthroscopy provides an effective, readily available technique for assessing the size, depth, and perhaps the etiology of traumatic and degenerative cartilage disorders. It should be noted, however, that while cartilage changes are among the most common arthroscopic findings in general, the clinical presentation frequently does not correlate with the cartilage morphology. Patients with massive cartilage changes often report very mild complaints, while an essentially "virgin" cartilage may be seen in patients with severe knee pain.

Large osteochondral fractures can usually be diagnosed by radiography. Arthroscopy is indicated when it is uncertain whether an osteochondral fracture is present or where the osteochondral fragment originates. Arthroscopy is helpful in deciding whether it would be feasible to attempt reattachment of the osteochondral fragment. Sometimes the fragment consists of multiple small pieces held together by small bridges of tissue. In these cases arthroscopic removal of the entire fragment will eliminate the need for an arthrotomy.

Osteochondral and chondral fractures are a frequent cause of hemarthrosis in pediatric knee injuries.

2.1.5 Pain of Unknown Etiology

Arthroscopy is indicated in both young and old patients for the evaluation of knee pain whose cause cannot be verified by other means. However, arthroscopy should be used very sparingly in young women with anterior knee pain. This condition usually resolves spontaneously after 20–25 years of age, and arthroscopy is warranted only if the pain is persistent and severe.

In adolescents with obscure knee pain, Glinz (1987) was able to confirm the presumptive clinical diagnosis in only 18% of cases. He identified meniscal injuries, cruciate ligament injuries, cartilage lesions, and a hypertrophic medial shelf as the causes of the pain. In over 15% of patients with unexplained knee pain, no definite evidence of pathology can be found. This leads some patients to regard the arthroscopic examination as pointless ("Then I shouldn't have had the operation after all!"). However, the normal findings can serve as a basis for reassuring the patient that there is nothing seriously wrong with the knee.

Knee soreness in children should never be dismissed as "growing pains," even with a negative arthroscopic examination. Instead, a selective radiographic study of the entire affected extremity and of the pelvis should be included in the differential diagnostic workup of pediatric knee pain. Blood studies that include a differential blood count can also be performed to exclude a rheumatoid disorder or a malignant systemic disease such as leukemia, whose first presenting symptom may be knee pain.

2.1.6 Meniscal Tears

If there is clinical suspicion of a meniscal tear, the meniscus should be evaluated arthroscopically prior to arthrotomy, even if an arthroscopic meniscectomy is not proposed. Only arthroscopic examination can accurately localize the tear and define its extent. The decision whether to resect or repair a torn meniscus is also based on arthroscopic findings.

It is not unusual for the symptoms of a lateral meniscus tear to project to the medial side. Preliminary arthroscopy is of great value in these cases, as it avoids arthrotomizing the wrong side of the joint. It is also common for retropatellar complaints or a medial shelf to produce meniscus-like symptoms that can be very difficult to interpret by clinical means.

2.1.7 Detection of Associated Injuries for Preoperative Planning

Before reconstruction of the anterior cruciate ligament in chronic instability, arthroscopy should be performed to evaluate for preexisting cartilage damage and involvement of the menisci by degenerative change or injury.

In patients with acute ligament injuries, arthroscopy can be used to check for associated injuries (posterior horn meniscus tears, contusions or flake fractures of cartilage). Findings in these cases may prompt the selection of a different arthrotomic approach.

Arthroscopy in patients with acute capsuloligamentous injuries should be performed briskly to minimize the leakage of fluid through ruptured portions of the capsule into subcutaneous tissues.

Diagnostic arthroscopy is also recommended before corrective osteotomy to evaluate the joint compartment that will be weight-bearing once the angular correction has been carried out. Significant cartilage disruption in that area may imply a reduced chance for a successful corrective outcome.

Arthroscopy before ligament reconstructions and corrective osteotomies can also help make patient expectations more realistic by identifying preexisting damage that may still be asymptomatic.

Secondary Baker cysts, especially in older patients, are frequently associated with severe intraarticular lesions that incite an increased production of synovial fluid and thus perpetuate the cyst. Curative treatment for this type of cyst must involve removal of the causative intraarticular lesion.

2.1.8 Arthroscopy in Children and Adolescents

Meniscal tears, cartilage lesions, trauma from patellar dislocation, and ruptures of the anterior cruciate ligament are common arthroscopic findings in children and adolescents. Not infrequently, the time elapsed between trauma and definitive diagnosis is so long that adequate treatment can no longer be provided.

Osteochondral fractures are significantly more common than in the adult population, and this must be taken into account when making a diagnosis. Surgical reattachment of the fragment in the hope of achieving anatomic healing is sensible only if a timely diagnosis has been made. In cases where diagnosis and postoperative functional exercises are delayed, the fragment often becomes entrapped between the joint surfaces, leading inevitably to fracturing of the fragment and further cartilage damage. Severe injuries should be excluded before a decision is made whether conservative treatment or postoperative functional exercises would be of greater benefit.

Thus, an indication for diagnostic arthroscopy is recognized in pediatric patients with obscure knee pain, unexplained swelling, recurrent locking, osteochondral fractures, and hemarthrosis.

2.1.9 Arthroscopy for Settling Liability Judgments

In rare cases diagnostic arthroscopy is indicated to establish causality, i.e., in insurance settlements or in patients contending for compensation benefits.

2.1.10 Control Arthroscopy

In patients who have residual complaints following a previous operation, arthroscopy can be used to check for deterioration or improvement of the initial findings. Arthroscopy can even be scheduled before the first operation in cases where, for example, an alloplastic or autologous material is to be implanted to reconstruct the anterior cruciate ligament. The synovial reaction in the joint, the width of the intercondylar notch, and the condition of the implant can be arthroscopically evaluated. Any factors that threaten the function or integrity of the implant, such as osteophytes, can be simultaneously removed.

2.2 Therapeutic Indications

Nearly all intraarticular disorders are amenable to arthroscopic treatment (see below and Chap. 16).

2.3 Contraindications to Arthroscopy

Arthroscopy is not a vitally important or life-saving procedure, so the candidate for arthroscopy should be in an optimum state of health. In elderly patients, specific medical and anesthesiologic preparation is recommended due to the higher incidence of local and systemic complications in that group (Sherman 1986).

In patients with an infectious disease (e.g., influenza, angina tonsillaris, hepatitis), arthroscopy should be postponed until the infection has cleared. Arthroscopy is also contraindicated in patients with skin eruptions or unhealed abrasions about the affected knee. Arthroscopy may be performed when all superficial signs of infection or inflammation have resolved.

An acute, extensive capsuloligamentous disruption is a relative contraindication to arthroscopy, as it may allow large amounts of irrigating solution to leak from the joint into the compartments of the thigh, posing a risk of compartment syndrome.

While bacterial contamination of the skin is a contraindication, arthroscopy is the method of choice for treating an intraarticular infection following, say, an intraarticular injection or an arthroscopic procedure (see Sect. 12.7).

3
Equipment

Considerable equipment and instrumentation are needed for diagnostic arthroscopy. The minimum requirements are as follows:

- sheath (trocar sleeve) with a sharp trocar and blunt obturator
- arthroscopic telescope
- light cable
- light source
- irrigation system for distending the joint
- probe

The equipment should allow for safe, smooth conduct of the arthroscopic examination. Continual refinements have been made in arthroscopic equipment in recent years, the most important development being the incorporation of video technology using increasingly compact, high-resolution cameras. Major improvements also relate to the development of improved arthroscope sheaths and of optical systems that provide an expanded field of view.

3.1
Arthroscope

The arthroscope consists basically of the optical component (telescope) and the sheath into which the telescope is inserted.

3.1.1
Sheath

The assembled sheath and trocar create the access portal for inserting the telescope into the joint. First the sharp trocar is used to pierce the fibrous capsule, then it is replaced with the blunt obturator (Fig. 3-1). To reduce the risk of cartilage injury, many arthroscopists have stopped using a pointed trocar and use only a blunt obturator. To facilitate insertion of the sheath and obturator, the fibrous capsule is incised with a pointed scalpel when the skin

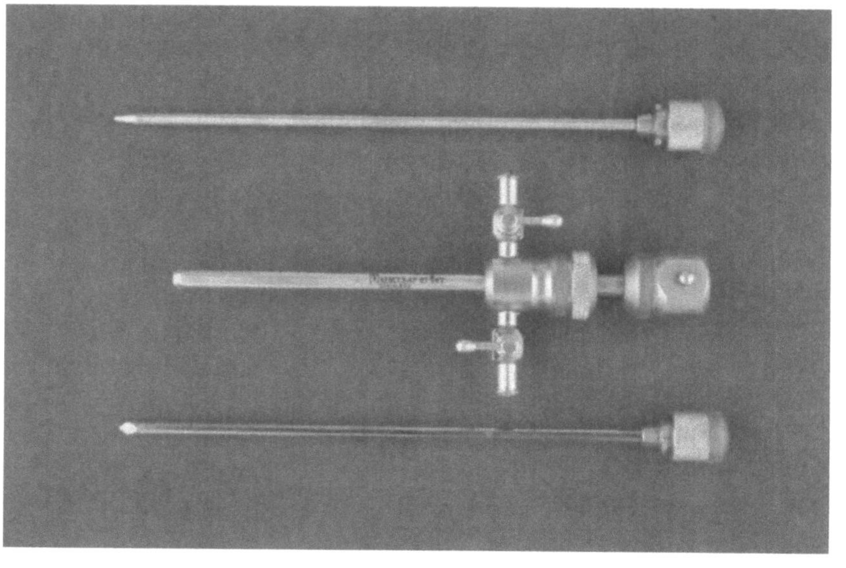

Fig. 3-1. Arthroscopic sheath with sharp trocar and blunt obturator (Aesculap)

incision is made. Once the sheath is inside the joint, the telescope is substituted for the obturator (see Sect. 6.1 for further details).

The sheath consists basically of a tube into which the telescope is inserted and locked in place. Spigots on the sheath regulate the inflow and outflow of the arthroscopic medium, usually a fluid. The difference between the inside diameter of the sheath (e.g., 6 mm) and the outside diameter of the telescope (e.g., 4 mm) determines the space available for inflow and outflow of the medium. Even a slight change in this difference has a major effect on the flow-through capacity (Hagen-Poissouille law). We find that a 6 mm sheath allows for ample fluid flow per unit time. In all but a few cases (e.g., arthroscopic synovectomy), the 6 mm sheath eliminates the need for a separate inflow cannula. Many sheaths are only 5.0 or 5.5 mm in diameter, and in these cases it is better to insert a separate, large-gauge inflow cannula so that the joint can be distended more rapidly (see Sect. 3.5.1).

The sheath should be designed such that, once the telescope has been inserted, the inflow and outflow systems can be separately controlled. This allows for simultaneous inflow and aspiration of the irrigating fluid (Fig. 3-2). There is no space with oscillating or regurgitant flow analogous to the dead space volume in the lung.

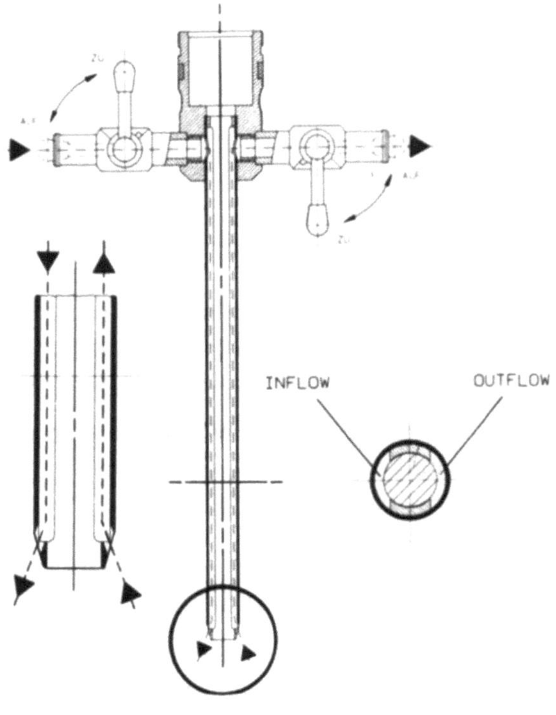

Fig. 3-2. Sheath and telescope assembly with separate inflow and outflow channels (Aesculap)

The spigots should be mounted on a collar that can be rotated relative to the sheath. This ensures that the inflow and outflow tubing will not become twisted or tangled when the arthroscope is moved about. Rotation of the spigots must not loosen any seals or adjusting screws on the collar or on the spigots themselves. Fluid dripping from the sheath during the procedure can be most annoying.

It is advantageous if both spigots can be controlled with one hand (Fig. 3-3), especially if the arthroscopist works without an assistant. One hand holds the arthroscope at the level of the spigots ("arthroscope hand") while the other hand operates the instruments: the probing hook in diagnostic arthroscopy, and operative instruments in surgical procedures ("instrument hand").

A loose or leaky connection between the telescope and sheath is another factor that can interfere with the smooth conduct of the procedure. Pausing to tighten the connection between the scope and sheath not only wastes time but can spoil an arthroscopic view that may have taken some effort to obtain. There is also a danger that the scope will bend if it slips partially out of the sheath with camera attached. Leakage of intraarticular fluid is another problem that can result from a loose connection between the scope and sheath. Although the locking mechanisms are simple in principle, in many systems the telescope can lock only when in a specific position relative to the sheath. In some systems the scope and sheath will fit together in any number of rotational positions, but there is only one position in which the components can lock. Snap-lock mechanisms that function in two positions perform very well and reduce the chance of accidental unlocking.

A criterion often neglected in selecting a sheath is the configuration of the arthroscope

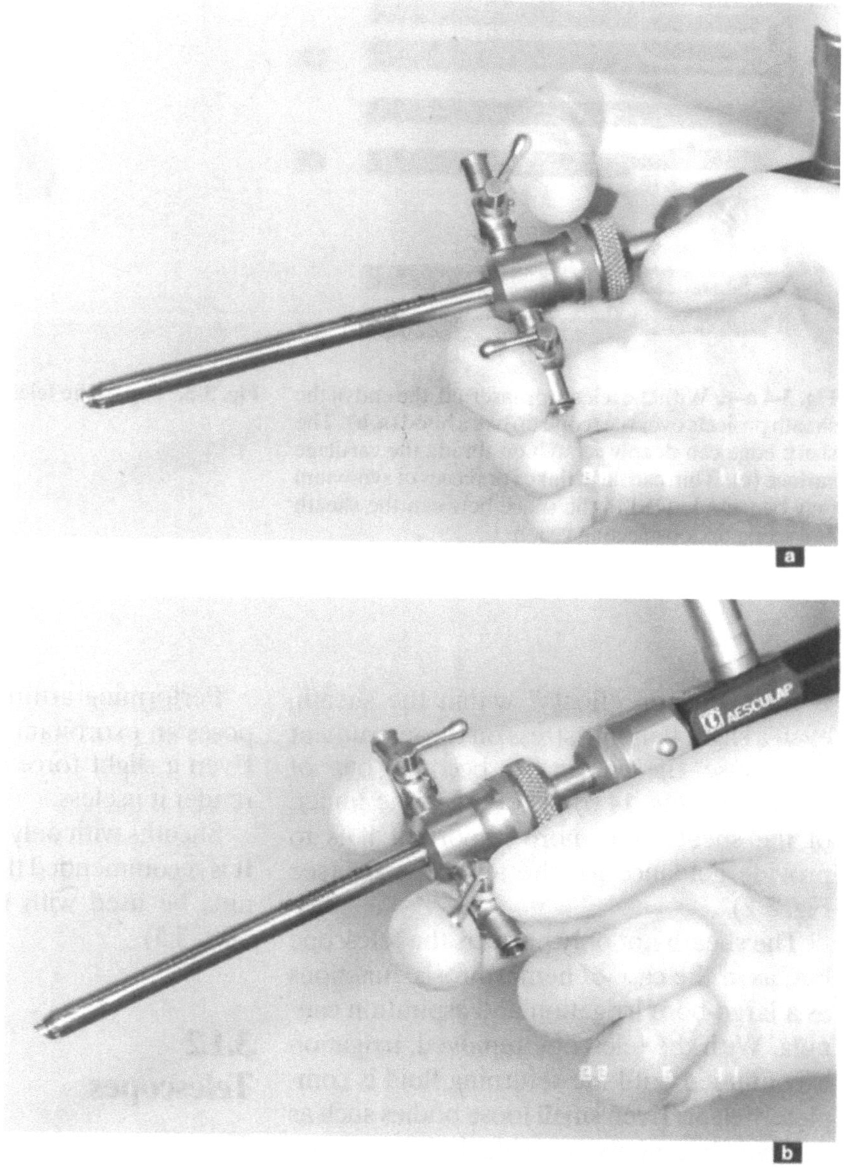

Fig. 3-3 a, b. One-hand operation of the inflow and outflow spigots ("arthroscope hand")

tip when the sheath and telescope are assembled. In many systems the distal sheath opening is oval-shaped so that when the telescope is inserted, a portion of the sheath projects over the scope tip like a hood (Fig. 3-4). Obviously this projection is intended to protect the scope tip, but from what? Brushing the cartilage surface with the scope tip, as any examiner may do repeatedly in the course of an examination, certainly poses a greater threat to the cartilage than to the arthroscope. When the "hood" touches the cartilage, it behaves like a gouge and may scratch, raise, or even scrape off portions of the cartilage surface. Excoriated cartilage flakes can easily become trapped in the space between the sheath and telescope and obscure vision. When the instrument tip touches the capsule, synovial villi also may become caught in the "trap," causing obstruction of vision (see also Chap. 11). The junction of the sheath and scope should be designed to eliminate this gouging and trapping effect. Multiple irrigation ports may be placed on the sides of the sheath (Fig. 3-5). When the telescope, and especially the telescope tip, is threaded into the sheath without a guide, the entire arthroscope becomes less stable against bending forces.

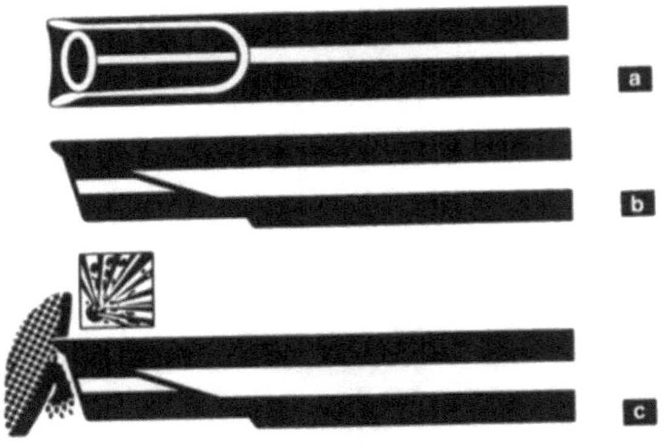

Fig. 3-4 a–c. With the telescope inserted, the end of the sheath projects over the scope tip like a hood (**a, b**). The sharp edge can deeply scratch or abrade the cartilage surface (**c**). Thin cartilage flakes or pieces of synovium may become lodged in the space between the sheath and scope tip, obstructing vision

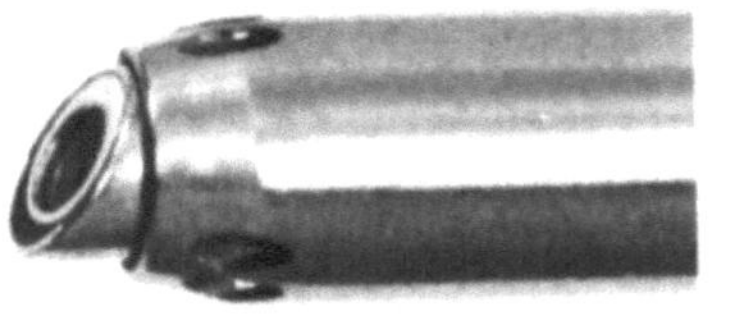

Fig. 3-5. Top of the telescope and sheath, saline ports

If the scope tip "floats" within the sheath, even a slight bending stress on the instrument can cause the image to become out of round (see Fig. 14-5). The larger the lumen of the sheath, the more important it is to provide guidance for the telescope tip (see Fig. 3-2).

The sheath not only protects the telescope but, as in the case of hemarthrosis, functions as a large-bore irrigation and aspiration cannula. With the telescope removed, irrigation is continued until the returning fluid is completely clear. Even small loose bodies such as cartilage fragments or residual pieces of meniscus left by a partial meniscectomy can easily be flushed from the joint through the sheath (Figs. 3-6 and 3-7). The irrigating and cleansing action can be enhanced by ballotting or massaging the compartment containing the debris.

With a longstanding hemarthrosis that is undergoing organization, large blood clots cannot be aspirated through the arthroscope sheath. They can be flushed from the joint through a separate instrument portal (see Sect. 6.2) or extracted with a grasping forceps. If this is unsuccessful, larger blood clots can be aspirated with a motorized instrument (shaver system with a synovial resector or Rosenberg resector).

Performing arthroscopy without a sheath poses an exorbitant danger to the telescope. Even a slight force can bend the scope and render it useless.

Sheaths with only one spigot are available. It is recommended that a separate inflow cannula be used with this type of sheath (see Sect. 3.5).

3.1.2 Telescopes

The arthroscopic telescope consists of a lens system and a system of optical fibers for transmitting light into the joint. Telescopes come in various lengths and calibers. While acromatic systems once dominanted the market, rod-lens systems are more popular today and offer significant advantages over the acromatic thin-lens scopes. Besides having a smaller diameter, they produce a wider visual field and a brighter image (Fig. 3-8).

The shape and size of the eyepiece should be considered when a telescope is purchased. Otherwise problems may arise later when the system is expanded by the addition of a camera for video or still photography.

Telescopes with an extended eyepiece are recommended only if there are no plans to

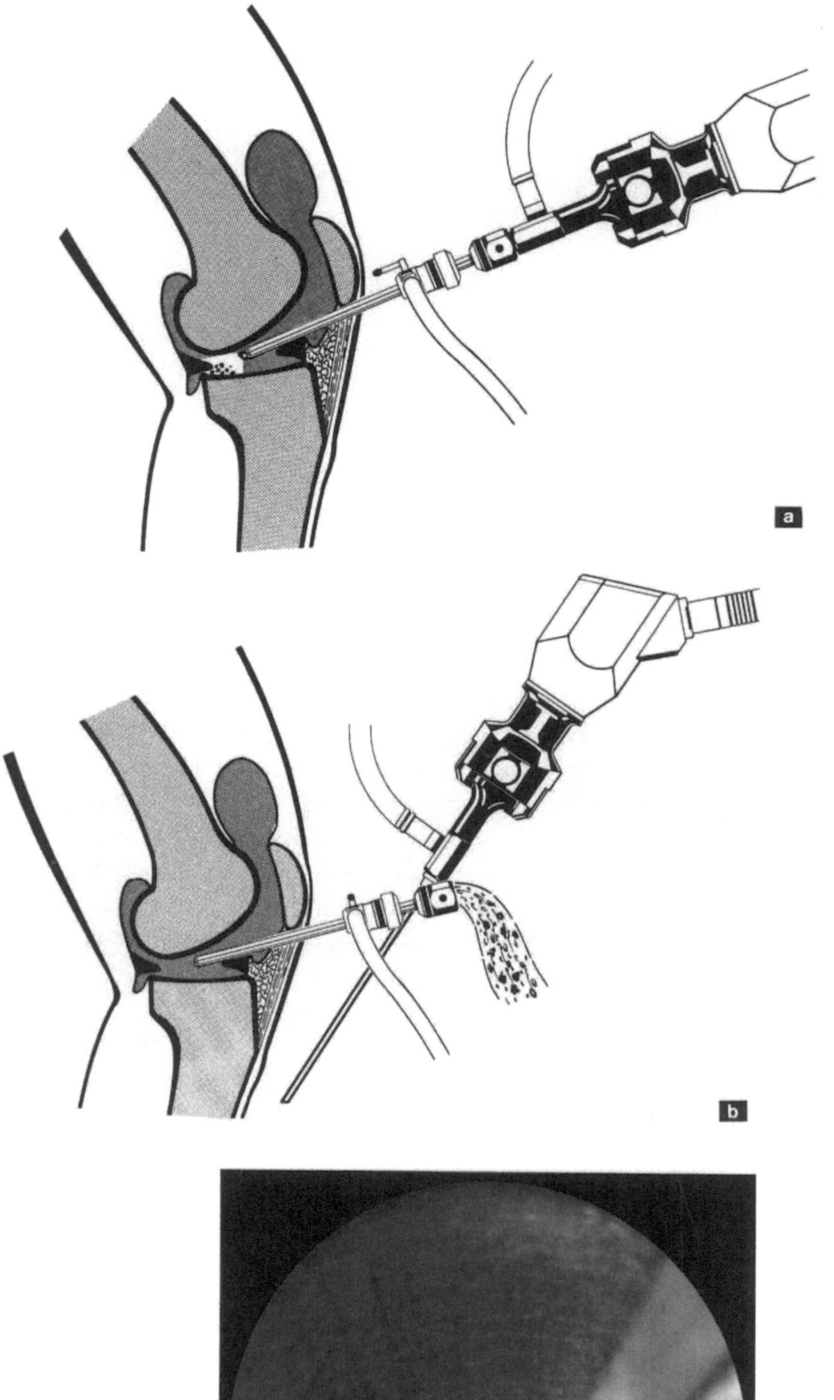

Fig. 3-6 a, b. Removal of small loose bodies lying in front of the posterior horn of the meniscus. The debris is visualized, and the joint is distended (**a**). With the scope removed from the sheath, the debris is flushed from the joint cavity (**b**)

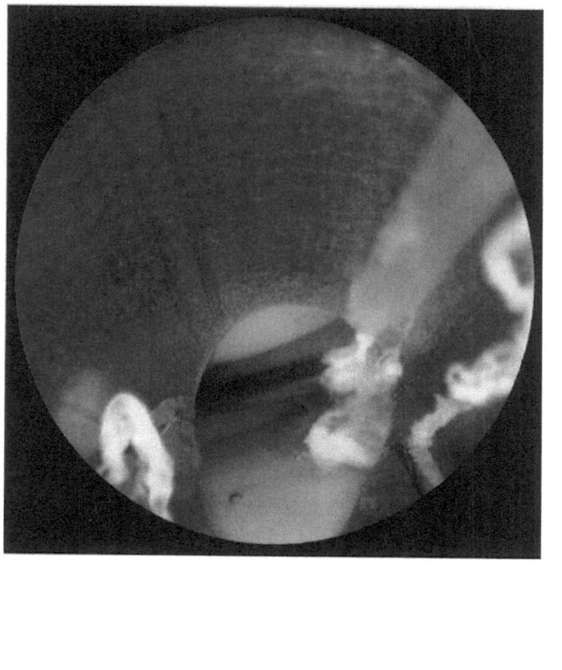

Fig. 3-7. Fibrin clots and small cartilage fragments are flushed from the joint after the telescope is unlocked and removed

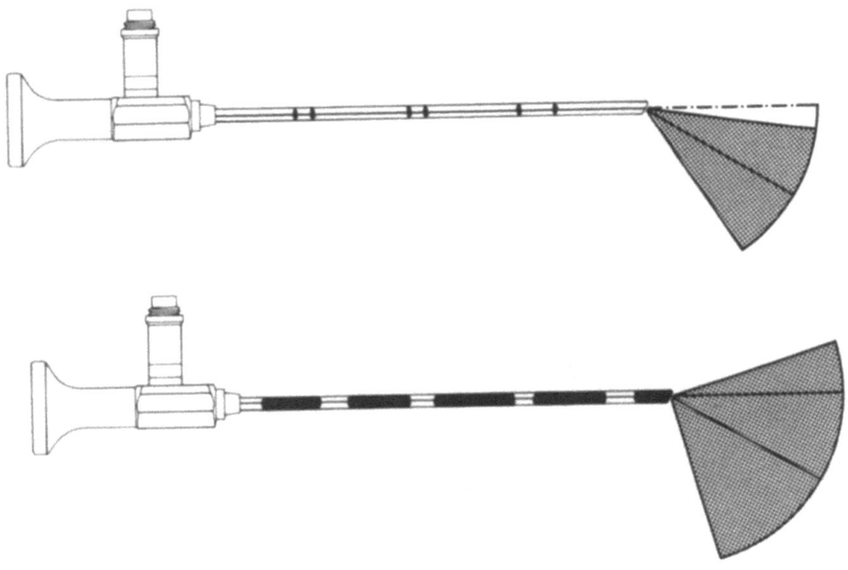

Fig. 3-8. Arthroscopic telescopes. The acromatic system (*top*) provides a significantly smaller visual field (shaded area) than the rod-lens system (*bottom*)

add a video camera in the forseeable future. The increased distance between the surgical mask and the sterile hand holding the arthroscope reduces the contamination risk. (Improved asepsis is one reason to consider the purchase of a video system; see Sect. 3.3.)

Three main types of telescope are available: the 0° direct-viewing ("straight-ahead") scope and the 30° and 70° oblique scopes (Fig. 3-9). In a 0° scope the direction of vision is directly in line with the long axis of the scope. In a 30° oblique scope, the direction of vision is inclined 30° from the scope axis; in a 70° scope, it is inclined 70°. The special arrangement of the lens systems and the use of rod lenses have led to the development of "wide-angle" telescopes that provide a 90° field of view (Fig. 3-10).

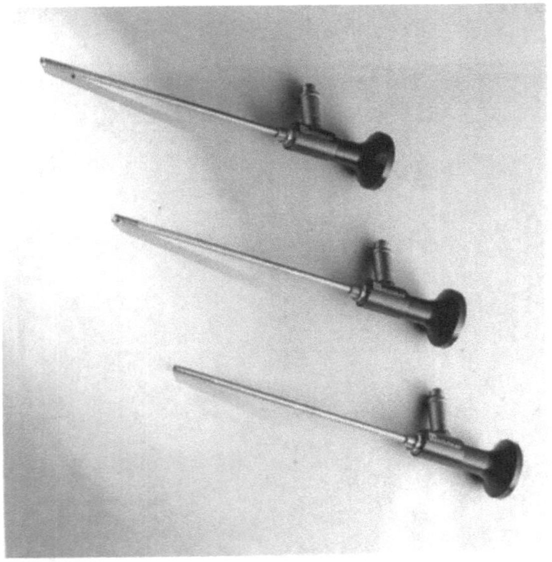

Fig. 3-9. From top to bottom: 0°, 30°, and 70° wide-angle arthroscopic telescopes (Aesculap)

The flexible light cable connects to the light post of the arthroscope. The light post is mounted at right angles to the sheath, and when an oblique-viewing scope is used, the direction of view always points away from the side carrying the post. Thus, if the light post of a 30° scope points *upward* (Fig. 3-11), the viewing angle is directed 30° *downward*. If the post points downward, the viewing angle is directed 30° upward.

The position of the light post is an important aid to orientation.

It is reasonable to consider which type of telescope is best suited for arthroscopy of the knee joint. If we accept that the goal is to inspect the entire joint cavity, and if we consider the physical capabilities of the various systems, we may draw the following conclusions:

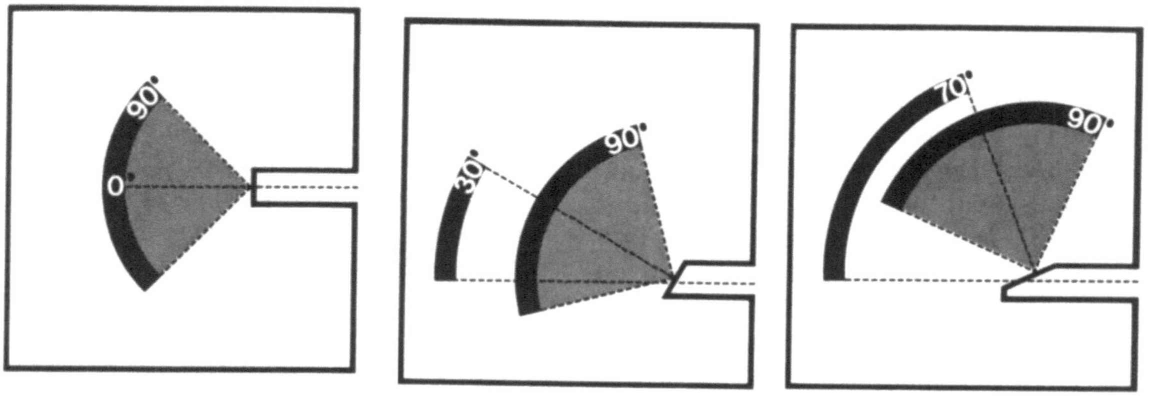

Fig. 3-10. Visual field (shaded) of 30°, 70°, and 0° wide-angle telescopes

1. The 0° direct-viewing scope "looks" straight ahead along a path directly in line with the sheath axis. The visual field can be changed only by advancing or retracting the arthroscope. As the scope is advanced toward a structure to be inspected, the visual field diminishes; as the scope is pulled back, the field expands (see Fig. 7-2). Only structures directly ahead of the scope can be visualized, and the only way to extend the visual field laterally is by sweeping the scope. Rotating the scope will not bring additional portions of the joint into view. A 0° telescope is excellent for examining a hollow tubular space, whose lateral walls can be inspected simply by retracting the instrument. However, a direct-viewing scope is not well suited for inspecting the angled and loculated compartments within the knee joint.

Perhaps the knee could be successfully examined with a flexible fiberoptic endoscope similar to the type used for gastroscopy, but tests with a flexible 3.5 mm cystoscope with a deflectable tip have not given satisfactory re-

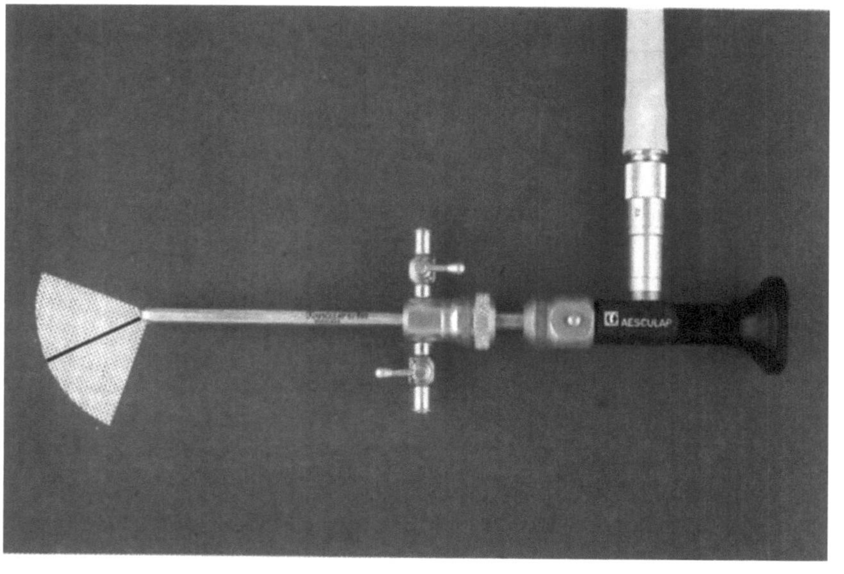

Fig. 3-11. The viewing angle of an oblique scope is always directed away from the side of the instrument that carries the light post. If the light post points upward, the viewing angle (black line) is directed downward. The rod-lens system provides a 90° field of view (light area)

sults in the knee. Aside from the small visual field, comparable to that of a very small-caliber arthroscope (Needlescope), the light transmission in a flexible system is so weak that a very powerful light source is required. Another serious disadvantage is the delicacy of the endoscope tip. The optical glass fibers, protected only by a thin rubber sheath, are too fragile for maneuvering within a space like the knee joint, which is bounded by firm tissues and cartilaginous structures. The tip is so susceptible to damage that multiple dark spots appear on the image after only a brief period of use (Brandenburg 1985). At present there is no evidence that a practical, flexible endoscope for arthroscopy of the knee joint will be developed in the near future.

2. The 30° wide-angle scope gives a foreoblique field of view, i.e., one directed straight ahead and also to the side. Retracting and sweeping the scope extends the visual field as in a direct-viewing instrument. But the 30° scope is advantageous in that the examiner can significantly extend the visual field (i.e., "look to the side") by rotating the instrument (Fig. 3-12, see also Chap. 7). This capability increases the field of view by approximately 300% compared with a straight-ahead scope.

3. The 70° wide-angle scope gives a field of view that is directed laterally and also backward. The scope is "blind" to the area directly ahead of its tip (Fig. 3-13).

The 30° wide-angle telescope is the mainstay of diagnostic knee arthroscopy owing to its foreoblique field of view. Able to inspect virtually the whole interior of the knee joint, the 30° scope represents the best compromise between the direct-viewing and oblique-viewing instruments. 70° wide-angle scopes

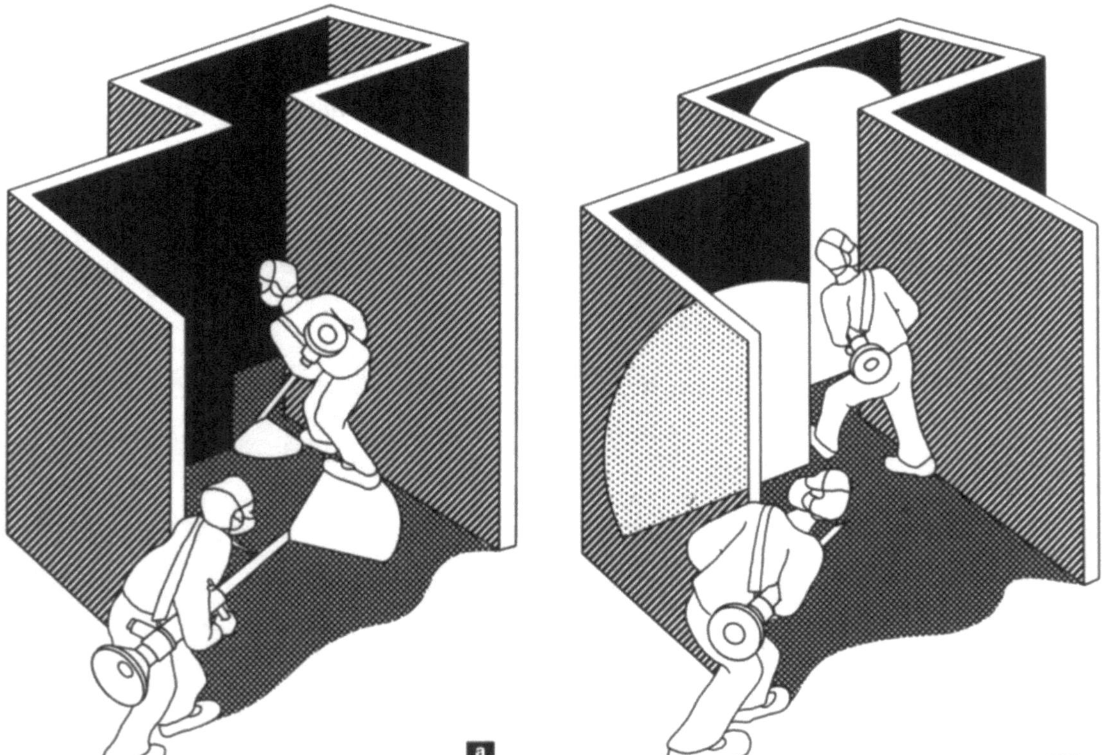

Fig. 3-12 a, b. If the arthroscope is used like a pocket flashlight, only the floor is illuminated (**a**). Rotating the oblique-viewing scope directs the beam onto the walls of the angled corridor (**b**) (modified from Johnson 1986)

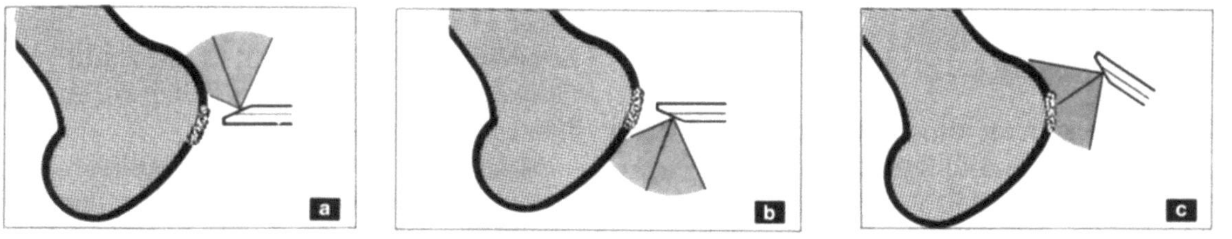

Fig. 3-13 a–c. Use of the 70° wide-angle scope. A structure directly in front of the lens cannot be visualized even by rotating the scope (**a, b**). The structure is brought into view by aiming the scope past it (**c**)

may be useful for special investigations but are unnecessary for routine examinations.

Arthroscopic telescopes are expensive and should be handled with care. Excessive bending stresses exerted during use or cleaning can easily damage the lens system (see Sect. 4.7.1).

3.2 Lighting System

The lighting system consists of a light source and a light cable (Fig. 3-14). The brightness and clarity of the arthroscopic image depend on the intensity (wattage) of the light source, the quality of light transmission through the cable, and the integrity of the arthroscopic lens system.

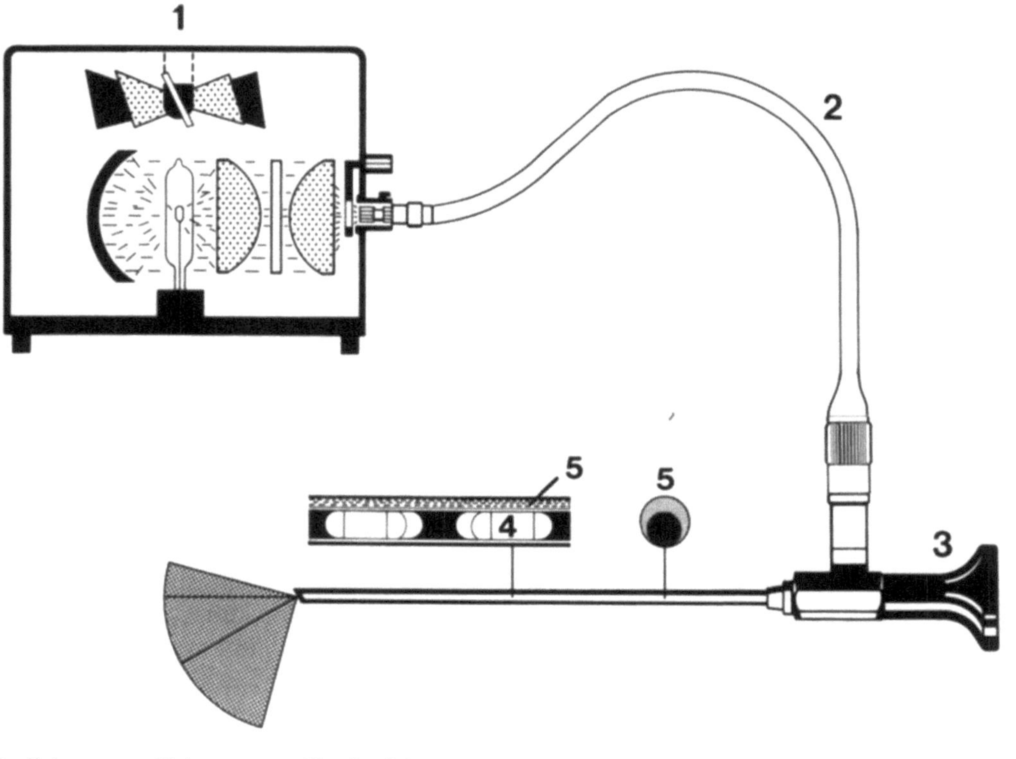

Fig. 3-14. The light source (1) is connected by flexible cable (2) to a 30° wide-angle scope (3). The scope transits light into the joint via a lens system (4) and fiberoptic bundles (broken lines, 5)

3.2.1 Light Source

The light sources most commonly used for arthroscopy are cold-light sources with a light intensity of 100–250 W (Fig. 3-15). Whereas 200-W and 250-W light sources were once required for video arthroscopy, the improved video cameras of today can deliver clear images at lower intensities. When a video system is purchased, the intensity of the light source should be matched to the requirements of the video camera, bearing in mind that older-model cameras require more light than modern video cameras. The latest generation of solid-state chip cameras require no more than 150 W to produce an image of acceptable brightness and clarity. A powerful light source is useful in that it provides a reserve capacity as the light-transmitting properties of the arthroscope and light cable deteriorate over time.

In many systems the light intensity can be varied by adjusting the brightness level at the source. In this way the lighting can be adjusted to meet the changing requirements in the joint. A brighter source is needed to illuminate the suprapatellar pouch, especially in large joints, since this compartment, containing no reflective surfaces, "swallows" light. Less illumination is needed to inspect the articular cartilage and menisci, which are strong reflectors of light.

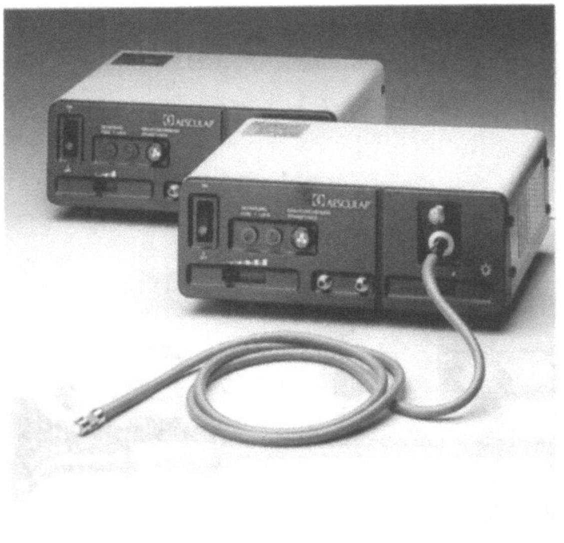

Fig. 3-15. Arthroscopic cold-light sources (150 W), one with 3 and one with 5 adjustable brightness levels. Each has a built-in reserve bulb. The 5-level model is shown with flexible light cable attached (Aesculap)

Modern arthroscopic light sources are equipped with reserve bulbs that can be switched on when needed by pressing a button.

Xenon light sources are more powerful (up to 300 W) but are considerably more expensive. As opposed to cold-light sources, which produce artificial light with a color temperature of 3400° Kelvin, xenon light is approximately 6000° Kelvin, comparable to full daylight. This type of light source is useful if high-quality intraarticular photographs and videotape recordings are desired.

Light sources may have one or two outlets for plugging in the light cable. In sources with two outlets, a twin-lead cable should be used (see below).

3.2.2 Light Cables

The light source is connected to the arthroscope by a flexible light cable. Two types of cable are used: fiberoptic cables and fluid cables.

Fiberoptic Cables

These cables transmit light through bundles of thin optical glass fibers (Fig. 3-16). The flexibility of the cable subjects the individual fibers to strong bending stresses, so the fibers tend to break with continued use. Image brightness is not noticeably affected until about 50% of the fibers are broken. Since breakage of the glass fibers is a "physiologic" process of aging and wear, the light cable should be checked every 3–4 months. This is done by shining a light into the end of the cable that plugs into the source (e.g., holding it up to a ceiling lamp) and inspecting the opposite end for dark spots (Fig. 3-17). The total darkened area is proportional to the percentage of broken fibers.

The main advantages of fiberoptic cables are their low purchase price and ease of steri-

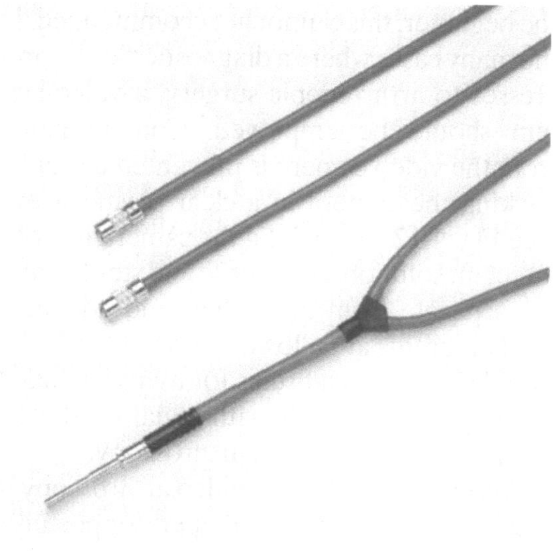

Fig. 3-16. Fiberoptic light cables: single-lead (top) and twin-lead types (bottom)

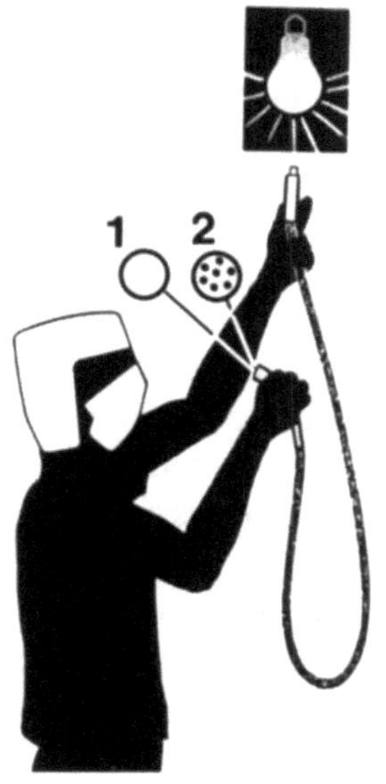

Fig. 3-17. Testing the light cable. When light is shined into the end of an intact cable, no dark spots are seen at the opposite end (1). Dark spots can be seen in a worn cable (2). The total area of darkening corresponds to the percentage of broken fibers

lization. These cables can be steam-sterilized at a pressure of 2 bar (134° C).

Fiberoptic cables are available in various lengths and diameters (3.5 and 4.8 mm). Large-diameters cables are preferable because they can transmit more light. The cable should be long enough to reach easily from the light source to the arthroscope during an operation. A tightly stretched cable is usually angled sharply at its ends, increasing the risk of breakage of the delicate glass fibers. The standard cable length is 180 cm, which is adequate for most operating situations. Longer cables are available if desired.

Fluid Cables

Fluid cables contain a gelatinous material that transmits light 40%–60% more efficiently than optical glass fibers. However, fluid cables are more rigid than fiberoptic cables and so are more difficult to handle. The gelatinous material cannot tolerate steam or gas sterilization, so the cable must be sterilized by soaking in an appropriate disinfectant solution.

More expensive than fiberoptic cables, fluid cables are for arthroscopists who want optimum light transmission and are willing to accept the disadvantages of high cost, cumbersome handling, and inconvenient sterilization. If the cable develops a defect, nonsterile light-conducting medium can leak out and contaminate the operative field.

Both fiberoptic and fluid cables are available in single- or twin-lead models for use with single- or double-outlet light sources (Fig. 3-16).

Problems. Scorching and perforation of the waterproof draping material by a hot light cable is an avoidable complication risk. Care should be taken that the light source is not switched on until the cable has been connected to the arthroscope. Meanwhile, adequate testing of the light source by the manufacturer is essential. If there is a defect in the protective heat filter built into most light sources (which filters out infrared radiation), there will be excessive heating of the light cable. This can damage not just the optical glass fibers but also any tissue that is touched by the scope tip, which be heated to 80° C. The arthroscope in effect becomes a coagulation instrument, casting doubt on the validity of the term "cold light source."

3.3 Video System

The development and miniaturization of video technology have made it possible to capture the intraarticular image with a video camera and display it on a monitor screen. A videocassette recorder or video printer can easily be added to the system for documentation purposes (see Chap. 14, Figs. 14-7 and 14-8).

Video arthroscopy offers several fundamental advantages over traditional arthroscopy in which the examiner views the joint directly through the eyepiece (Fig. 3-18).

Preservation of Asepsis. In direct arthroscopy, often only a few centimeters separate nonsterile areas (eyes, mask, arthroscope hand) from the sterile field (instrument hand, knee joint) (Fig. 3-18). While the careful operator can probably avoid accidental contact between these areas in diagnostic arthroscopy, such contacts occur frequently in arthroscopic surgery.

Asepsis in arthroscopic operations is constantly jeopardized as long as the operator looks directly through the arthroscope.

Of course, an experienced arthroscopist can perform virtually any arthroscopic procedure without the use of a video system. But for the beginner, this cannot be recommended. In the many cases where a diagnostic "look" progresses to arthroscopic surgery, a video system should be employed. Contamination from the video camera is prevented either by packing the camera in a clear plastic sleeve (see Fig. 4-12) or soaking the camera in a disinfectant solution. Nonsterile and sterile areas are separate from one other, and adequate safety margins are allowed. It need hardly be stated that the usual rules for asepsis in open knee operations apply with equal validity to diagnostic and operative arthroscopy.

Another advantage of video arthroscopy is that it avoids the contorted operator postures of traditional arthroscopy (Fig. 3-18) by permitting the arthroscopist to sit comfortably while working from the monitor (Fig. 3-19).

Ease of Documentation. Intraarticular findings displayed on the monitor can be documented as needed with a videocassette recorder or video printer. By contrast, direct documentation with a still camera coupled to the arthroscope eyepiece involves complicated steps to ensure that asepsis is preserved (see Chap. 14).

Participation of Others. Video arthroscopy enables the procedure to be witnessed by the operator, assistant, surgical nurse, anesthesiologist, visitors, and even by the patient him-

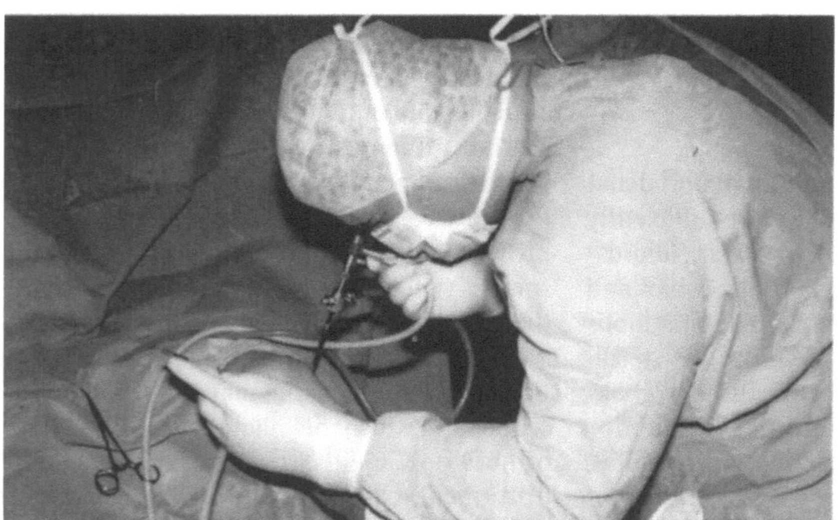

Fig. 3-18. Arthroscopy with the operator looking directly through the eyepiece of the telescope. Often the operator must assume a very uncomfortable position

self (Fig. 3-19). Significant findings can be discussed with the operating room staff and with the patient. More fully integrated into the procedure, the surgical nurse can be more efficient in having operating instruments ready as they are required.

By contrast, arthroscopy performed through the eyepiece is an "one man show." Only the arthroscopist can see the intraarticular structures in the darkened operating room. All others are excluded and may have trouble keeping their eyes open in a lengthy operation. If the arthroscopist is kind enough to demonstrate a "particularly interesting" finding, the untrained eye of the assistant may not be able to interpret it. Moreover, the scope may be tipped or rotated in the process of transfering the eyepiece to the assistant, who may then receive undeserved criticism for his inability to see the feature of interest.

Better Teaching and Learning Opportunities. During video arthroscopy the assistant, patient, and visitors can watch the procedure on the monitor as it takes place. The operator can explain, for example, why he is positioning the arthroscope one way rather than another, why the instrument portal should be placed somewhat more distally, or how extensive the cartilage damage is.

Videotaped findings and operative techniques can be edited together on one video cassette for demonstration purposes (conferences, lectures, patient information). For those present in the operating room, the video system makes the arthroscopic procedure a shared experience. Video arthroscopy also makes it easier for the expert observer to spot any deficiencies in the operating technique of the arthroscopist.

Disadvantages of video arthroscopy are its high cost, its technical complexity, and its space requirements (multi-tiered cart, see Sect. 4.5). While the success of direct arthroscopy depends only on the integrity of the light source, the light cable, and the arthroscope, video arthroscopy additionally requires that the video camera, camera cable, and monitor function flawlessly. Initial difficulties in setting up and operating a video system are only temporary, however, and today video arthroscopy has established itself as the technique of choice for arthroscopic procedures.

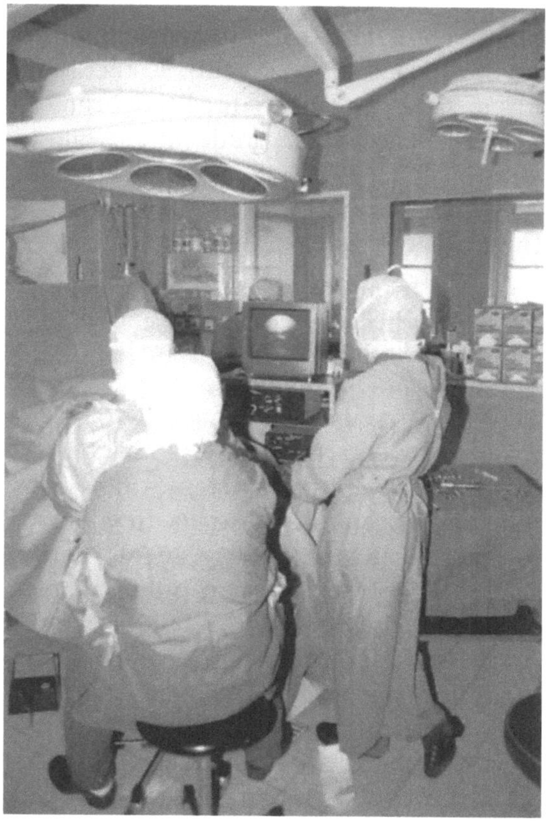

Fig. 3-19. Video arthroscopy allows everyone in the room to see what is happening inside the knee

3.3.1 Video Camera

Three-Tube Camera

In all color television systems, white light is broken up into the video primary colors of red, green, and blue (RGB). A three-tube camera contains one pickup vacuum tube for reading each of the video primaries and converting the color information into electrical signals. These signals are modulated and transmitted by cable to the monitor as video signals. Each tube integrates 584 active image lines, each of which is resolved on the monitor into 833 picture elements. The even- and odd-numbered lines are scanned alternately at a rate of 50 half-frames per second. This high-frequency image generation process by half-frames causes less flicker than scanning 25 complete frames per second at the same transmission rate. The three-tube camera gives excellent color reproduction owing to the 486,500 color picture elements or 1,459,400 individual picture elements that are generated per frame.

On the negative side, three-tube cameras have a high price tag and are somewhat difficult to use with an arthroscope. The typical three-tube camera weighs several kilograms, stands on a tripod, and is connected to the arthroscope by an articulated coupling that itself must be covered with a sterile drape. This arrangement seriously restricts freedom of movement. Also, three-tube cameras require a higher light intensity than ordinary cold-light sources can deliver.

These disadvantages have spurred industry to develop miniaturized cameras that are more consistent with arthroscopic requirements. Compact, easy-to-handle video cameras are now available that connect directly to the eyepiece of the arthroscope. Both single-tube and chip (CCD) cameras are available.

Single-Tube Camera

With a one-tube camera, the video primaries (RGB) are all read by a single pickup tube. The 350 active image lines, each with 833 pixels, give 291,550 color picture elements or 874,650 individual picture elements per frame. While this results in a somewhat lower resolution than a three-tube camera, the advantages of easier handling and lower cost have contributed to the great popularity of single-tube cameras for video arthroscopy (Fig. 3-20).

Chip Camera

In a chip camera (solid-state or CCD camera), the vacuum tube is replaced by a photosensitive semiconductor, but otherwise the principle of color image generation remains the same. Chip cameras can be made even smaller than single-tube cameras. They require less operating voltage, and their lower power consumption causes less intrinsic heating of the device. Chip cameras are relatively insensitive to mechanical vibrations and have a good signal-to-noise ratio. Unlike tube cameras, in which the image line represents a continuous signal, the image of a chip camera is made up of discrete spots, each of which corresponds to the signal from one photodetector.

The process for manufacturing chip cameras is similar to that for making integrated electronic circuits. The circuit elements, integrated on a semiconductor, provide for simultaneous digitization and serial readout of the image information.

The first color video camera with a semiconductor sensor was produced by Bell Laboratories in 1972. It contained three image sensors that employed CCD (charge-coupled device) technology with a 128–by-106 imaging array.

Further miniaturization led to the "one-chip camera," in which color images are produced by masking the individual photosensitive elements with appropriate color filters. Today chip cameras are available that are about the size of a matchbox and weigh less than 30 g.

Several years ago it was claimed that chip cameras were still lacking in resolution, color fidelity, and sensitivity. But the latest generation of chip cameras have a sensitivity of 10 lux with a horizontal resolution of 350 lines and a vertical resolution of 400 lines (Fig. 3-21). The color temperatures range from 2100° to 9500° Kelvin. Compared with tube cameras, chip cameras offer the advantages of lighter weight, easier white balance (set automatically or by pressing a button), faster "warm-up," less smearing, no burn-in, and good resolution. Tube cameras, on the other hand, offer better color reproduction in borderline situations.

Another advantage of chip cameras is that the housing can easily be designed to fit the arthroscopist's hand (see Fig. 3-21).

Other Criteria for Selecting a Video Camera

Because neither tube cameras nor solid-state cameras are autoclavable, they must either be covered with a sterile wrapping or rendered relatively germ-free by soaking in a disinfectant solution.

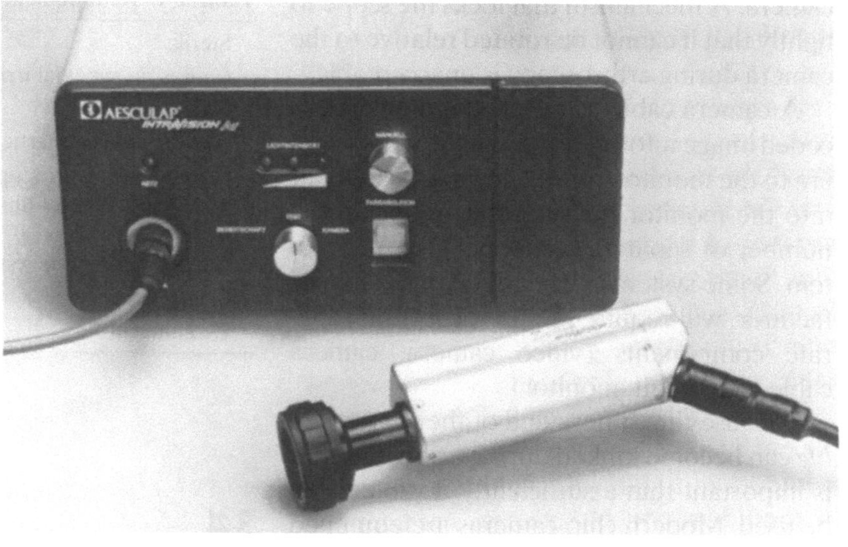

Fig. 3-20. Single-tube camera (Aesculap)

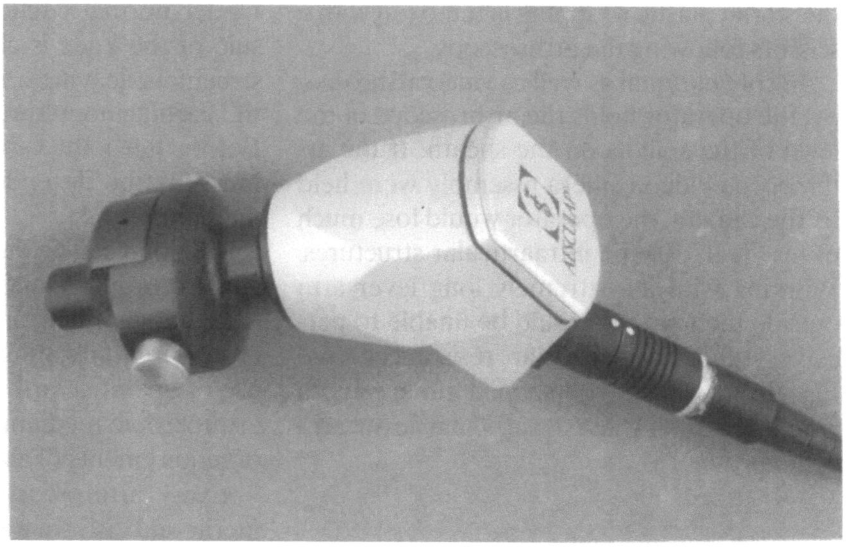

Fig. 3-21. Solid-state chip camera (Aesculap)

Another important consideration in the acquisition of a video camera is the *suppression of radio interference* in the video system as a whole and especially in the video camera. Otherwise significant image distortion can occur during the use of electrosurgical instruments.

Another, frequently neglected factor is the *coupling mechanism* between the video camera and telescope. Since it is often necessary to rotate the video camera relative to the telescope during arthroscopy so that the orientation of the monitor image conforms to anatomy (e.g., a horizontal joint space), the mechanism should be secure yet easy to loosen and refasten as needed. Some mechanisms lock according to the "all or nothing" rule: Either the telescope is secured against rotation, or it is free to wobble in relation to the camera, creating a troublesome "wandering" or shaking of the monitor image. Better camera models allow the examiner to rotate the telescope against a slight resistance even when the scope is securely coupled to the camera. A mechanism that locks the scope so tightly that it cannot be rotated relative to the camera during arthroscopy is unacceptable.

A camera cable transmits the digitally encoded image information from the video camera to the monitor. Some electronics are built into the monitor housing, thus reducing the number of separate components in the system. Some systems, depending on the manufacturer, will require the use of several separate components (video camera, camera cable, video unit, monitor).

Because the camera end of the *camera cable* can become kinked during arthroscopy, it is important that a sufficiently flexible cable be used. Modern chip cameras are equipped with a flexible, interchangable transmission cable. The thinness of the cable, however, makes it susceptible to damage in cases where the sterile plastic wrapping is removed with a scissors following the arthroscopy.

In conventional as well as video arthroscopy, the operator holds the arthroscope at the level of the spigots on the sheath. If the arthroscope-video camera assembly were held by the camera, the operator would lose much of his "feel" for the intraarticular structures. Working with an extremely long lever arm outside the joint, he would be unable to perceive subtle intraarticular resistances (see Fig. 7-6). Using a rod-shaped tube camera would lengthen the extraarticular lever arm even further.

3.3.2 Monitor

The visual image captured by the camera is transmitted to the video monitor for display. Arthroscopy requires a high-resolution monitor with an antiglare screen. The monitor should have output jacks for a second monitor, a videocassette recorder, and/or a video printer.

Many video monitors have a splash-proof housing and are shielded against radio interference so that picture quality is not affected by the use of high-frequency instruments (electrosurgery).

Table 3-1. Requirements of an arthroscopic medium

- Sterile
- Causes no synovial irritation
- Nontoxic
- Allows good intraarticular vision
- Suitable for arthroscopic operations (including electrosurgery and the use of motorized instruments)
- Causes no local or systemic side effects
- Convenient to use
- Economical

3.4 Arthroscopic Media

Under normal circumstances the joint capsule of the knee is closely apposed to bony structures, leaving a minimal space between the cartilaginous surfaces and joint capsule. Before the joint can be inspected, then, it must first be distended with an appropriate medium.

The joint can be distended with a *fluid* or a *gas*. Accordingly, arthroscopists may be classified as "gas men" or "water men," the latter group predominating due to the increasing use of operative arthroscopy. An acceptable arthroscopic medium must satisfy a number of requirements (Table 3-1).

Every arthroscopic medium has specific merits and disadvantages. Because diagnostic arthroscopy in the knee is typically followed by arthroscopic surgery, we prefer to distend the joint with fluid since most arthroscopic operations require a fluid medium.

3.4.1 Fluid

When arthroscopy is performed with a fluid medium, the "aquarium effect" described by Henche (1978) must be taken into account (Fig. 3-22). The aquarium effect causes all intraarticular structures to appear larger and closer than they really are. In addition, pedunculated structures such as cartilage shreds and synovial villi float within the joint like aquatic plants in a water-filled aquarium (Fig. 3-23 a). Gas distention produces a quite different environment in which these structures lie flat like an aquatic plant in an empty aquarium (Fig. 3-23 b).

The joint may be distended with Ringer's solution, sterile water, or physiologic saline. Increasingly popular fluid media are nonelectrolytic solutions (e.g., Purisole SM), which are supplied in conveniently large containers (3, 5, and 10 liters) and are compatible with electrosurgical procedures.

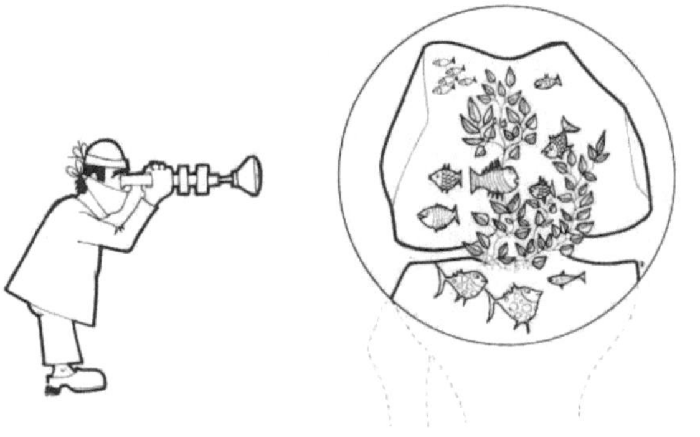

Fig. 3-22. "Aquarium effect" in a fluid-distended joint (from Henche 1978)

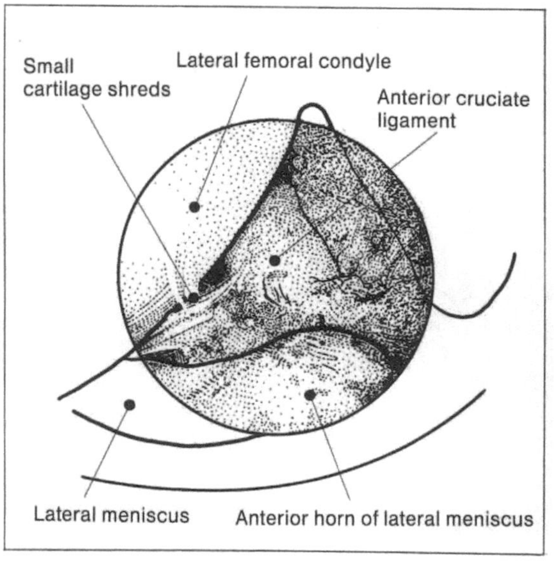

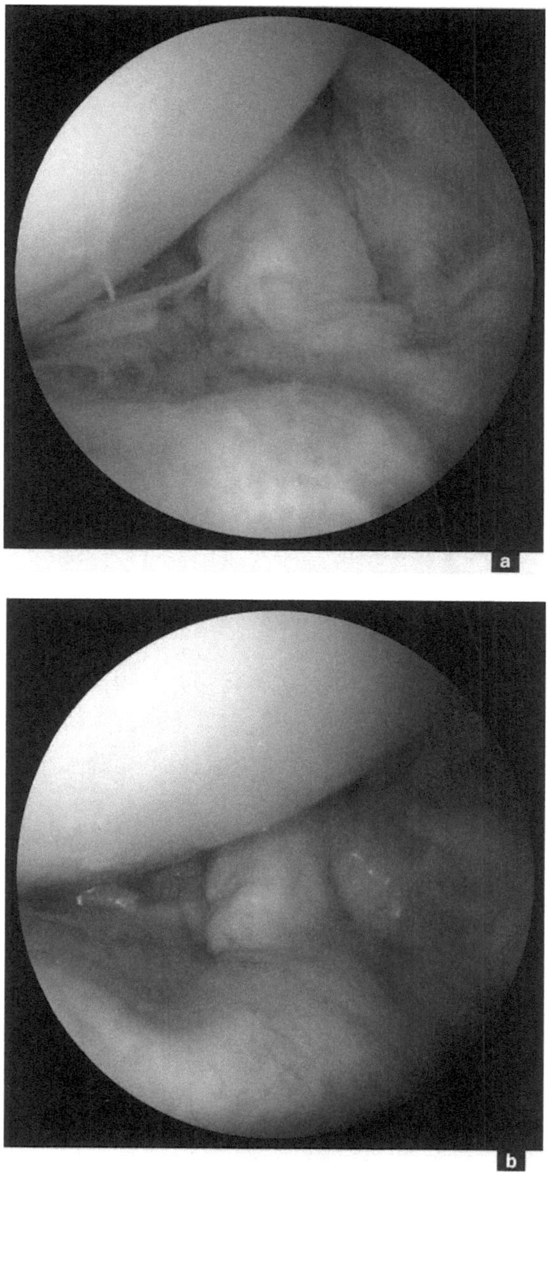

Fig. 3-23 a, b. Arthroscopy in fluid versus gas. In a fluid medium, small, superficial cartilage flakes and synovial fronds are plainly seen floating in the joint (**a**). Gas distention flattens these structures out. Anatomic surfaces have a glistening appearance, and the angle of vision is somewhat wider than in fluid (**b**)

Because we very often proceed from diagnostic arthroscopy to arthroscopic surgery in the same sitting and employ electrosurgical instruments, we always use a nonelectrolytic irrigating solution (Fig. 3-24).

Fluid distention of the joint is easy and requires no special instruments or equipment. Roller pumps are available that can maintain a designated intraarticular fluid pressure and flow rate through the joint, but these devices are costly and delicate and must be handled with great care.

An equally effective but more economical solution is to suspend the fluid bags from a tall i.v. pole or preferably from a motorized ceiling lift and introduce the fluid into the knee by gravity. The bags should be suspended at least 1.5 m above the level of the knee.

If the bags are hung from an ordinary i.v. pole, extreme caution is advised. These poles cannot be extended very far and, when fully extended and loaded, they can easily tip over. It is safer to use a ceiling lift which adjusts the bag height electrically (Fig. 3-25) or a specially reinforced i.v. pole.

A major advantage of fluid arthroscopy is the irrigation effect that is achieved by passing several liters of fluid through the joint. Cellular debris, small cartilage flakes, and lysosomal enzymes released from the damaged cartilage are washed from the joint cavity. In older patients with degenerative joint changes, it is common for irrigation of the joint alone (lavage) to provide substantial pain relief during the arthroscopy.

When arthroscopy is performed in patients

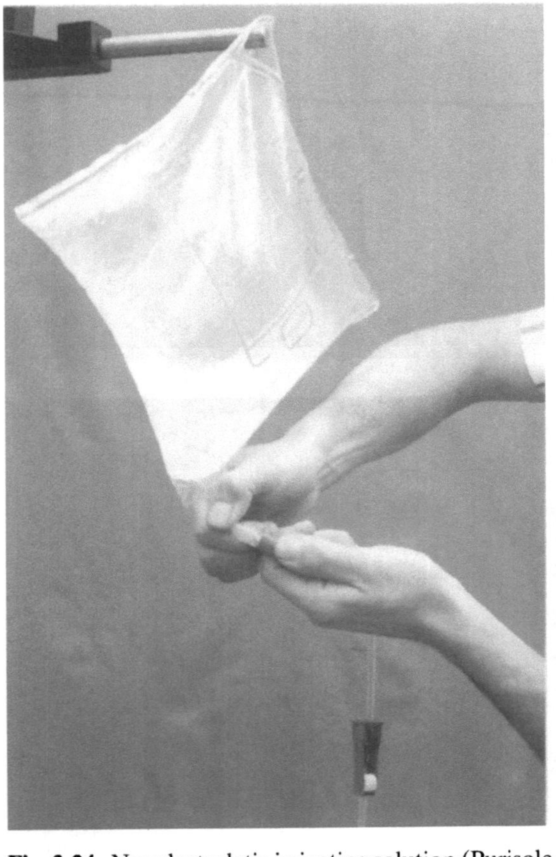

Fig. 3-24. Nonelectrolytic irrigating solution (Purisole SM, Fresenius). A Safe-lock adapter connects the infusion tubing to the fluid bag. The locking tab must be bent back to initiate flow

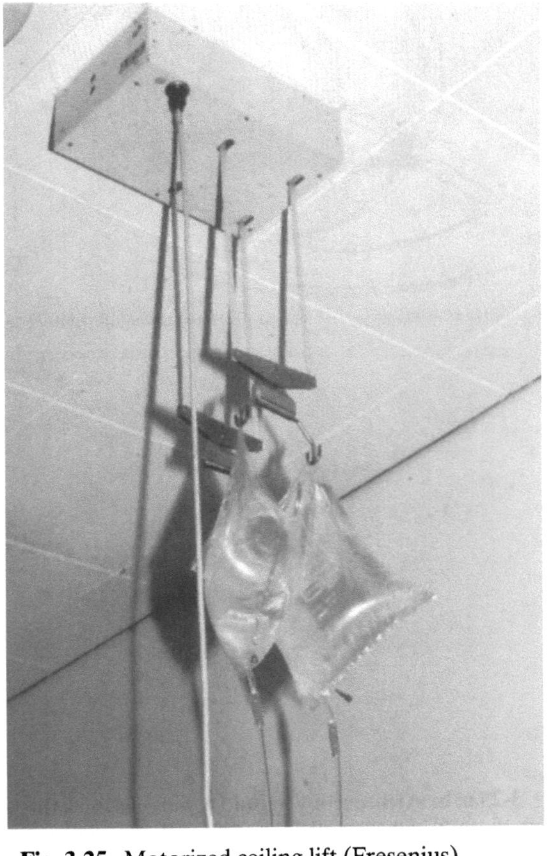

Fig. 3-25. Motorized ceiling lift (Fresenius)

who have previously had a hepatitis B infection, the hepatitis B antigen can be demonstrated in the aspirated irrigating solution, though at much lower levels than in the blood. This is possible if the joint shows no evidence of an inflammatory reaction at the time of the examination (Koorneef 1987). In the arthroscopic irrigation of an infected knee joint, all the irrigating fluid is considered to be contaminated (see Chap. 12.7).

3.4.2 Gas

For arthroscopy in a gas medium, the joint may be distended with CO_2, nitrous oxide, or air. While gas arthroscopy has several advantages, it is also associated with numerous risks and disadvantages (Tables 3-2 and 3-3).

Indeed, the presumed advantage of easier diagnosis in the presence of hemarthrosis represents the greatest potential danger of gas arthroscopy. Two cases of death following arthroscopy with air were reported at the Second Congress of the German-Speaking Association of Arthroscopy (AGA) in 1987. Both patients had a fresh bony injury, and both died from pulmonary embolism.

Distention of the joint with air is contraindicated in the presence of hemarthrosis.

In acutely injured patients with hemarthrosis, a fracture cannot always be excluded with complete confidence even by radiography, and some fractures are overlooked. With primary gas distention, the advantage of easier cruciate ligament evaluation is secured at the cost of a potentially lethal embolism risk.

Other serious complications have also been observed in gas-distended knee joints. Lotman (1987) reported two life-threatening complications following arthroscopy in CO_2. One patient developed a massive pneumoperitoneum, and the other developed acidosis with a pH of 7.02. In both cases arthroscopy had been performed without a tourniquet.

Since an insufflation device is required, gas does not satisfy the requirement than the arthroscopic medium be convenient to use.

Table 3–2. Advantages of gas distention

- Good image quality
- Rapid inflation of the joint
- Easy to differentiate between recent and old ruptures of the anterior cruciate ligament
- Joint is easy to evaluate in the presence of hemarthrosis

Table 3–3. Disadvantages of gas distention

- Gas escapes through incisions, leading to deflation
- Vision is obscured by bubbles in residual intraarticular fluid
- Blood and synovial fluid stick to the lens, obscuring vision
- Steam may fog the lens, especially when a high-power light source is used
- Escaping gas can cause cutaneous emphysema
- Gas insufflation device is required
- Risk of fatal pulmonary embolism

A gas medium can accommodate only a limited range of arthroscopic operations. Procedures involving the use of motorized or electrosurgical instruments cannot be performed.

Another problem is the tendency of the gas medium to escape through the instrument portals. This requires the creation of very small portals, adding to the difficulty of instrument insertion. Gas also sacrifices the lavage effect obtained with a fluid medium (see Sect. 3.4.1).

Arthroscopy in a gas medium alone can be recommended as long as its limitations are understood and precautions are taken. It is imperative that a tourniquet or exsanguinating bandage be applied prior to gas arthroscopy. The complications described to date (air embolism, pneumoperitoneum) occurred in cases where a tourniquet or Esmarch bandage was not used.

3.4.3 Combination of Gas and Fluid

Alternate gas and fluid distention has produced good results at some centers. Following application of an Esmarch bandage, the joint is first irrigated with fluid, then distended with gas and inspected with the arthroscope. If arthroscopic surgery is required, the gas is evacuated and the joint redistended with fluid.

Fresh bony injuries, such as a fracture of the proximal tibia, are a contraindication to primary air arthroscopy. Primary fluid distention is required.

3.5 Irrigation System

Distending the joint once with fluid is not sufficient to obtain optimum viewing conditions for arthroscopy. Often there are tissue fragments (meniscus, cartilage, loose bodies) floating within the joint, or a bloody effusion may be present. To ensure unobstructed vision, copious irrigation is required to clear the joint of loose tissue fragments and effusion, especially when hemarthrosis is present. The joint may be filled and aspirated through the arthroscope sheath or through a separate irrigation cannula.

3.5.1 Fluid Inflow

The fluid may flow into the knee joint directly through the arthroscope sheath (see Sect. 3.1.1) or through a separate inflow cannula. A separate cannula is rarely needed when a large-bore sheath is used.

Inflow Through the Sheath

The fluid flows from the plastic bags to the arthroscope sheath through a large-bore tube or Y-shaped tubing system (infusion set) like that originally developed for urologic surgery (Fig. 3-26). The infusion set is attached to the fluid bags by a special, easy-to-handle *Safe-lock connector* (Fresenius). With its simple rotary connector, the Safe-lock system protects against contact contamination and maintains an effective seal through integrated microbe barriers. Flow from the bag is released by bending back a lock tab on the bag connector (Fig. 3-24).

All air bubbles are removed from the infusion system. Bubbles in the joint obstruct vi-

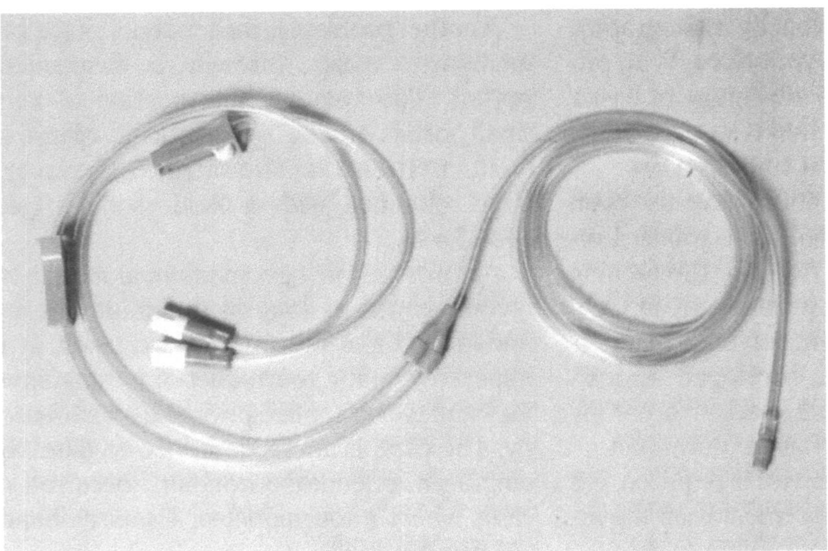

Fig. 3-26. Y-shaped infusion set with a Luer adapter that connects the tubing directly to the arthroscope sheath (Fresenius)

sion and can even lead to the misinterpretation of findings. The Y-tube infusion set is sufficiently long and has Luer lock fittings that connect it directly to a stopcock on the sheath. A separate inflow tube is not required.

Inflow Through a Separate Cannula

Following distention of the joint through the sheath, a separate inflow cannula can be easily inserted into the joint under arthroscopic vision. Inserting the large inflow cannula before distending the joint is less reliable, and faulty placement of the cannula can hamper the rest of the procedure.

Advantages. A separate inflow cannula is advantageous in that it produces a good, rapid irrigating effect so that a good-quality image can be quickly achieved. Placement of the arthroscope portal is made easier by previous distention of the joint through a separate cannula, although since the knee is a large joint, primary placement of the arthroscope portal is scarcely a problem. In the arthroscopy of other joints such as the ankle, shoulder, elbow, or wrist, it is helpful to distend the joint with fluid before making the portal for the arthroscope.

Problems. Failure of the joint to distend after the cannula is inserted and the inflow turned on may be due to faulty placement of the cannula or an anatomic variant such as a complete suprapatellar plica (Fig. 3-27). If there is only one opening at the cannula tip, it may be occluded by hypertrophic synovial villi.

Besides positioning errors (Fig. 3-27), the inflow cannula also may slip out of the joint cavity. Or inflow may be blocked by flexing the knee past 60°–80° or by moving the leg to the figure-four position (see Fig. 8-79). This degree of knee flexion flattens the suprapatel-

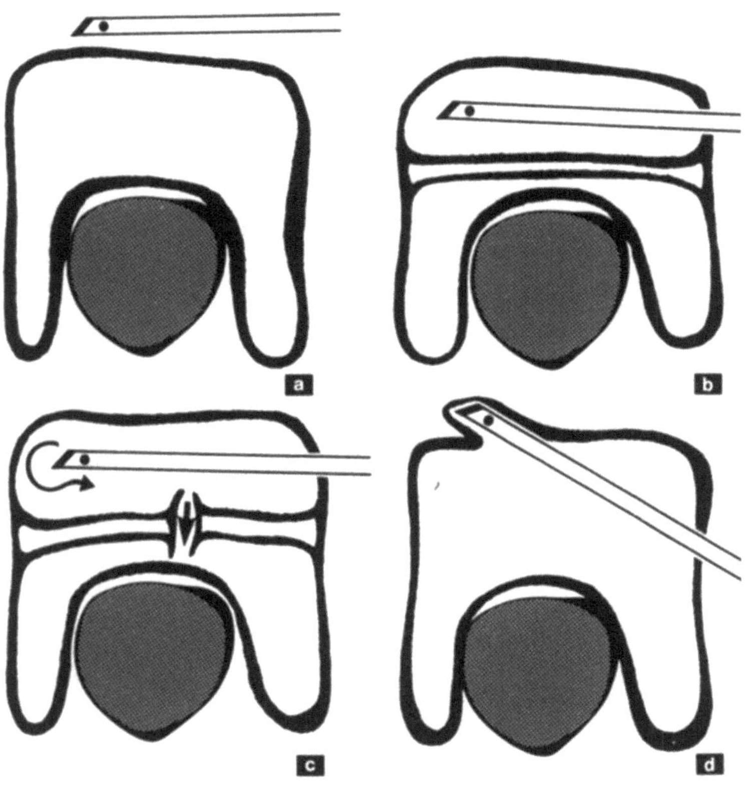

Fig. 3-27 a–d. Insufficient distention of the knee joint through a separate inflow cannula. Potential causes are extrasynovial placement (**a**), a suprapatellar septum (**b**), adhesions in the suprapatellar pouch or a minimal opening in the suprapatellar septum (**c**), or obstruction of the cannula opening by synovium (**d**)

lar pouch, obliterates the communication between the pouch and the femorotibial joint space, and occludes the cannula outlets. In such situations it may be necessary to irrigate directly through the arthroscope sheath.

Indications. A separate inflow cannula is indicated for arthroscopic operations in which motorized instruments (shavers) are used for an extended period of time. Motorized instruments require a copious fluid stream as they simultaneously break up and aspirate tissues. If there is insufficient flow to keep the joint distended, portions of the synovium will be drawn against the cutter and damaged, causing the joint to collapse. This produces a "yellow out" on the monitor (see Sect. 11.3), and the procedure must be interrupted until the joint can be redistended.

A large-bore arthroscope sheath delivers an adequate fluid volume (see Sect. 3.3.1) and usually obviates the need for an inflow cannula. If an instrument portal has been created, it can also serve as a portal for the inflow cannula.

Positioning. Like the sheath, the inflow cannula is inserted into the extended knee joint with the aid of an obturator following incision of the skin and fibrous capsule. Since a diagonal irrigation path is supposed to be advantageous, a medial suprapatellar portal has been recommended for the irrigation cannula when the arthroscope is introduced through a lateral portal. But in this approach the cannula passes directly through the vastus medialis obliquus muscle, and we have found that this frequently results in lingering postoperative pain. Occasional partial or even complete atrophy of the vastus medialis is also observed. Thus, in cases where a separate inflow portal is needed for joint distention, we introduce the cannula just medial to the medial patellar border through the tendinous insertion of the vastus medialis obliquus (Fig. 3-28) or, if possible, through a lateral suprapatellar approach.

With a high medial portal, there is risk of injury to the femoropatellar articular cartilage, especially if the knee joint is flexed.

3.5.2 Fluid Outflow

We aspirate the irrigating fluid through a Y-shaped tubing system (Fig. 3-29). The princi-

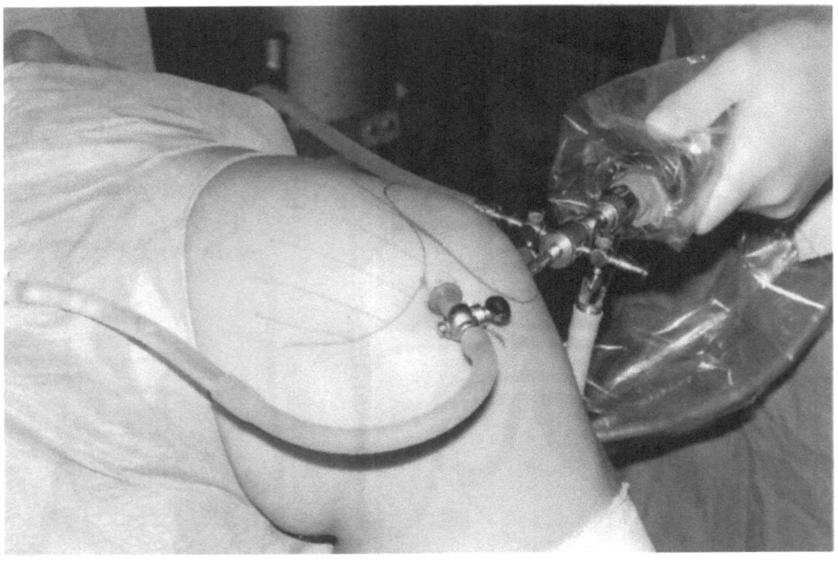

Fig. 3-28. The inflow cannula is inserted through the tendinous insertion of the vastus medialis obliquus (muscle fibers indicated by hatched lines) following distention of the joint through the arthroscope sheath

ple of this aspiration system is easy to understand once the problems are recognized. During arthroscopy in an aqueous medium, the irrigating fluid is drawn out of the joint through the arthroscope sheath, which is connected by tubing to the suction apparatus in the operating room.

In principle, however, additional suction devices would be needed to remove the fluid that leaks continuously from the instrument portals and collects between the patient's legs, as well as the outflow from motorized instrumentation (shaver system). A sensible alternative to multiple suction devices is to combine the various outflows (sheath, shavers, leaking fluid) in one system. We do this by connecting a *Y piece* to the approximately 150 cm length of tubing from the suction apparatus. To each arm of the Y piece, we attach a 40 cm length of tube, one of which has an adjustable stopcock at its center (see Fig. 3-29). The tube without a stopcock is connected to the arthroscope. The tube with a stopcock is placed between the patient's legs in a closed position; it is used to selectively remove leaking irrigation fluid from the waterproof draping sheet. When a motorized instrument is used, this tube is connected to the aspiration port of the shaver. An assistant can adjust the stopcock to regulate the level of suction, or switch it off, as required.

The fluid is aspirated intermittently, or in rare cases continuously, through the arthroscope sheath or through a separate outflow cannula, which is similar to a large-gauge inflow needle. The outflow cannula, which has a diameter of 5–7 mm, is inserted through an instrument portal with the stylet in place. The cannula tip is then directed under arthroscopic vision to the portion of the joint where cartilaginous or meniscal debris will collect during the arthroscopic surgery. In this way the particles can be selectively aspirated from the joint.

The alternating use of aspiration and inflow can be utilized diagnostically. By positioning the scope tip in front of the hard-to-see posterior horn of a meniscus and aspirating fluid, the free inner border of the meniscus can be drawn toward the scope so that it can be inspected more easily. Sometimes this maneuver is necessary to detect the presence of a tear, although it is no substitute for palpation with the probing hook (see below).

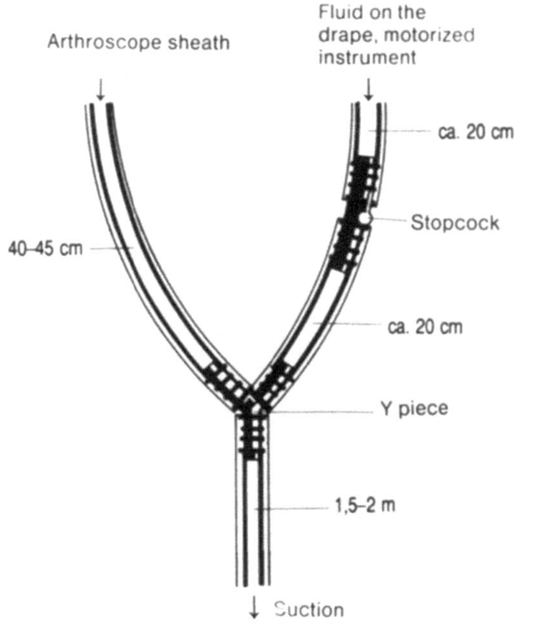

Fig. 3-29. Y-tube fluid aspiration system

Some arthroscopists use an irrigation cannula passed into the superior pouch through a suprapatellar portal as an outflow drain.

3.6 Probing Hook

Since the arthroscopist cannot insert his finger into the joint to check the integrity and consistency of the cartilage, menisci, and anterior cruciate ligament, he must use a slender instrument, the probing hook, which represents an extension of his palpating finger (Fig. 3-30).

The probing hook is of fundamental importance in diagnostic arthroscopy. Once the basic technique for using the probe has been learned in a model knee, routine arthroscopic work offers ample opportunities to perfect the visualization and selective palpation of anatomic structures within the arthroscopic field.

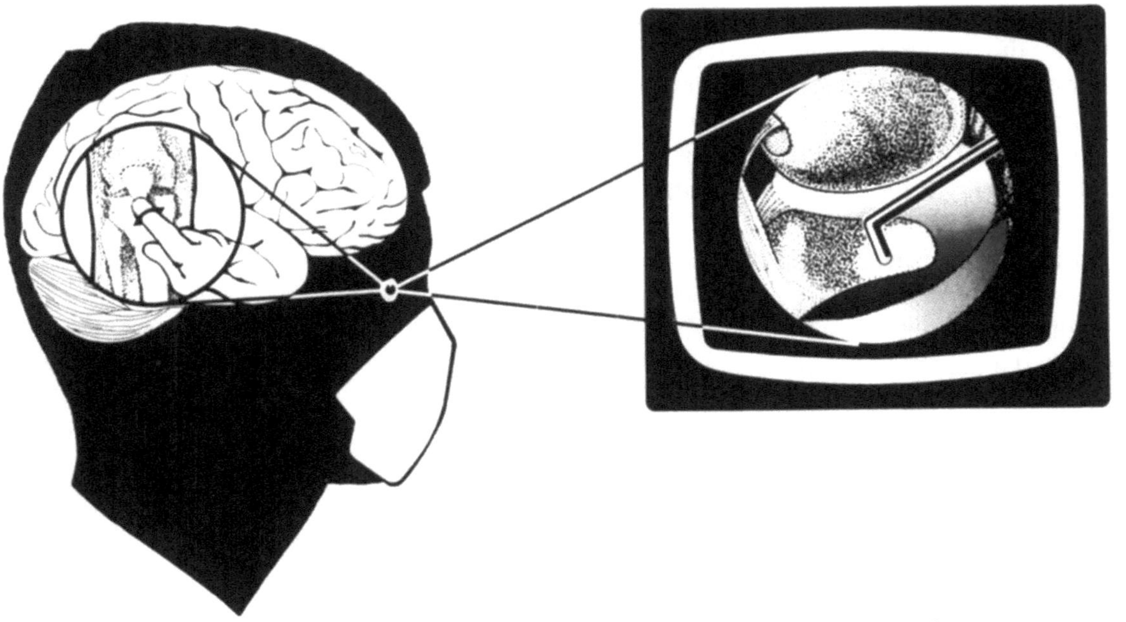

Fig. 3-30. The probing hook functions as a thin extension of the arthroscopist's palpating finger

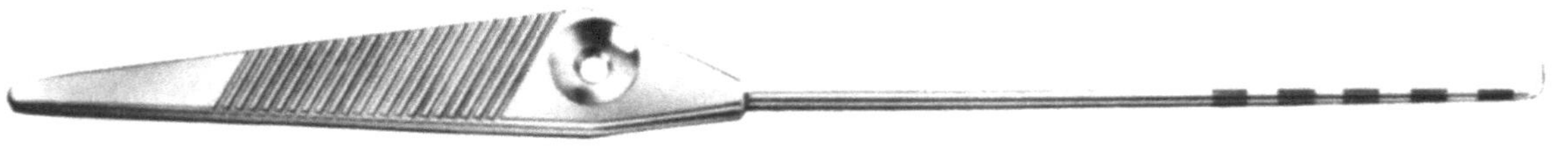

Fig. 3-31. Arthroscopic probe with length markings (Aesculap)

Selective probing is a basic prerequisite of operative arthroscopy.

The probe is inserted into the knee through a separate instrument portal whose location is determined by the cannula technique (see Sect. 6.2).

The shaft of the probe has markings at 5 mm intervals to help the operator determine the size of intraarticular structures. The hook itself is 3 or 5 mm long. Knowing this, the operator should be able to estimate the size of a cartilage lesion or meniscal tear without difficulty (Fig. 3-31).

Some determinations during arthroscopy, such as the exclusion of a meniscal tear (Fig. 3-32 a), require more than simple inspection through the arthroscope. Neither should palpation be limited to touching or stroking tissues with the probe. Rather, the

Fig. 3-32 a–d. Probing the posterior horn of the medial ▶ meniscus.
History: The patient, a 16–year-old girl, fell 4 weeks ago while playing soccer. Her family doctor aspirated 30 ml of blood from the knee joint. The knee was subsequently immobilized in plaster for 3 weeks, followed by functional exercises. Effusion recurred, the knee showing a positive Lachman test with a soft end point and a negative pivot shift.
Arthroscopic findings: The posterior portion of the medial meniscus appears completely normal (**a**), but selective probing with pressure on the meniscal surface reveals a posterior longitudinal tear with inbulging of the free border of the meniscus (**b**). The extent of the tear is difficult to discern but can be defined by additional probing (**c**). Elevation of the meniscus clearly demonstrates the peripheral extent of the tear (**d**). Swollen remnants of the completely ruptured anterior cruciate ligament were found in the intercondylar area.
Procedure: Repair of the torn meniscus (the posterior horn performs an important stabilizing and proprioceptive function). If repair is not possible, partial meniscectomy is indicated. A cruciate ligament reconstruction is indicated

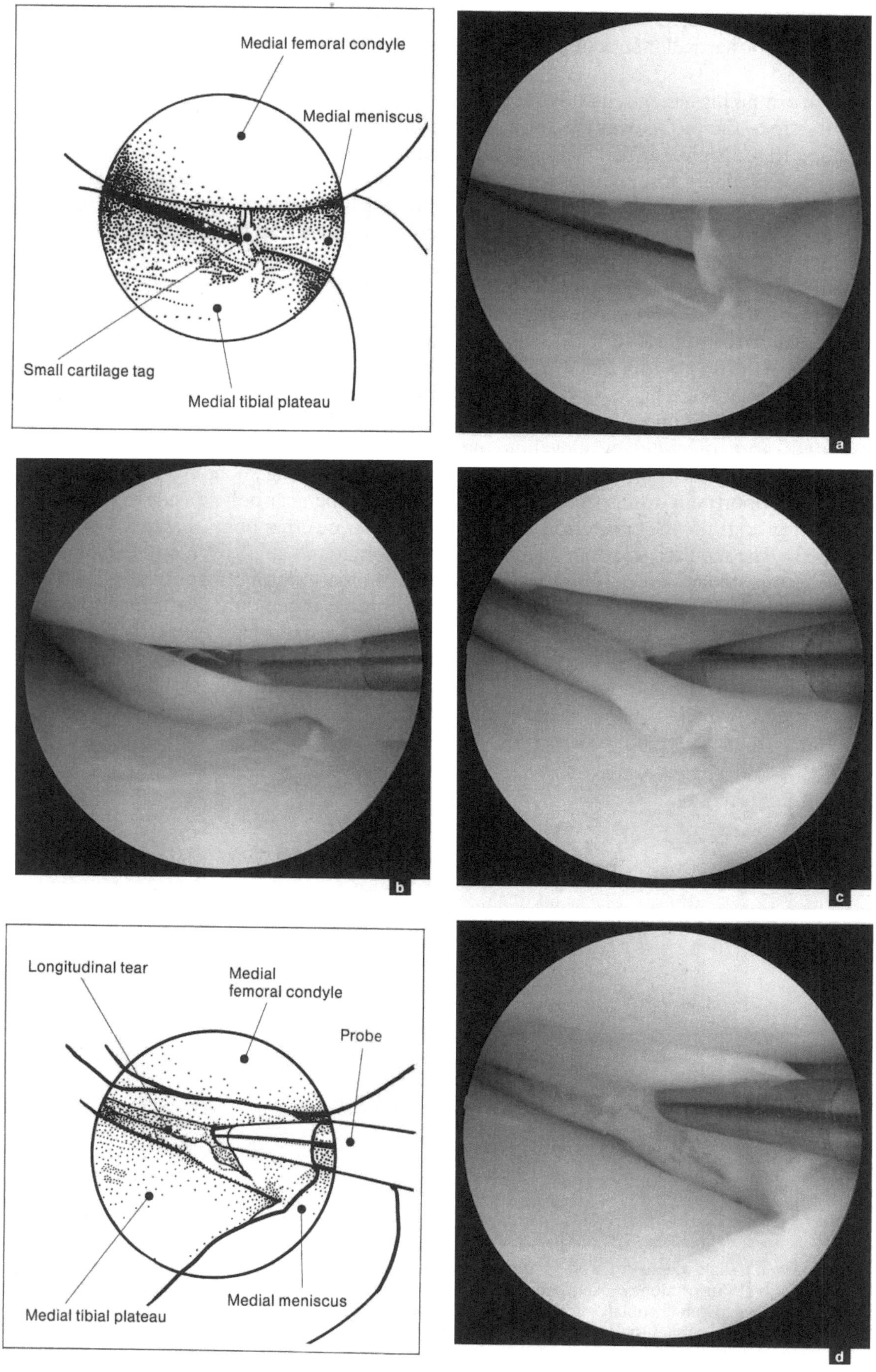
Medial femoral condyle
Medial meniscus
Small cartilage tag
Medial tibial plateau
a
b
c
Longitudinal tear
Medial
femoral condyle
Probe
Medial tibial plateau
Medial meniscus
d

probe should exert selective tension and pressure on the intraarticular structures of interest.

When examining a meniscus, it is not sufficient to stroke the probe over the surface in the hope that an unseen tear will pop into view. The examiner must actively search for meniscal lesions. He should apply tension to the base of the meniscus to detect any peripheral longitudinal tears or separations at the meniscosynovial junction. He should elevate the meniscus to inspect its inferior surface and apply pressure to its upper surface to look for elevations of the free border that would signify a submeniscal tear (Fig. 3-32 b-d). Sometimes the configuration of the tear can be evaluated more precisely by elevating the meniscus from below (Fig. 3-32 d). This also affords an opportunity to inspect the meniscotibial portion of the posterior capsule (Fig. 3-33). The menisci are probed to evaluate their consistency. Areas of degenerative change will be hard or so fibery that the hook can sink into the tissue. Healthy meniscus tissue has a tense, springy consistency.

The integrity of the anterior cruciate ligament is tested by pulling on the ligament with the probing hook. Sometimes ruptured portions of the anterior cruciate ligament can be pulled through small tears in the synovium.

Selective probing is also essential for ascertaining the depth and extent of cartilage lesions. If cartilage fissures or cartilage flaps are found, they are probed to determine whether the adjacent cartilage is detached or adherent. Probing is the only way to confirm or exclude chondromalacic softening (see Figs. 9-1 and 9.4).

The probing hook can also be used as a retractor to hold aside an infrapatellar plica or adhesive bands that obscure vision. Sometimes an infrapatellar plica must be retracted before the anterior cruciate ligament can be assessed. With a torn anterior cruciate ligament, it is important to determine whether portions of the ligament are still intact. Torn ligament fibers can be held aside with the probe tip to expose other fibers that may be intact.

Though still used by many examiners, a thin blunt obturator does not make a satisfactory probe. It can only exert direct pressure on structures; it cannot exert traction on the menisci or anterior cruciate ligament, nor can it explore fine cartilage fissures to establish their depth and extent. A probing hook is essential for these manipulations.

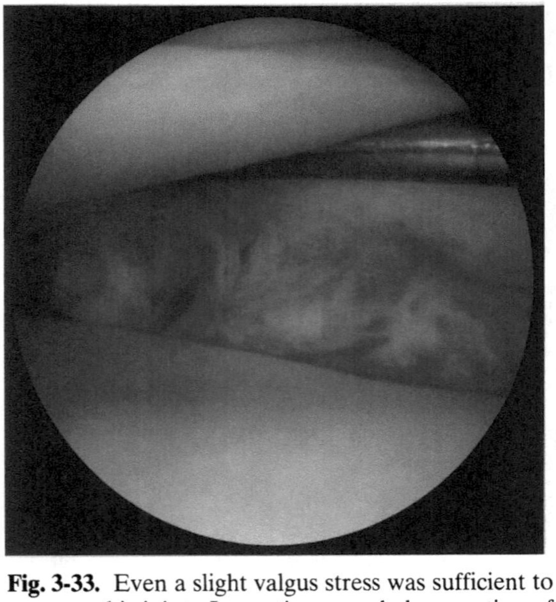

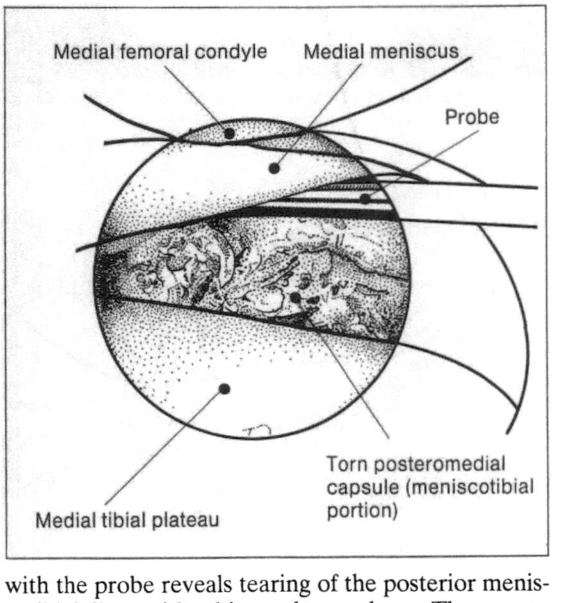

Fig. 3-33. Even a slight valgus stress was sufficient to open up this joint. Inspection revealed separation of the medial meniscus from the tibial plateau, implying a meniscotibial ligamentous injury. Lifting the meniscus with the probe reveals tearing of the posterior meniscotibial fibers with subjacent hemorrhage. There was a coexisting rupture of the anterior cruciate ligament

4
Preparation of the Patient and Equipment

4.1
Anesthesia

Besides general anesthesia, regional forms of anesthesia (spinal and peridural) may be used for arthroscopy of the knee. Depending on the type of anesthesia used, the preoperative workup includes an ECG, chest radiograph, and laboratory blood studies (electrolytes, hemoglobin and hematocrit, white blood count, platelets). It is imperative that the major plasma coagulation parameters-partial thromboplastin time and prothrombin time-be determined. These values are not only important for the anesthesiologist but also provide the arthroscopist with valuable information. In juveniles with hemarthrosis following an apparently trivial injury or with unexplained knee pain, more serious disorders (hemophilia, malignant or rheumatoid systemic disease) may be causative. In these cases the examiner should be alert for pathologic blood and coagulation values. In patients with chronic complaints, further information can be obtained by determining the ESR and possibly by testing for rheumatoid factors.

The patient must be fasted for the operation, regardless of the type of anesthesia used.

4.1.1
General Anesthesia

General anesthesia represents the simplest and most convenient form of anesthesia for the operator. The complete muscular relaxation permits a more thorough arthroscopy, including the accurate testing of ligamentous laxity. Also, the patient feels no discomfort when the tourniquet on the thigh is inflated. One disadvantage of general anesthesia is that the patient cannot watch the procedure on the monitor, so he must rely on the postoperative description of the operator. However, prior arrangements can be made to give the patient a videotape of "his" arthroscopy upon discharge.

4.1.2
Regional Anesthesia

Spinal and peridural anesthesia are forms of anesthesia, besides local (see below), that allow the patient to witness his own operation. Spinal anesthesia is recommended for older patients, and peridural anesthesia for younger patients. Continuous peridural anesthesia is induced by passing a thin catheter into the peridural space and injecting a local anesthetic. The great advantage of this technique is that the peridural catheter can be left indwelling for several days to control pain in the immediate postoperative period. We prefer this form of anesthesia following arthroscopic arthrolyses, as it allows for painless postoperative mobilization on a continuous passive motion device. Management of the patient with a peridural catheter requires close cooperation among the arthroscopist, anesthesiologist, and nursing staff. The catheter site should be checked daily for signs of inflammation (redness?).

Spinal anesthesia, unlike peridural, induces complete muscular relaxation. While it is technically easier to perform, a "spinal" headache may persist for several days postoperatively. This is an especially common sequel in younger patients.

4.1.3 Local Anesthesia

Local anesthesia is technically easier than general or regional anesthesia, and the examiner can induce it himself, although a standby anesthesiologist should be available. The preparations (blood work, chest radiograph) are the same as those for general or regional anesthesia. It is necessary that ECG monitoring be maintained during the procedure.

Significant disadvantages of local anesthesia are lack of muscle-relaxing effect; in tight joints it can be very difficult to visualize the posterior horns of the menisci. A tourniquet or Esmarch bandage cannot be applied in every patient. Moreover, the duration of anesthesia is limited, and this can place the less experienced arthroscopist under time pressure. If the patient complains of pain, the beginner will tend to hurry the procedure to get through.

Although most arthroscopic operations can be performed under local anesthesia, we use a local anesthesic only in exceptional cases where general or regional anesthesia is contraindicated.

As noted above, standard preoperative preparations are carried out. The patient is fasted, and an intravenous line is placed as in the regional forms of anesthesia. In the few patients who experience nausea or even an anaphylactic response, the i.v. line provides a route for administering drug therapy.

Technique of Local Anesthesia
Following skin preparation, the entry site for the arthroscope is infiltrated with a local anesthetic (1% mepivacaine with epinephrine) from the skin to the synovium. When the needle tip enters the joint cavity, it becomes easier to depress the plunger. The needle is left in that position, and a syringe containing 20 ml of a long-acting local anesthetic (0.5% bupivacaine) is attached. When the solution is injected into the joint cavity, a slow dripping of the administered solution from the hub confirms intraarticular placement of the needle tip. If the infrapatellar fat pad is injected by mistake, the patient will describe a strong feeling of anterior knee pressure during the injection. A distended fat pad can make the rest of the procedure more difficult. The operator waits for the anesthetic to take effect (5–10 min) before proceeding with the arthroscopy.

Problems
If the patient moves his leg during the arthroscopy, the scope tip can easily damage the articular cartilage (Glinz 1987). Due to the disadvantages of local anesthesia – no exsanguination (see Sect. 4.3), time pressure, lack of complete muscular relaxation – general or regional anesthesia is strongly recommended for the less experienced arthroscopist.

General rule of thumb: A patient who is relaxed and cooperative during the clinical examination is a good candidate for local anesthesia. If the patient is anxious or tense, local anesthesia is contraindicated.

4.2 Positioning

The leg should be positioned so that the knee joint is accessible from the medial and lateral sides. It should be easy to manipulate instruments inserted through a medial or posteromedial portal. Additionally, it should be possible to examine the knee in various flexion angles, to apply a varus and valgus stress, and to move the leg to the figure-four position.

Whether the knee is extended on the table or flexed over the table edge, the patient should be in the supine position.

4.2.1 Extended Leg Position

A padded *lateral post* is attached to the side of the table a handswidth proximal to the superior patellar border (Fig. 4-1). The thigh can be placed against this post for the application of valgus stress during examination of the medial compartment.

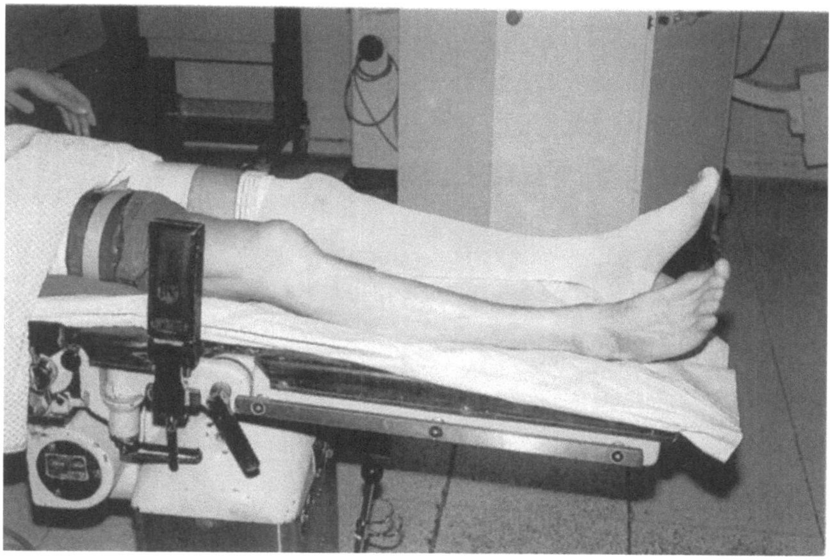

Fig. 4-1. Positioning the leg in extension. The lateral post is attached to the table about a handwidth proximal to the patella

The unaffected leg is slightly lowered and abducted so that irrigation fluid draining from the portals can collect where the drape sags between the legs, where it is easily removed by suction. The knee can be flexed by placing the foot flat on the operating table or by flexing the leg over the edge of the table.

Extending the operated leg next to a side post is a simple, time-saving positioning technique. No special table adjustments are needed, and padded side posts are readily available.

Problems. Placing the side post too far proximally (i.e., at the center of the thigh) results in a very unfavorable lever arm for opening the medial compartment. The thigh can easily rotate internally, making it difficult to stress open the medial joint space. Adjustable, articulated side posts have not proven satisfactory as they tend to give way when a strong valgus force is applied.

4.2.2 Flexed Leg Position

This position requires the use of a *leg holder* (Fig. 4-2). Otherwise the thigh would tend to rotate at the hip, and a specific knee position could not be maintained.

A lateral post like that used for the extended knee is inadequate since it can stabilize the knee against valgus but not against rotation.

The foot of the operating table is broken 90° or removed on the side where the arthroscopy is to be performed (Fig. 4-3). The opposite leg is laterally abducted, either extending the lower leg or flexing it about 60°. The leg holder is applied so that it is flush with the edge of the table. It must not press against the inside of the opposite thigh or pinch the genitals. Abducting the healthy leg avoids this positioning complication while allowing free instrument manipulations through medial and posteromedial portals.

Before the leg is fixed in the holder, it is confirmed that the thigh is in a position of neutral rotation. Otherwise the joint space cannot be adequately stressed open during arthroscopy.

The tourniquet should be positioned as far proximally on the thigh as possible. Integrating the tourniquet into the leg holder (Fig. 4-2) is helpful in that it increases available working space about the knee-a particular advantage in cruciate ligament operations. The tourniquet is secured in the leg holder with a velcro fastener to increase its resistance to thigh rotation. The position of the thigh in the holder is personally checked by the operator and adjusted as needed.

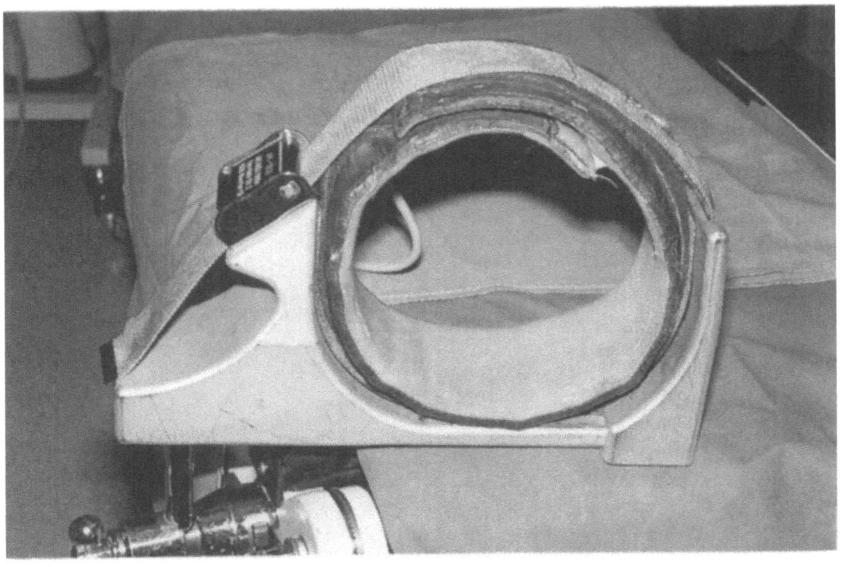

Fig. 4-2. Leg holder with integrated tourniquet, used when the knee is flexed over the edge of the table

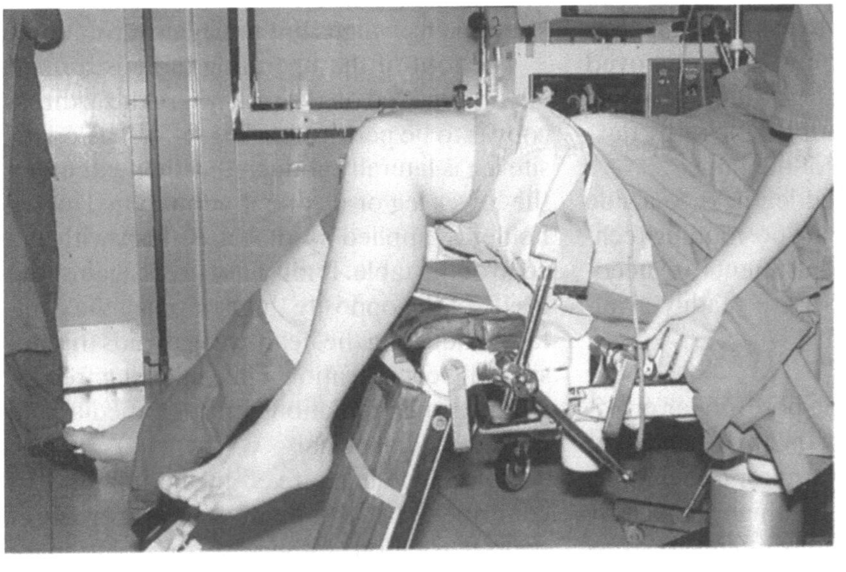

Fig. 4-3. The foot of the operating table is lowered for use of the leg holder. Before skin preparation is begun, the leg holder and proximal thigh are draped off from the operative site with a waterproof sheet

Just distal to the leg holder with integrated tourniquet, a waterproof drape is taped about the circumference of the thigh to prevent alcohol from running back beneath the tourniquet and thigh during the skin preparation (Fig. 4-3). Without this precautionary measure, alcohol pooling might cause caustic burns to pressure-bearing sites on the thigh and buttock.

For visualization of the medial meniscus, the arthroscopist places the distal part of the patient's lower leg against his own iliac crest, using his body weight as a convenient means to stress open the medial joint space. The slight flexion required for this maneuver is optimized as needed by adjusting the height of the operating table. For examination of the lateral compartment, the leg may be held by an assistant, or the lower leg may be crossed over the contralateral thigh (figure-four position, see Fig. 8-81). If the knee must be kept extended for a prolonged period, the foot is braced against the instrument table.

Both positioning methods restrict terminal flexion of the knee, but this is of no consequence since the anterior portions of the joint cannot be evaluated in any case due to pressure from the fat pad and patella. The posteromedial compartment is accessible by both the intercondylar and posteromedial routes when the knee is flexed to just 70°–90°.

4.3 Bloodless Field

The necessity of a bloodless field for arthroscopy of the knee joint can no longer be questioned. The use of a tourniquet or Esmarch bandage prevents troublesome bleeding from the portals, from capsuloligamentous tears, and from the synovium. The joint can be cleared of hemarthrosis much more rapidly since there is no afterbleeding to sustain it. Without tourniquet control or exsanguination, acutely injured knees are often very difficult to examine arthroscopically. Adequate anesthesia is necessary whenever a tourniquet or exsanguinating bandage is applied. When local anesthesia is used, the patient can tolerate tourniquet inflation only if the femoral nerve is concurrently blocked.

Before the skin prep is begun, the tourniquet is placed on the thigh and secured circumferentially with adhesive tape to prevent accidental loosening. When a leg holder is used, care is taken that the tourniquet is fixed at the level of the holder (see Fig. 4-2).

Exsanguination is accomplished by wrapping the leg with an *Esmarch bandage* and inflating the tourniquet to the desired pressure (500 mm Hg for adults, 300–400 mm Hg for adolescents, 100–300 mm Hg for children) (Fig. 4-4).

The tourniquet may be kept inflated for *no longer than 120 min* (see Sect. 12.4). While less experienced operators tend to use the fully allotted tourniquet time, seasoned arthroscopic surgeons require an average of 15–60 min, although more time is needed for complicated procedures such as anterior cruciate ligament reconstruction or synovectomy.

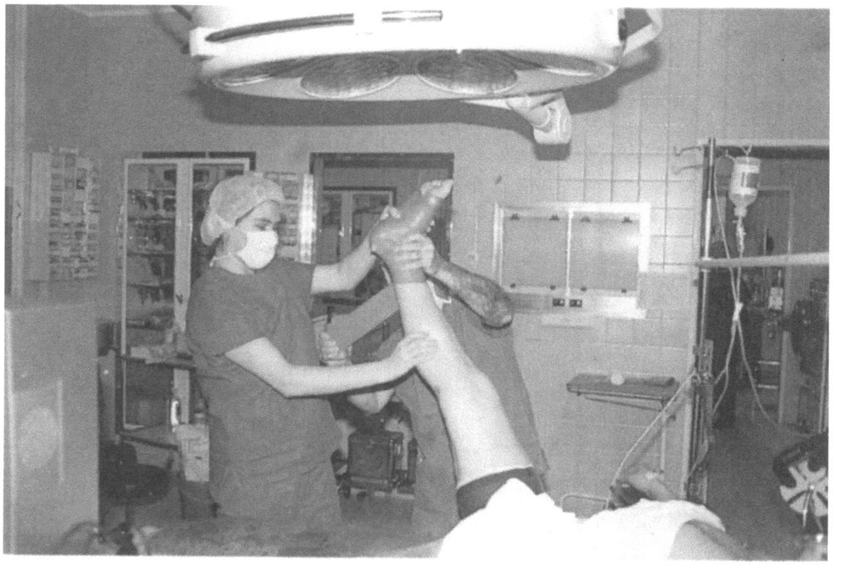

Fig. 4-4. The leg is exsanguinated with an Esmarch bandage

4.4 Draping

For arthroscopy in a fluid medium, the operative area must be draped with a waterproof material. Waterproof disposable drapes and gowns are available for this purpose. The instrument table, the leg to be arthroscopied, and the operator must be covered with waterproof materials. The many preoperative preparations are too time-consuming for OR personnel if all the draping materials have to be individually unwrapped. It is far more efficient to use an arthroscopy pack (several are available on the market) that includes all the materials needed for a complete arthroscopic draping procedure (Fig. 4-5, Table 4-1). Cloth drapes are used for arthroscopy in a gas medium.

Following application of the tourniquet or Esmarch bandage and the skin preparation, the unaffected leg and the operating table are draped with a large sheet, and a medium sheet is placed over the patient's upper body. The lower leg on the operative side, held by a sterile assistant during the preliminary draping, is covered with a stockinette or adhesive drape to just below the tibial tuberosity. The stockinette is secured with adhesive tape to form a watertight seal (Fig. 4-6).

Next the foot is drawn through the opening in the large aperture sheet. The sheet is pulled up to the desired level, slightly proximal to the femoral condyles, and unfolded. This draping procedure creates a sterile, waterproof seal that completely encompasses the operative site, isolating it from the operating table and screening it off from the anesthesiologist (Fig. 4-7).

Generally we no longer use an incise drape on the knee. About a half-dollar-size area of the drape must be removed in any case over the arthroscopic and instrument portals. If the drape is only incised, there is a danger that instrument changes or pistoning of the arthroscope will tear off small pieces of film that may contaminate the joint cavity. Sometimes we use an incise drape for arthroscopic reconstructions of the anterior cruciate ligament.

Before draping is begun, the operator again checks the position of the lateral post or leg holder and makes any final adjustments that are needed.

Table 4-1. Contents of a draping set for arthroscopy

– Large sheet (e.g., 150 x 200 cm)
– Small or medium sheet (e.g., 100 x 150 cm)
– Instrument table cover
– Stockinette for foot and lower leg
– Large aperture sheet (e.g., 200 x 300 cm)
– Adhesive tapes
– Surgical gown

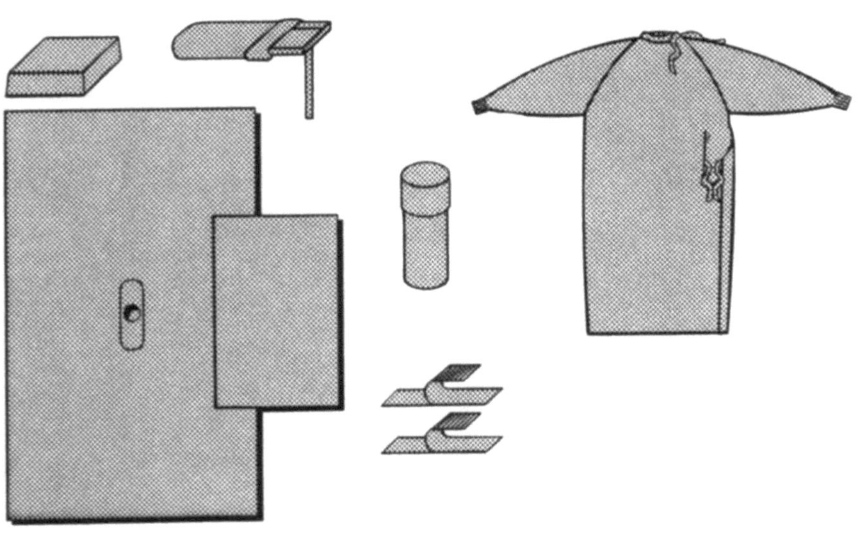

Fig. 4-5. Draping set for diagnostic and operative arthroscopy (e.g., Klinidrape 100 from Mölnlycke)

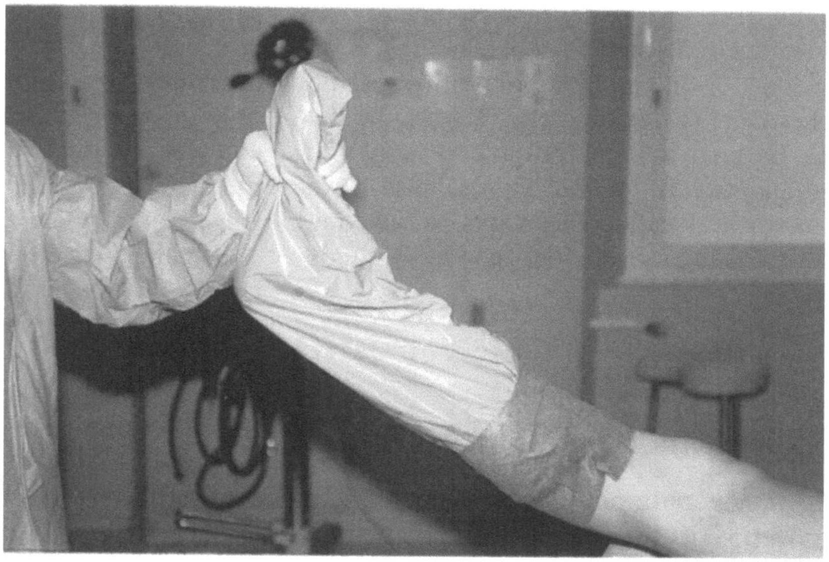

Fig. 4-6. The foot and lower leg are covered with a waterproof stockinette (Mölnlycke)

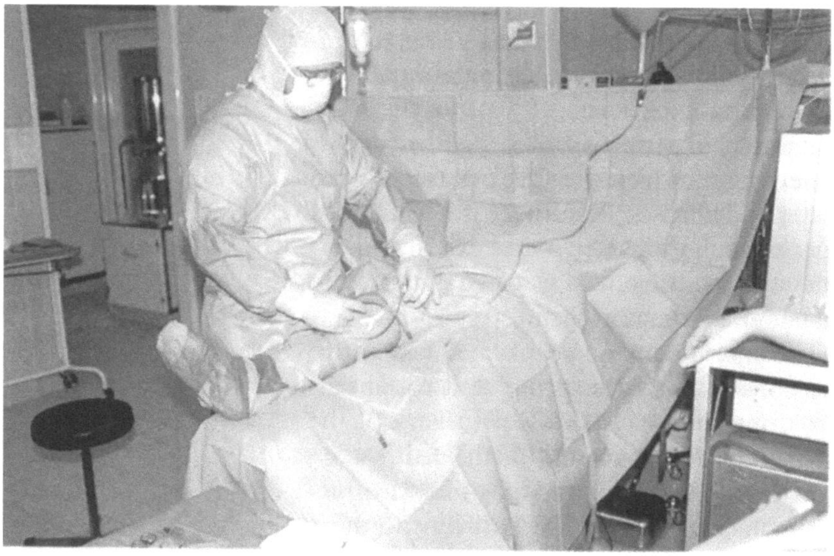

Fig. 4-7. The operative site is completely draped off with water-repellent materials, to which the inflow and aspiration tubing (Y tubing) are secured

4.4.1 Problems with Fluid Runoff

Even diagnostic arthroscopy in a fluid medium is rarely a "dry" procedure. In arthroscopic operations, it is common for multiple portals to be established and alternately used. The uncontrolled drainage of irrigating fluid is unavoidable, yet it is also desirable for its lavage effect in the joint cavity. Puddles of water collect on the drape and sometimes on the floor of the operating suite. Fluid pooling in the sterile field is removed with the suction line of the arthroscope (after disconnecting it from the spigot) unless Y-shaped aspiration tubing is used (see Fig. 3-29).

Towels may be spread on the floor of the operating suite, or an industrial vacuum may be used. If a particularly "wet" operation is anticipated, a separate collecting and drainage bag, or one integrated into the aperture sheet, can provide for continuous fluid drainage. Even so, wet feet continue to be an occupational hazard for the arthroscopist. If wet socks are objectionable, socks or stockings should be removed before the procedure begins.

4.5 Equipment Preparation and Layout

For the operator and OR personnel, the introduction of arthroscopy means a significant departure from traditional surgical practices. While in open knee operations the field of operation is frequently visible to the whole operating team, and the instrumentation is reasonably well known, it was only the advent of video arthroscopy that has given the arthroscopic examination the similar quality of a "common experience." Even so, the high-technology nature of video arthroscopy is something to which the OR personnel must adapt. If arthroscopic surgery is additionally performed, various new types of instruments enter the picture, and this can easily lead to misunderstandings in the initial phase.

The instrument nurse plays a less active and consequently less prominent role in arthroscopy than in traditional surgery of the extremities. Many nurses find the arthroscopic anatomy unfamiliar and may find the monitor image, or indeed the entire procedure, difficult to comprehend. Initially, then, it is not unusual for nurses to take a somewhat disparaging attitude toward arthroscopy and arthroscopic surgery.

The arthroscopist should make an effort to establish close cooperative ties with the rest of the operating team. Special problems relating, say, to the draping procedure or selection of instruments should be discussed and resolved with the participation of the OR team.

Given the high technical complexity of arthroscopic equipment and procedures, practices must be standardized. Devices that require a power supply (video monitor, light source, video recorder, shavers, electrocauteries) should all be placed on one mobile cart or arranged on a special multilevel arthroscopy cart (Fig. 4-8). Any number of customized equipment setups may be devised to meet the needs or preferences of the operator (Fig. 4-9).

Whether the arthroscopy cart is specially purchased or homemade, it should be equipped with a power outlet strip; this will help greatly to sort out the tangled mass of cables. All devices on the cart are powered from this central strip, which is bolted to the cart and has a single main cable that plugs into an electrical outlet.

In cases where the operated leg is flexed over the end of the table (see Sect. 4.2.2) and the arthroscopist stands at the foot of the table and faces the anesthesiologist, it may be convenient to mount the equipment on a gantry above the anesthesia screen (Fig. 4-10).

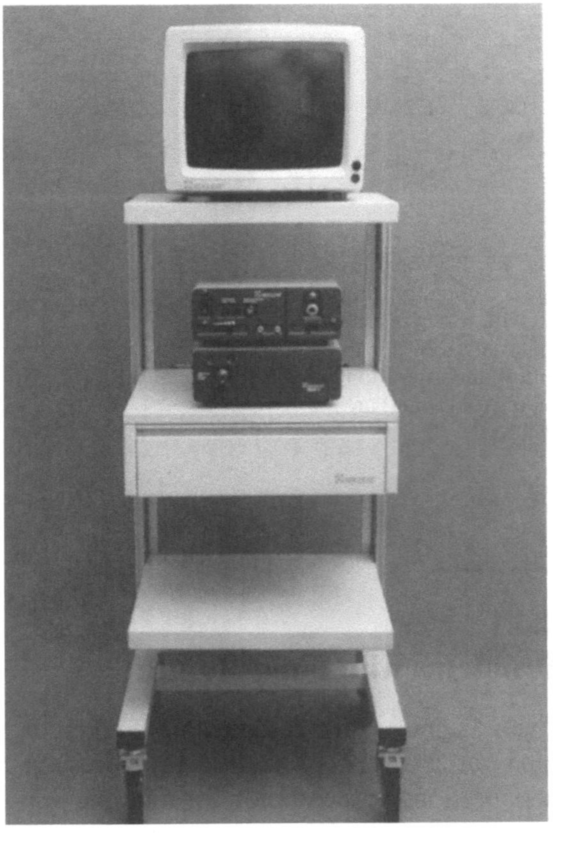

Fig. 4-8. Multi-tiered arthroscopy cart with monitor, light source, and shaver system (Aesculap)

The positions of the operator, assistant, and nurse at the operating table depend on how the leg is positioned. When an extended leg position is used, the nurse, operator, and assistant sit on the lateral side of the leg, with the arthroscopy cart standing on the opposite side at the level of the knee joint (Fig. 4-11). With this arrangement, all participants in the operation can comfortably watch the events on the monitor screen. The instrument table is placed at the foot of the operating table.

Placement of the cables and tubing likewise should be standardized. We find it convenient to route all the cables and tubes into the operative area from the same direction. The suction line, light cable, camera cable, and (in arthroscopic operations) the shaver and electric knife cables from the arthroscopy cart all enter the operative field at a site proximal to the knee joint (see Fig. 4-11). Fluid inflow comes from the anesthesia area, since the i.v. pole or ceiling suspension is usually placed by the patient's head.

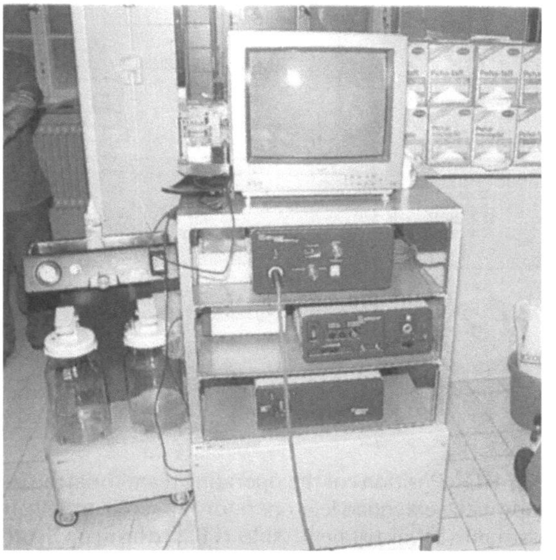

Fig. 4-9. Homemade arthroscopy cart

All cables and lines are secured to the waterproof drape with a blunt clamp or a strip of adhesive tape. It should be possible to adjust the cable lengths slightly if required.

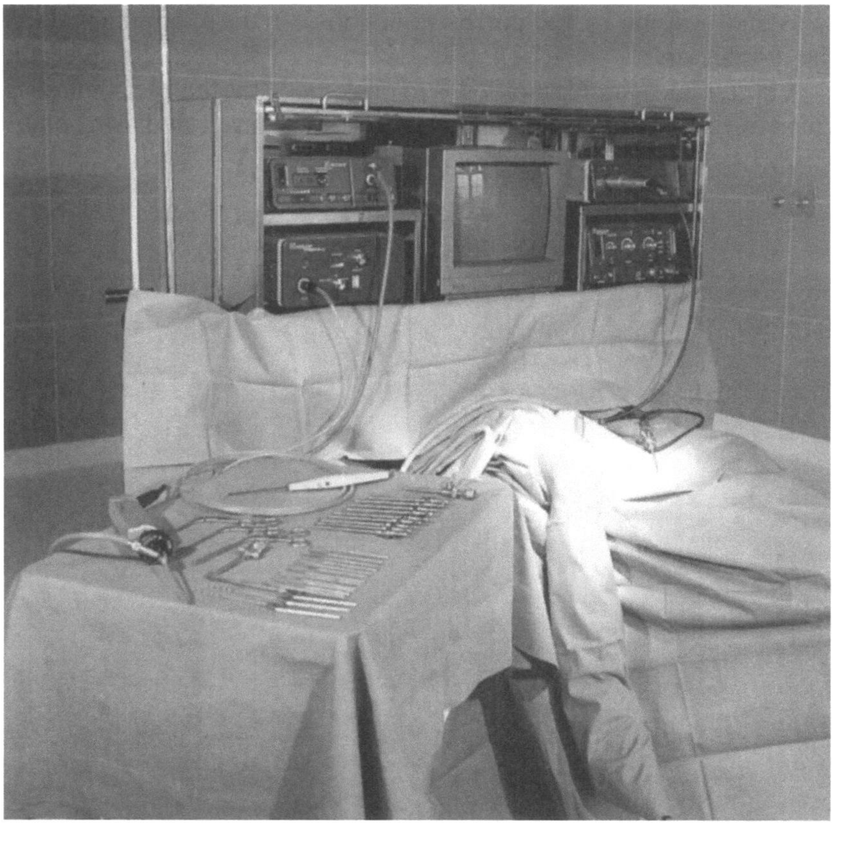

Fig. 4-10. Equipment gantry (Aesculap)

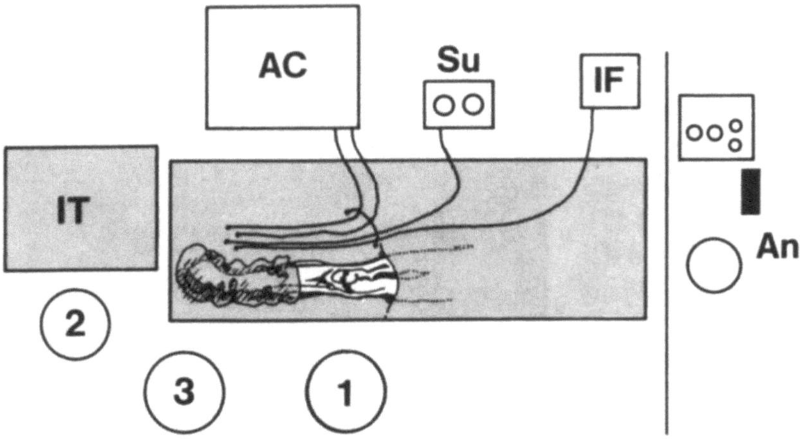

Fig. 4-11. Positions of the operating team for arthroscopy in the extended leg: operator (1), scrub nurse (2), assistant (3), instrument table (IT), arthroscopy cart (AC), suction (Su), suspension for irrigating fluid (IF), anesthesia area (An)

4.5.1 Preparation of the Video Camera

Most video cameras, especially the solid-state chip cameras, can be made relatively sterile by soaking them in a disinfectant solution. However, this risks damage to the camera seals and housing by the corrosive action of the disinfectant.

A better and simpler method is to pack the video camera into a sterile, transparent plastic sleeve (commercially available). First the sleeve is taped to the eyepiece of the telescope, then the camera is placed into it (Fig. 4-12). This method is advantageous as it allows the video camera to be readied quickly for arthroscopy while ensuring absolute sterility during use. A potential disadvantage is that the wrapping makes it difficult to change telescopes. However, this objection is weakened by the fact that all parts of the joint can be inspected using one 30° wide-angle telescope.

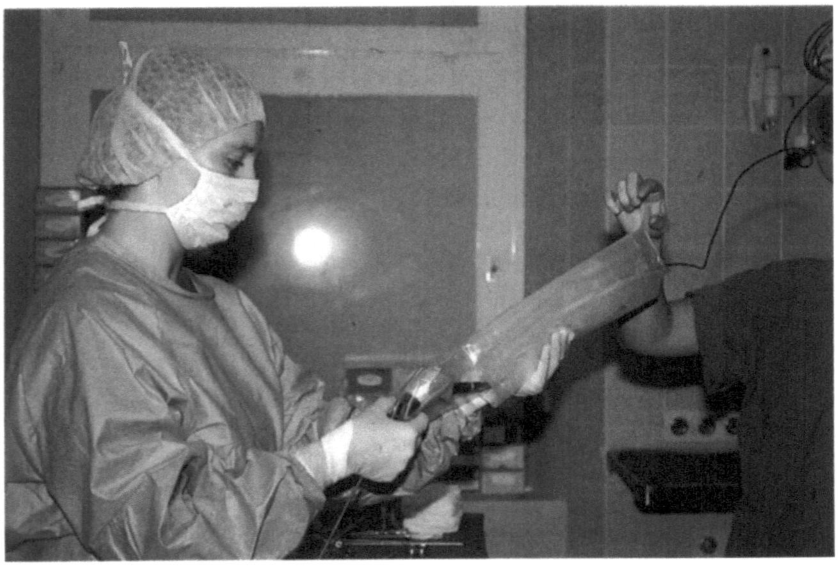

Fig. 4-12. The video camera is packed in a sterile plastic sleeve

For cases where a change of scopes is desired, Kohn (1985) has developed a special adapter to which the sterile plastic sleeve is attached. The telescope can then be changed without violating sterile technique.

4.6 Facilities

An operating room for arthroscopy, whether in a hospital or an outpatient facility, should meet the same requirements in terms of floor space, asepsis, and layout as an operating suite in which open knee surgery is performed. Consideration should also be given to the space requirements for video equipment (see arthroscopy cart, Sect. 4.5) and any additional documentation equipment that is desired (videocassette recorder, extra monitor).

4.7 Care and Maintenance of Arthroscopic Instruments

All arthroscopic instruments are very costly and, because of their small size, are more delicate than comparable instruments for conventional limb or abdominal surgery. Consequently these instruments must be handled with very great care. Careless handling can easily bend or scratch an arthroscopic telescope, necessitating its replacement, or can so damage a fine surgical instrument that it becomes useless. Besides careful handling, the regular care and maintenance of telescopes and operating instruments are extremely helpful in prolonging their useful life.

4.7.1 Telescopes

Arthroscopic telescopes are precision instruments composed of various materials (steel, glass, plastic, air, adhesive), each having a specific coefficient of expansion. Steam sterilization at 134° C (frequently higher) would impose large stresses on these materials and might cause them to disintegrate. That is why gas sterilization, though more time-consuming, is recommended. Since several hours' aeration is required after sterilizing, it is necessary to have several telescopes on hand. Newly developed telescopes that can be sterilized in autoclaves are now available.

The number of telescopes needed is determined by the formula: number of arthroscopic procedures per day + 1 = number of telescopes.

Thus, if 4 telescopes are available, 3 arthroscopic procedures per day can be performed. One back-up telescope should be kept in reserve in the event that the scope in use becomes nonsterile.

The telescopes should be inspected at regular intervals, giving attention to the image quality, geometry (bent scope), eyepiece, and attachment sites to the light cable and sheath. Damage to the scope tip is a common occurrence, especially when operating in anterior joint areas with motorized instruments (Fig. 4-13). The useful life of a telescope is approximately 70–120 arthroscopic procedures.

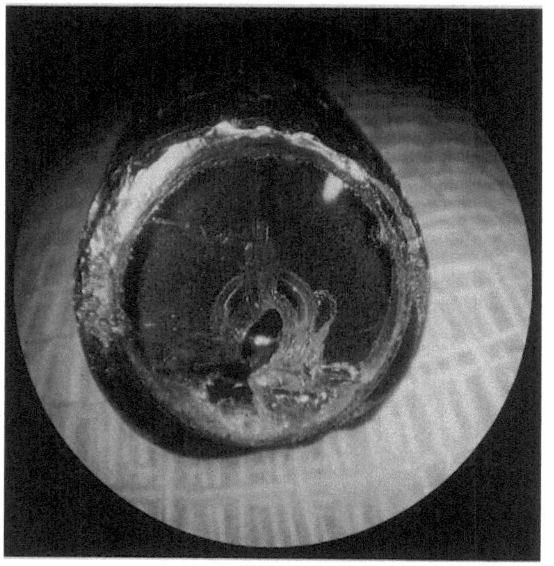

Fig. 4-13. Damaged telescope tip

Regular steam sterilization is the surest way to ruin scopes quickly.

The monitor image is determined essentially by the telescope. Telescopes that give a dim or cloudy image should no longer be used because they endanger the patient (the operation is like wandering in the fog or even in the dark) and present the operator with formidable problems. If the telescope is damaged or its lens system is clouded, most manufacturers have a repair/exchange policy by which the old scope can be exchanged for a reconditioned scope at approximately 30%–50% the cost of a new instrument.

4.7.2 Operating Instruments

Cutting instruments should be tested for the sharpness of their cutting edge. Blunt cutting instruments contuse the wound margins and increase the risk of iatrogenic instrument breakage.

Particular care must be given to motorized instruments (shaver systems) and their attachments. Even slight bending of the internal rotary blade will cause the instrument to function poorly. The thorough but careful manual cleaning and maintenance of shaver instruments reportedly is preferable to the more convenient use of a "washing machine."

4.8 Basic Equipment Requirements

By continuing to develop new and more advanced instrumentation, industry has made operative arthroscopy easier while extending the range of available arthroscopic operations. Frequently, however, new operating instruments are marketed and sold which subsequently are found to have very limited uses, if any. The following basic principle should be noted in the acquisition of instruments for arthroscopic surgery:

An arthroscopist needs fewer instruments than he thinks.

An experienced arthroscopist is distinguished not by his ownership of many different kinds of instruments but by his proficiency in the use of a few instruments.

The basic instruments recommended for diagnostic arthroscopy are listed in Table 4-2.

Table 4–2. Basic equipment needed for diagnostic arthroscopy

- Wide-angle telescope (30°) (2)
- Sheath with blunt trocar
- Cold-light source
- Light cable (2)
- Probing hook
- Video system with video camera and monitor, video cassette recorder if desired

5
Preoperative Examination under Anesthesia

Before arthroscopy is begun, the affected knee joint is examined with the patient anesthetized (peridural, spinal, or general anesthesia). The thigh tourniquet is not inflated until after this examination is completed.

The anesthesia should eliminate or markedly reduce the reflex, largely pain-induced muscular guarding response that can mask the presence of a true pathologic instability.

The following examinations and laxity tests are performed:

Passive Mobility. A preoperative extension loss raising suspicion of, say, a meniscal tear may turn out to be a pain-induced reflex extension deficit caused, for example, by a stretched or partially torn medial collateral ligament. In these cases the knee can be easily extended under anesthetic conditions.

If the degree of the extension deficit is not altered by anesthesia, it may be caused by extensive intraarticular adhesions, an entrapped bucket handle, or a loose body. Hyperextensibility is tested to exclude an injury of the posterior capsule and cruciate ligaments.

Spontaneous Posterior Drawer. Both knees are flexed 90°, and the feet are placed flat on the operating table. The examiner sights across the tibial tuberosity from the side, watching for a posterior sag that would raise suspicion of a ruptured posterior cruciate ligament.

Varus and Valgus Laxity. These are tested with the knee in extension and slight flexion (20°). As in the clinical examination, the end-point resilience is noted. A hard end point is consistent with an intact or partially ruptured ligament, while a soft end point implies a complete rupture.

Lachman Test. The Lachman test is an anterior drawer test performed with the knee flexed to only 20°–30°. Unlike the traditional 90° drawer test, the Lachman test is almost always positive with an isolated rupture of the anterior cruciate ligament (a frequent injury). The end-point resilience is always evaluated when the Lachman test is performed (see Sect. 2.1.1).

When the test is performed in muscular or obese patients, it is difficult to steady the femur and tibia simultaneously with the hands alone. One solution is for the examiner to hold the patient's thigh against his own thigh, which he places beneath the patient's thigh to form a stable "knee bench." With the other hand he grasps the proximal tibia and attempts to pull it forward.

The Lachman test is the most important test for evaluating the integrity of the anterior cruciate ligament.

Pivot-Shift Test. Patients with an acutely ruptured anterior cruciate ligament frequently manifest a false-positive pivot-shift test on clinical examination. Even with a chronic capsuloligamentous instability, the anterior subluxation is difficult to elicit. The patient is very fearful of having his knee subluxate (pivot) while slightly flexed, as this reproduces the disturbing phenomenon that he may be experiencing daily. The muscular guarding provoked by this fear makes the pivot shift an extremely difficult sign to elicit.

In the anesthetized patient, however, the pivot-shift test is usually positive when there

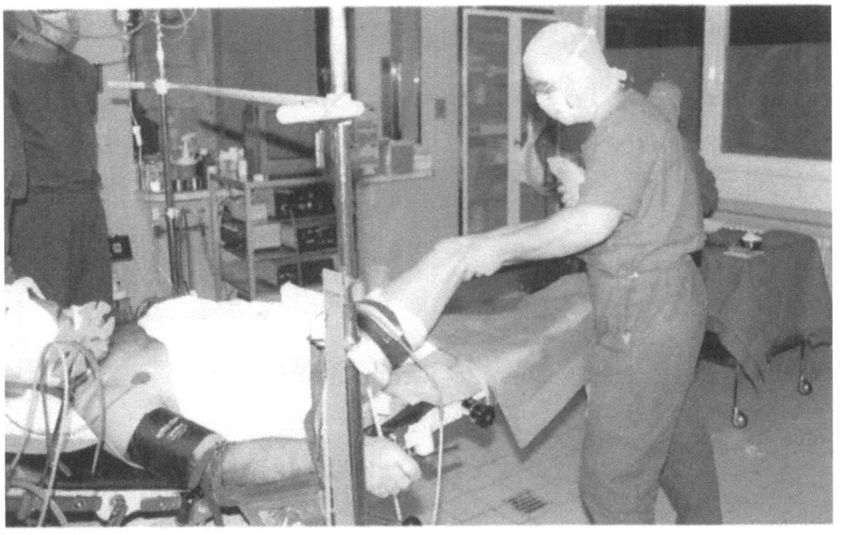

Fig. 5-1. Preoperative pivot-shift test in the anesthetized patient

is either a fresh or old rupture of the anterior cruciate ligament. Only muscle-relaxing anesthesia can provide optimum conditions for eliciting the pivot-shift sign (Fig. 5-1). This opportunity should not be missed.

Performing the pivot-shift test with the tibia in external, neutral, and internal rotation (graded pivot shift test of Jakob) is also much easier in the anesthetized patient.

Anterior Drawer Test in 90° Flexion. The traditional drawer test is performed with the knee flexed 90° and the tibia in internal, neutral, and external rotation.

The patient with an acute knee injury is usually unable to flex the knee joint to 90° due to pain, so the 90° anterior drawer test is very unreliable in the acutely injured knee. Patients with chronic instabilities, on the other hand, tolerate the 90° drawer test without difficulty.

Posterior Drawer Test in 90° Flexion. It is often difficult to distinguish between the anterior and posterior components of drawer mobility. It is helpful in these cases to check for sagging of the upper tibia (spontaneous posterior drawer) and evaluate the end-point resiliency. With a ruptured posterior cruciate ligament, a soft posterior end point will be noted.

Skin preparation and draping for arthroscopy are begun only after the examination under anesthesia is completed.

The standard radiographic views of the knee joint (biplane and patellar sunrise projections) should be available to the examiner. Attention is given to bony abnormalities, degenerative signs such as joint-space narrowing and lipping, recent or old fractures, ligament calcifications, and intraarticular loose bodies. If the patella is low- or high-riding (patella baja, patella alta), this must be taken into account when determining the location of the arthroscope portal (see Sect. 6.1).

The results of the examination in the anesthetized patient should be entered on the operation report and also on a standard documentation form, if available (see Sect. 14.1.2).

6
Portals

For proper evaluation of the knee joint, optimum sites must be selected for insertion of the arthroscope and probe. Because the creation of the instrument portal (for the probe and operating instruments) differs fundamentally from the insertion of the arthroscope, the portals for the arthroscope and instruments are discussed separately.

Every arthroscopic approach to the knee joint should:

- preserve important anatomic structures,
- cause minimal traumatization,
- be easy to locate.

A knowledge of anatomy is essential for meeting the first, most important requirement. Because nerves and blood vessels course on the flexor side of joints, it is safest to place arthroscopic portals on the extensor side. There are sites on the anterolateral and anteromedial aspects of the knee, adjacent to the patellar ligament, that are not traversed by essential stabilizers, nerves, or blood vessels. If a posteromedial or posterolateral approach is required, the portal must be created with extreme care (see Sect. 6.2.5).

Since the classic approaches for open knee operations are in the anteromedial and anterolateral regions, these sites are already reasonably familiar to the surgeon. Nevertheless, the unaccustomed "blind" penetration of the joint capsule in arthroscopy, so different from the meticulous dissection and broad exposure of an arthrotomy, may at first cause uneasiness among surgeons used to performing open operations.

The feared complication of iatrogenic damage to the articular cartilage (see Fig. 12-4) can be avoided by following the basic rules for creating the arthroscope and instrument portals.

6.1 Arthroscope Portal

With the knee flexed approximately 70°, the triangle formed by the lateral femoral condyle, the lateral tibial plateau, and the lateral border of the patellar ligament is located by palpation (Fig. 6-1). This site must be positively identified before the arthroscope portal is created.

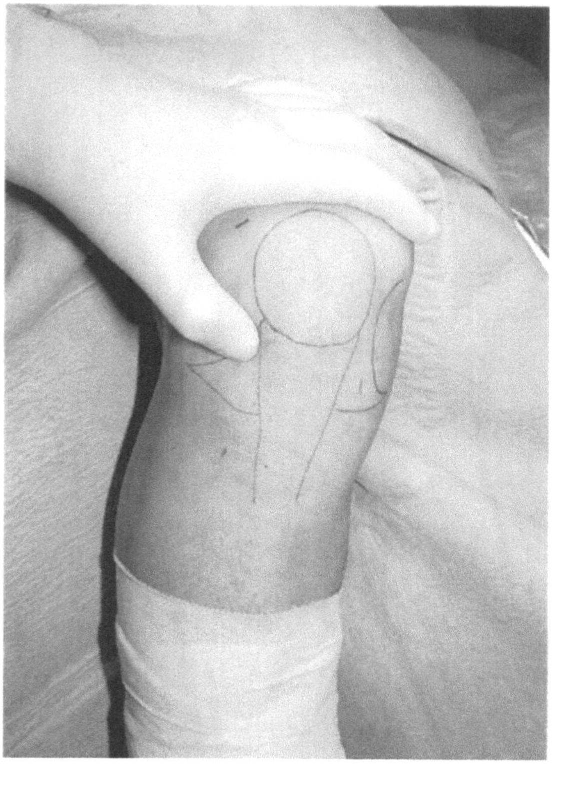

Fig. 6-1. Palpation of the anterolateral triangle in the flexed knee

Optimum placement of the arthroscope portal is essential for a successful arthroscopy.

Initially it is best to employ one *standard approach* rather than switch between two or more approaches. Although the differences between different portals are minimal in terms of the ability to visualize intraarticular structures, these differences may confuse the inexperienced arthroscopist and lead to needless uncertainty.

6.1.1 High Anterolateral Approach (Standard Approach)

Our standard approach is the *high anterolateral portal,* which has proved advantageous not only for diagnostic arthroscopy but also for most arthroscopic operations.

Localization
With the knee flexed 70°, the patellar apex is palpated, and a longitudinal stab incision is made just lateral to the border of the patellar tendon using a No. 11 or No. 15 knife blade (Fig. 6-2). Placing the incision close to the lateral border of the patellar ligament facilitates inspection of the intercondylar area (cf. Gillquist's approach, Sect. 6.1.3). The patellar tendon itself is not perforated.

The skin incision is approximately 0.8 cm long, aiming the cut in the direction of the anterior cruciate ligament. If an incise drape is used, a circle about the size of a half dollar is cut out of the drape before the incision is made (see Sect. 4.4).

If too short, the incision will lead to skin tension and hamper manipulations of the arthroscope. If too long (> 1 cm), the skin incision will allow leakage of irrigating fluid, resulting in inadequate joint distention.

The anterolateral portal is placed lower *(low anterolateral portal)* if a lateral retinacular release is proposed. In this case the viewing portal becomes an instrument portal through which the cutting instruments are introduced. Care is taken to place the arthroscope portal close to the patellar ligament if

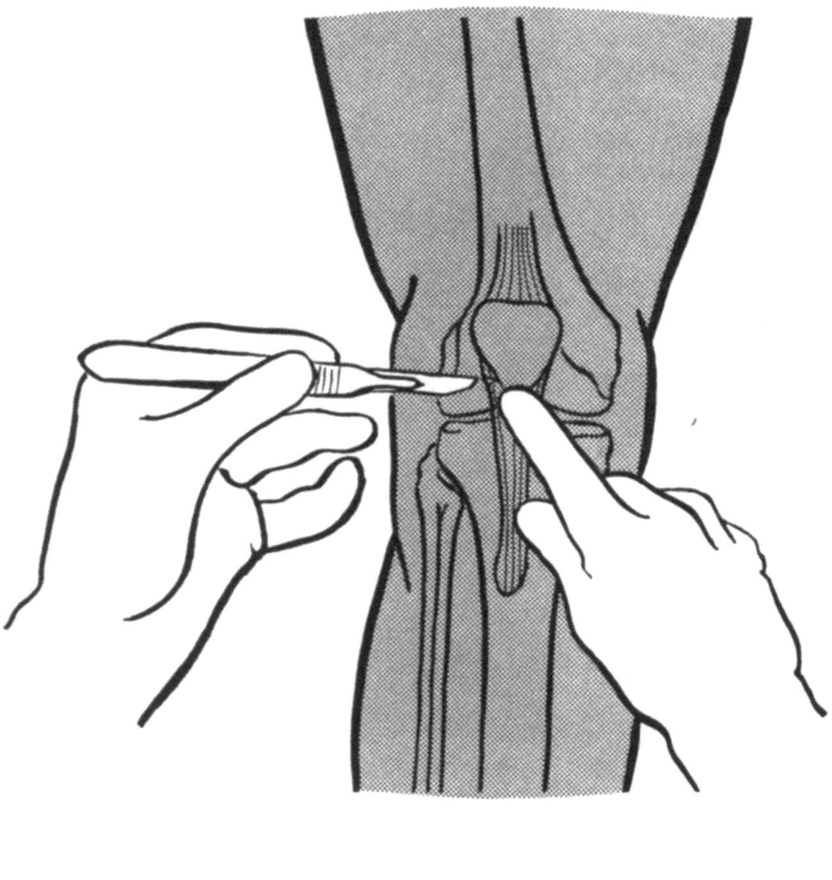

Fig. 6-2. The patellar apex is palpated with the knee flexed approximately 70°–90°. A stab incision is made just lateral to the patellar apex

an arthroscopic procedure on the anterior cruciate ligament (repair or reconstruction) is planned. The closer the portal is placed to the patellar ligament and thus to the midline, the easier it is to evaluate the sites of origin and insertion of the anterior cruciate ligament.

Introduction of the Sheath

Insertion of the sheath (trocar sleeve) is a four-step process, regardless of which approach is used:

Step 1. Having made the stab wound, the (right-handed) operator takes the assembled sheath and blunt obturator into his right hand, placing the tip of his index finger firmly on top of the sheath about 2 cm from the end (Fig. 6-3). Tissue resistance varies from one patient to the next, and if resistance to arthroscope insertion suddenly gives way, the extended finger will prevent plunging that could damage the articular cartilage.

Holding the assembly perpendicular to the skin surface, the operator advances the sheath and blunt obturator with a *careful rotating motion* while aiming the tip toward the anterior cruciate ligament (Fig. 6-4). Once the fibrous capsule layer has been penetrated, the operator will notice a decreased resistance to passage of the sheath. If a sharp trocar has been used up to this point, it is now changed for a blunt obturator. Meanwhile pressure is kept on the sheath so that it does not slip out of the fibrous capsule.

If the sheath is inserted forcibly and without a rotating motion, it can plunge suddenly into the joint and inflict severe cartilage damage, especially if a sharp trocar is used (see Fig. 12-4).

Aiming the tip toward the anterior cruciate ligament is an important safety measure. This will ensure that, if plunging occurs despite rotation and careful insertion, damage will be confined to the synovial investment of the anterior cruciate ligament. Insertion toward the medial joint space or medial femoral condyle can result in severe cartilage damage (Fig. 6-5).

Many arthroscopists have stopped using a sharp trocar, prefering to use only a blunt obturator. If the sheath-obturator assembly presents a smooth, reasonably pointed contour when the blunt obturator is inserted, this "point" will be sufficient to penetrate the subcutaneous tissue and capsule (Fig. 6-6). Insertion of the sheath and blunt obturator into the joint is made even easier by incising the fibrous capsule slightly at the time the skin incision is made (directing the cut toward the anterior cruciate ligament). This eliminates the need to change the sharp trocar for a blunt obturator, and the absence of a sharp trocar

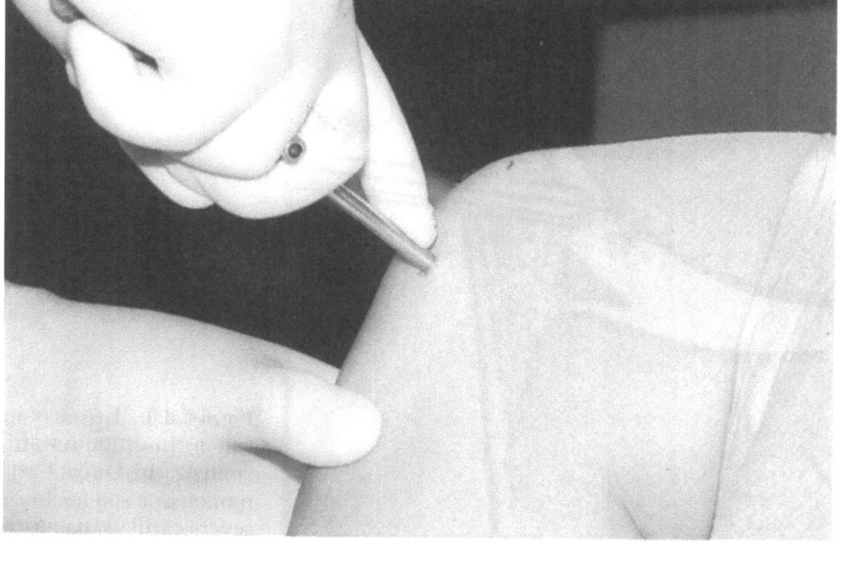

Fig. 6-3. The index finger on the sheath serves as an "emergency brake"

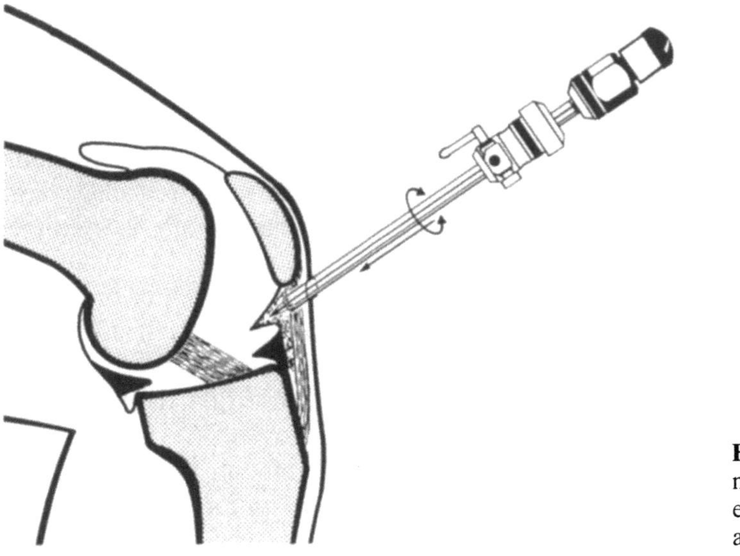

Fig. 6-4. With a careful rotating motion, the sheath with trocar inserted is advanced in the direction of the anterior cruciate ligament

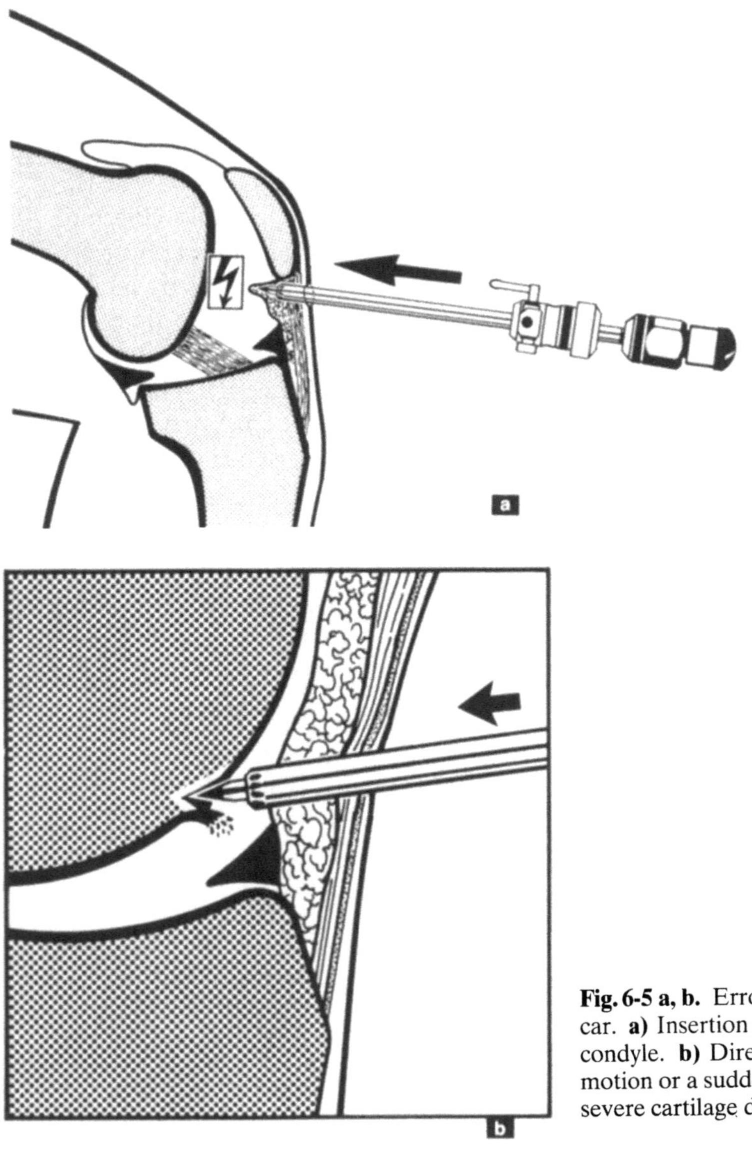

Fig. 6-5 a, b. Errors of insertion of the sheath and trocar. **a)** Insertion toward the medial or lateral femoral condyle. **b)** Direct, "wild" insertion without a rotary motion or a sudden loss of tissue resistance can lead to severe cartilage damage by the misdirected trocar

provides an additional safety factor. Even the plunging of a blunt obturator is unlikely to inflict deep cartilage lesions.

Step 2. After the sharp trocar has been replaced with the blunt obturator (if necessary), care is taken that the obturator is locked securely in place-for if the obturator becomes loose, the lumen of the sheath may gouge out synovial tissue or cartilage.

As the synovial membrane is penetrated with a steady rotating motion of the sheath and obturator, the leg is simultaneously extended to open up the femoropatellar space, which the sheath must traverse. The instrument is aimed toward the medial portion of the suprapatellar pouch (Fig. 6-7).

Directing the sheath toward the superomedial pole of the patella in the extended knee allows the force of the insertion to dissipate in the spacious suprapatellar pouch.

Step 3. When the sheath can be swept easily from side to side without resistance, this confirms its entry into the joint cavity (Fig. 6-8).

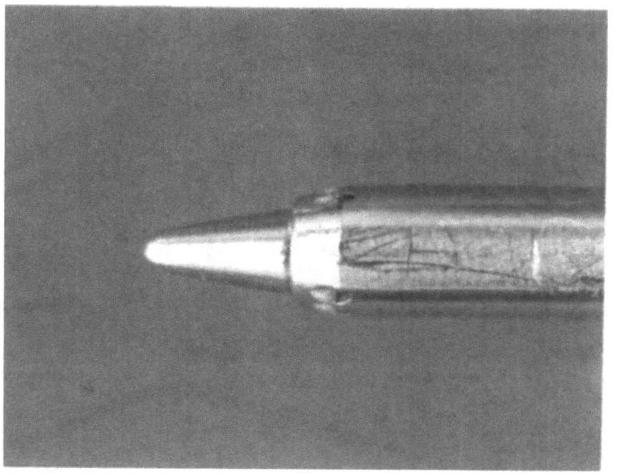

Fig. 6-6. Homogeneous "point" of the assembled sheath and blunt obturator (Aesculap)

Step 4. The blunt obturator is removed and replaced by the telescope. The inflow and outflow tubes for the irrigating fluid are attached, and the light cord is connected. Once the intraarticular space has been distended, the instrument is ready for use.

First the arthroscope is slowly retracted with a careful rotating motion until the light

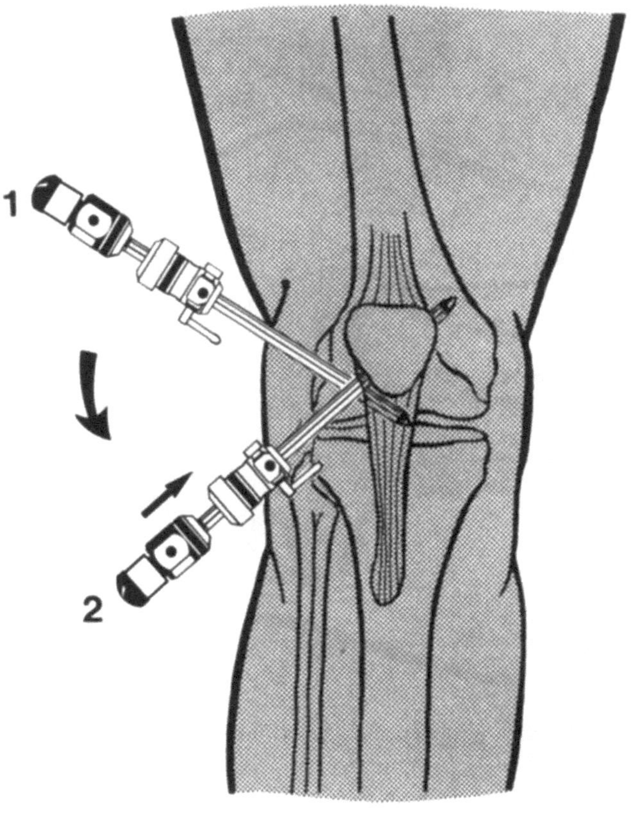

Fig. 6-7. Redirection of the sheath during insertion. The sheath is advanced toward the anterior cruciate ligament in the flexed knee (1). As the knee is extended, the sheath is advanced further in the direction of the medial suprapatellar recess (2)

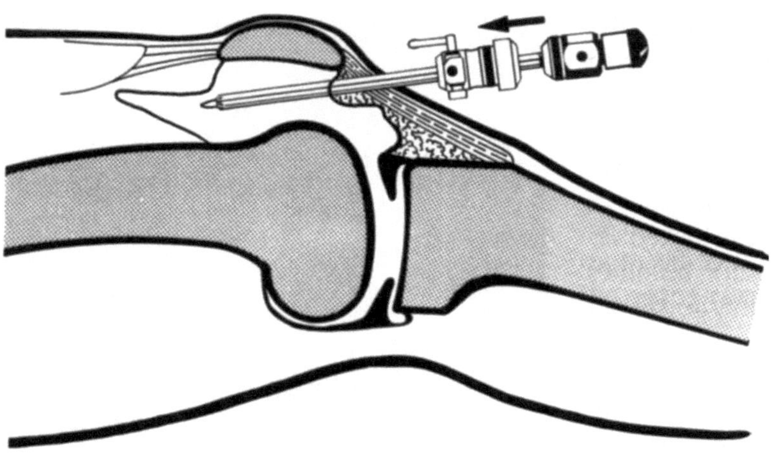

Fig. 6-8. Sheath and blunt obturator in place within the suprapatellar pouch

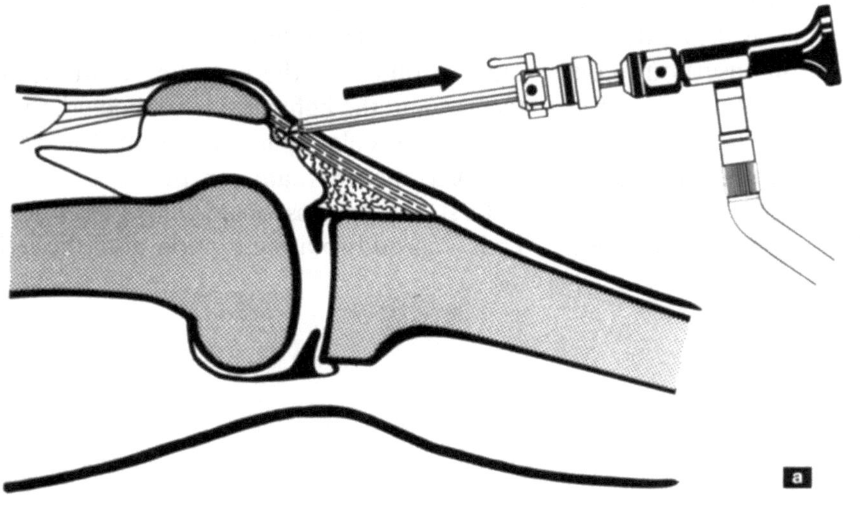

a

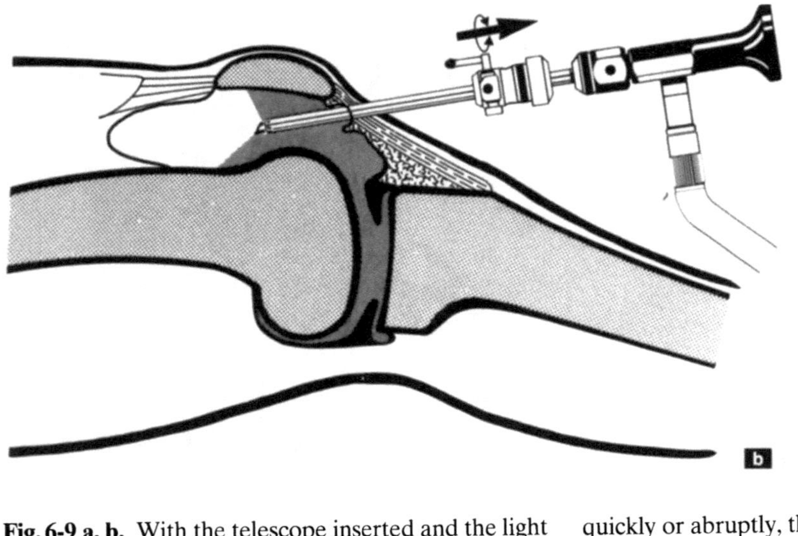

b

Fig. 6-9 a, b. With the telescope inserted and the light post in the 6:00 position, the arthroscope is slowly retracted with a rotating motion (**a**). If retracted too quickly or abruptly, the arthroscope tip may enter the subcutaneous tissue, causing a yellow-out and preventing further inspection of the joint (**b**) post points downward (6:00 position) (see Sect. 7.1) (Fig. 6-9 a). The scope should not be retracted abruptly, as this might move the tip into the subcutaneous tissue (Fig. 6-9 b), causing a "yellow-out" on the monitor (see Sect. 11.3). The continued infusion of irrigating fluid at that point would greatly distend the subcutaneous tissue, making reinsertion of the arthroscope more difficult.

6.1.2 Anterolateral Approach

The anterolateral approach is made at the center of the palpable lateral triangle (see above). The technique of sheath insertion is the same as described for the standard high anterolateral approach.

The classic anterolateral portal gives somewhat poorer visualization of the intercondylar notch and the posterior horn of the medial meniscus than the high anterolateral portal. An arthroscope inserted just above the tibial plateau may be deflected by a high medial intercondylar tubercle, a tertiary intercondylar tubercle (inconstant), or by osteophytes. This approach also requires perforation of the intrapatellar fat pad. Consequently, arthroscopists are increasingly abandoning the classic anterolateral portal in favor of the high anterolateral portal described above.

A low anterolateral portal is indicated when an arthroscopic lateral release is proposed. After the diagnostic phase of the procedure is accomplished, the scope is moved to a medial portal while the low anterolateral portal is used for insertion of the cutting instrument.

6.1.3 Transligamentous Approach (Gillquist's Approach)

In 1976 Gillquist described insertion of the arthroscope at a site approximately 1 cm below the patellar apex on the midline, directly through the patellar ligament. Compared with the anterolateral approach, this approach makes it easier to inspect the intercondylar space and the posterior compartments. On the other hand, the lateral recess with the popliteal hiatus is far more difficult to evaluate.

Although the central transligamentous approach is popular in Scandinavian countries, we do not believe it offers any significant advantages.

6.1.4 Midpatellar Lateral Approach

The anterior horns of the menisci are difficult to visualize from low anterolateral and transligamentous portals. This led Patel, in 1980, to describe a midpatellar lateral approach through the middle third of the lateral patellar border. This portal gives an excellent view of the anterior joint compartment, especially the anterior horns of the menisci, but it has not gained widespread acceptance.

6.1.5 Problems of Arthroscope Insertion

A number of factors can hamper or complicate insertion of the arthroscope sheath. The most important basic rule is:

Never enter the joint forcibly!

- ***Extension deficit.*** With an extension deficit greater than 30°, caused for example by adhesions in the suprapatellar pouch or retropatellar degenerative arthritis, even forced extension of the knee will not maximally open the femoropatellar space. This situation calls for a very careful technique, especially when creating the arthroscope portal. The sheath and blunt obturator are advanced slowly. When a resistance is felt, the operator carefully maneuvers the sheath past it. It may even be necessary to advance the sheath initially toward the medial joint space, although this increases the risk of iatrogenic cartilage injury.
- ***Portal placed too far distally.*** If the portal is placed too low or directed at too caudal

an angle toward the lateral tibial plateau, the arthroscope will be difficult to advance and may damage the lateral tibial plateau or the anterior horn of the lateral meniscus.

- ***Large mediopatellar plica.*** A hypertrophied (type III) mediopatellar plica may impinge on the medial femoral condyle in extension as well as in flexion. This makes it more difficult to advance the sheath toward the medial suprapatellar recess, as the plica hampers its passage through the femoropatellar space.
- ***Misdirected sheath.*** Inserting the sheath at too low an angle toward the medial joint space leads to perforation of the infrapatellar fat pad. The sheath may even hang up on the fat pad itself. Inserted at too high an angle, the sheath can easily dissect between the fibrous and synovial layers of the capsule (Fig. 11-4). In both cases the sheath cannot be maneuvered within the joint, and a yellow-out is seen when the telescope is inserted.
- ***Osteophytes.*** Osteophytes projecting from the lower edge of the patella can obstruct passage of the sheath toward the medial suprapatellar recess, making it necessary to alter the direction of insertion. They can also interfere with arthroscope maneuvers during the examination and the operation.

6.2 Instrument Portals

Simple inspection of the joint interior is not sufficient to detect all pathologic conditions. Selective palpation with a probing hook is necessary to establish the true location, depth, and extent of cartilage and meniscal lesions. Thus, in every arthroscopic examination a probing hook (see Sect. 3.6) is introduced into the joint through a separate instrument portal. This portal also provides access for the various operating instruments.

Every target structure, such as the medial meniscus, should be accessible without having to touch the articular cartilage. This applies to probing and especially to instrumentation during arthroscopic surgery.

Intraarticular structures and ligamentous laxity vary among different individuals. While the medial joint space is easily stressed open in one individual, in another it can scarcely be opened even by a strong valgus force. Pathologic findings, too, vary greatly in their location and extent. Accordingly, there is no "standard" instrument portal that gives optimum access to all intraarticular structures.

There is no standard instrument portal.

The creation of a separate instrument portal represents the greatest departure from traditional surgery of the extremities, in which access can be increased merely by extending the skin incision a few centimeters. In arthroscopy, extension of the original incision would cause an exorbitant loss of distention medium leading to rapid collapse of the joint cavity. For arthroscopy in fluid, the leakage would not only drench the feet of the operator and his assistants but, more importantly, would sacrifice the essential advantages of arthroscopic surgery (minimal traumatization, preservation of proprioception).

Another basic difference between the arthroscope and instrument portals is that the arthroscope portal is made without benefit of visual guidance from inside the joint, whereas the instrument portal is *always* made under arthroscopic vision using the *"cannula technique."*

6.2.1 Cannula Technique

Creation of the instrument portal is accomplished in three steps:

Step 1–General orientation. The arthroscope is trained on the area of the capsule from which the target structure (e.g., the posterior horn of the medial meniscus) can be reached most easily and safely. This area is marked by transilluminating it with the arthroscope beam (Fig. 6-10). The examiner than applies

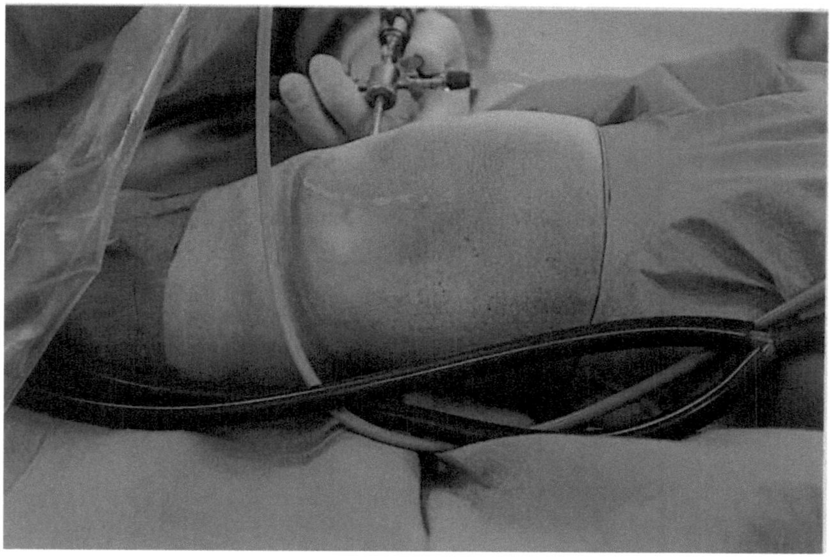

Fig. 6-10. The proposed site for the instrument portal is transilluminated for general orientation

digital pressure to the joint capsule in that area while watching for the corresponding indentation on the monitor (Fig. 6-11).

Step 2–Introduction of the cannula. At the site marked by the examiner's finger, a spinal needle or infusion cannula (Ch 18) is inserted through the skin (Fig. 6-12 a) until the tip of the cannula is visible on the monitor (Fig. 6-12 b).

The efficacy of the portal is tested by attempting to reach the target structure with the cannula (Fig. 6-13). If this is difficult to do with the thin cannula, it will be much more difficult with the thicker probe. And if arthroscopic surgery is required, the operating instruments will either be unable to reach the area or reach it with an exorbitant risk of iatrogenic cartilage damage.

If the cannula cannot reach the target structure optimally, it should be removed and reinserted at a slightly different site. If possible the needle should reach the target site without touching the femoral condyle, which

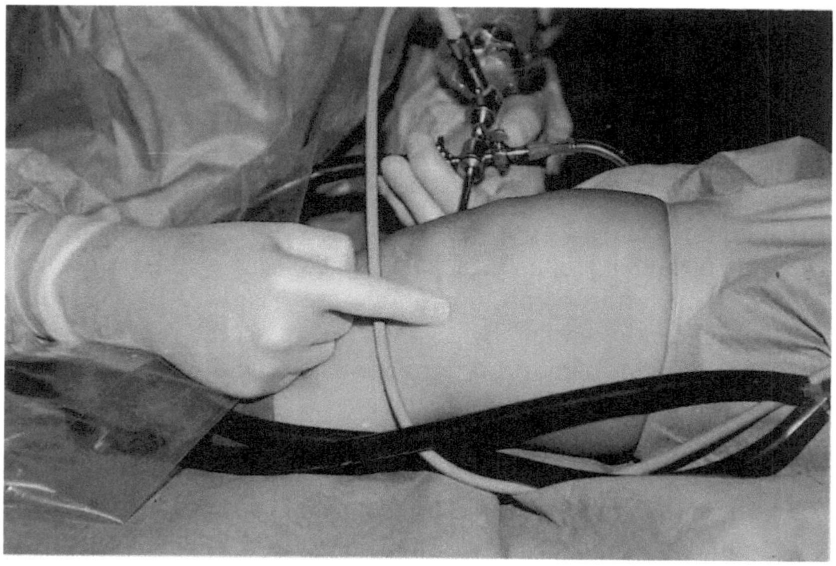

Fig. 6-11. Palpation of the proposed site for the instrument portal

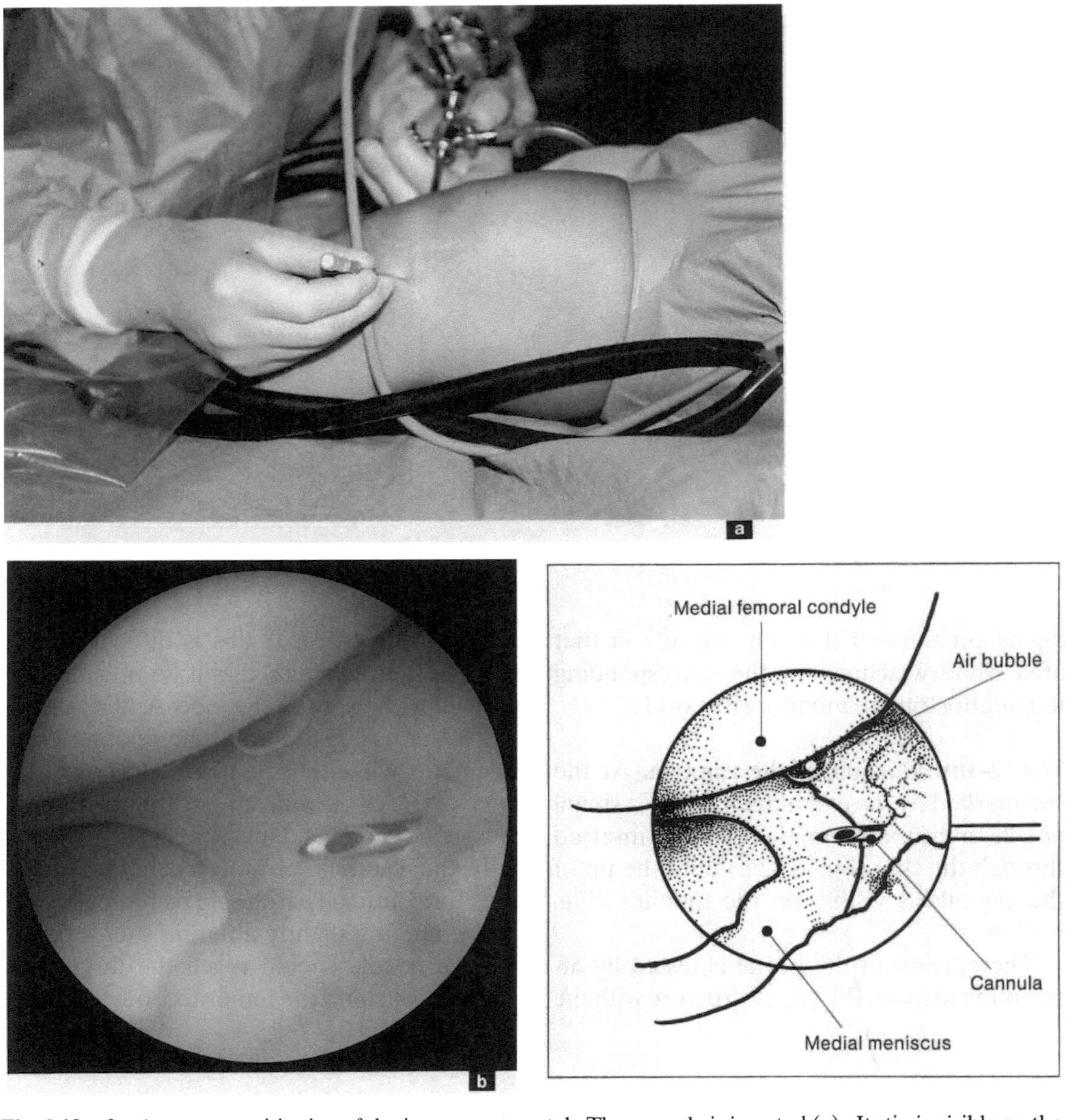

Fig. 6-12 a, b. Accurate positioning of the instrument portal. The cannula is inserted (**a**). Its tip is visible on the monitor (**b**)

presents the greatest obstacle to probing the posterior horns of the menisci.

Multiple reinsertions of the cannula are less traumatizing than a poorly positioned instrument portal that jeopardizes the cartilage surfaces. Most arthroscopic operations are made significantly easier by a favorably placed portal, and many procedures cannot be successfully accomplished without an optimum portal.

Step 3–Incision of the skin and capsule. Once the optimum location for the instrument portal has been determined, a scalpel (No. 11 or No. 15 blade) is introduced along the upper surface of the still-indwelling cannula. Superficial veins delineated by the transilluminating beam should be preserved. Venous injury can lead to bleeding that obscures arthroscopic vision. Also, damage to the fine cutaneous nerves that accompany the vessels can cause sensory disturbances or a painful scar neuroma.

The sharp edge of the blade should point upward so that if it slips, it will not damage the superior rim of the meniscus (Figs. 6-14 and

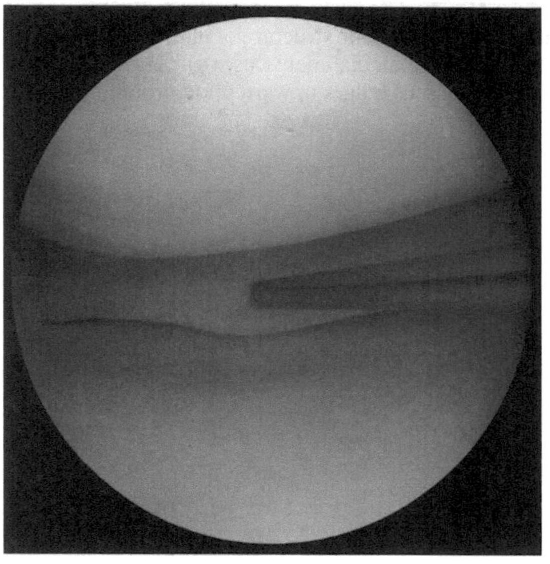

Fig. 6-13. The target structure (here, the posterior horn of the medial meniscus) is reached with the cannula

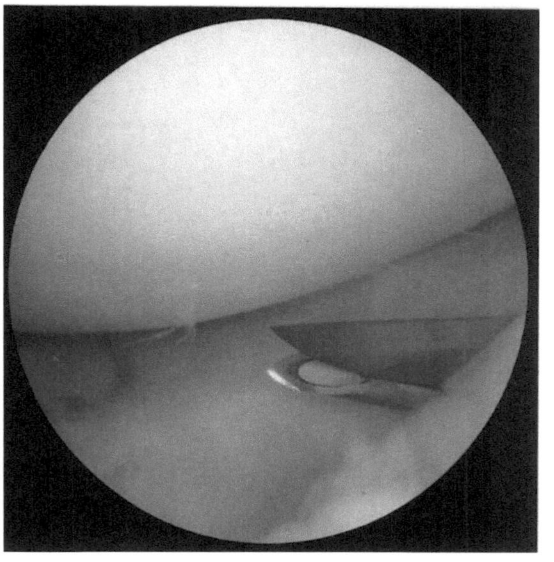

Fig. 6-15. The capsule is incised under visual control

6-15). As soon as the tip of the blade appears within the joint, "riding" atop the cannula, the latter may be withdrawn.

Now, under vision, a longitudinal incision approximately 0.5–0.8 cm long is made in the joint capsule, perpendicular to the base of the meniscus. The incision is made using short, sawing motions of the blade. During this time the operator may rest the ulnar side of his hand on the patient's knee or lower leg to control the blade movements more precisely, for uncontrolled cutting movements can produce large capsulotomies that allow excessive fluid leakage to the outside or into subcutaneous tissues.

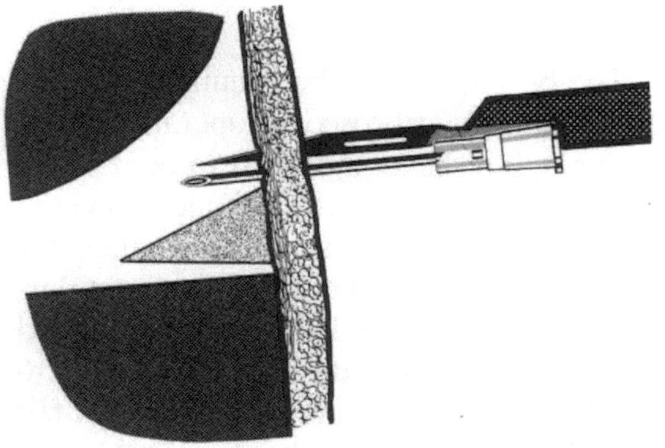

Fig. 6-14. During incision of the capsule, the knife blade slides along the surface of the cannula, its cutting edge directed upward

Care is taken that incisions of equal length are made through the skin, subcutaneous tissue, and joint capsule. A capsulotomy that is too small in relation to the skin incision will make it difficult to insert the probe and operating instruments, while a small skin incision over a large capsulotomy will allow copious leakage of irrigating fluid into the subcutaneous tissue, making the rest of the procedure more difficult. Changing the flexion angle of the knee during the incision will result in incisions of different lengths in the skin, subcutaneous tissue, and capsule. The portal should be made in the exact joint position in which the target structure is visualized. If the joint position is changed even slightly after the incision is completed, the tissue layers will shift relative to each other and hamper free instrument passage through the portal.

Introduction of the Probe. Following incision of the capsule, the probe is inserted (Fig. 6-16). Before larger operating instruments are introduced, it may be necessary to widen the portal carefully with the aid of a Kocher forceps or similar instrument.

Before the knee joint is moved to a new position, the probe is inserted in the initial joint position and visualized with the arthroscope. Then the knee joint is slowly and carefully re-

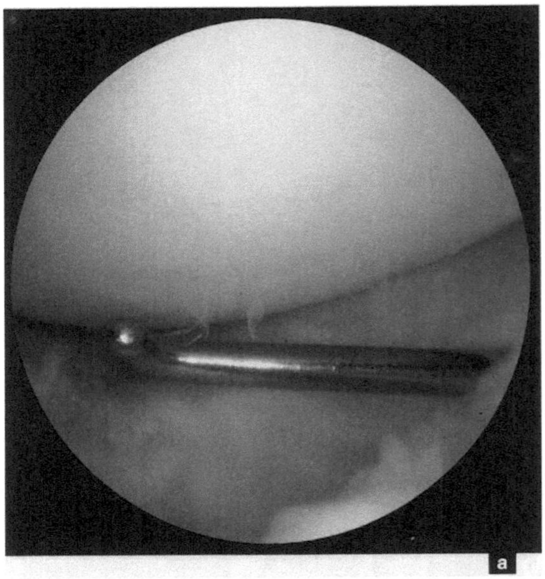

Fig. 6-16 a, b. The probe is inserted through the instrument portal (**a**) to the structure of interest (the posterior horn of the medial meniscus) (**b**). The free border of the meniscus bulges upward upon probing

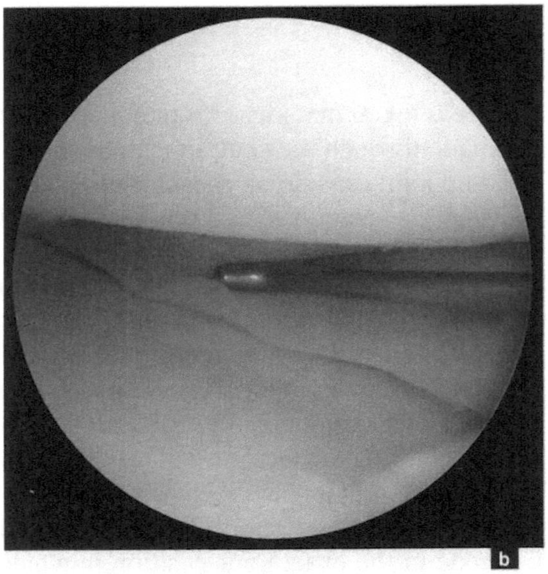

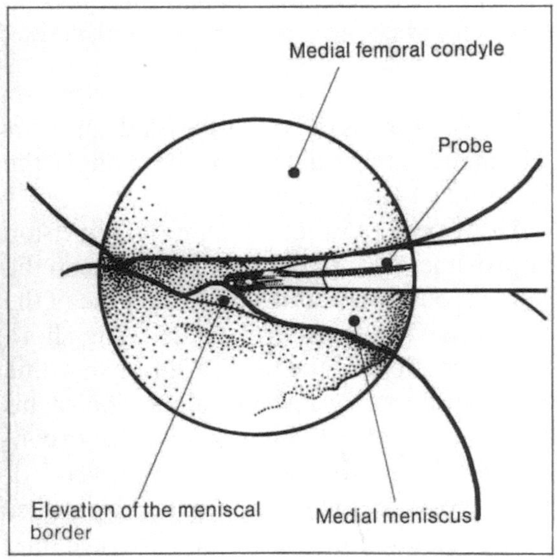

positioned, always keeping the tip of the probe within the field of view. After the repositioning maneuver is completed, the examiner attempts to palpate the now-visible structures with the probe. The same technique can be used to direct operating instruments into sites that are difficult to reach.

In arthroscopic operations, favorable placement of the instrument portal can eliminate the need for some instruments.

The beveled tip of the cannula can assist orientation in arthroscopic operations. For example, if a shaver system is to be used on the articular cartilage, the obliquely directed cannula opening can serve as a guide for matching the position of the instrument portal to the shaver head. Thus, for a shaver head whose orifice is angled 45° or 60° relative to the shaver shaft, a cannula with a 45° or 60° bevel is used to see whether the portal gives optimum access to the cartilage area requiring treatment (Fig. 6-17).

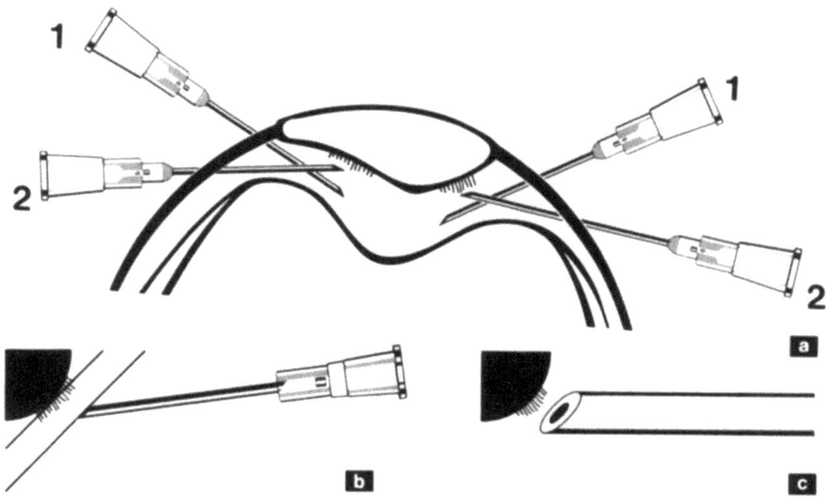

Fig. 6-17 a–c. A beveled cannula can be used to determine the optimum insertion angle of a motorized instrument, e.g., for shaving the retropatellar cartilage. Cannula 1 is improperly angled, so its beveled tip does not appose to the fibrillated cartilage area. Cannula 2, inserted at a more oblique angle, apposes correctly to the target area (**a**). Thus, when the instrument portal is created, it is helpful to match its placement to the bevel of the cannula tip (**b**) and the obliquity of the shaver head (**c**)

6.2.2 Medial Suprameniscal Approach

The medial suprameniscal portal – the most commonly used instrument portal – should pass just above the peripheral rim of the meniscus without cutting or penetrating the meniscal tissue (Figs. 6-15 and 6-18).

The medial suprameniscal portal is used for probing the posterior portions of the medial meniscus (and possibly the lateral meniscus). The posterior portions of the meniscus are most easily reached through a portal just anterior to the medial collateral ligament. This is especially important in a tight joint that cannot be widely opened. A route must be sought that bypasses the "obstructing" medial femoral condyle. If the joint space can be satisfactorily opened, the portal may be placed farther anteriorly (Figs. 6-19 and 6-20 a,b). In a joint with very high valgus laxity, the posterior horn may even be accessible from an anterior suprameniscal portal (Fig. 6-20 c), although this approach involves perforation of the infrapatellar fat pad. The high medial approach provides more direct access to the posterior horn of the medial meniscus (see Sect. 6.2.3).

If the lateral joint compartment is not accessible through the suprameniscal approach, it may be advantageous to add an accessory, high medial instrument portal for probing and instrumentation of that compartment. However, the operator may first attempt to probe the lateral compartment from the suprameniscal portal. For this the probe is passed through the existing medial portal and visualized on the monitor within the lateral triangle (lateral femoral condyle, lateral tibial plateau, anterior cruciate ligament) ("rendezvous technique," see Sect. 7.7). While the probe is kept in view, the leg is carefully moved to the figure-four position (see Sect. 8.8). If the intercondylar eminence is flat and if the portal is slightly anteromedial rather than directly suprameniscal, it should be possible to probe the lateral joint compartment. Frequently the intercondylar eminence will act as a ramp, deflecting the probe upward toward the lateral femoral condyle (Fig. 6-21). When present, this "ramp effect" necessitates use of a high medial instrument portal for selective probing of the lateral compartment.

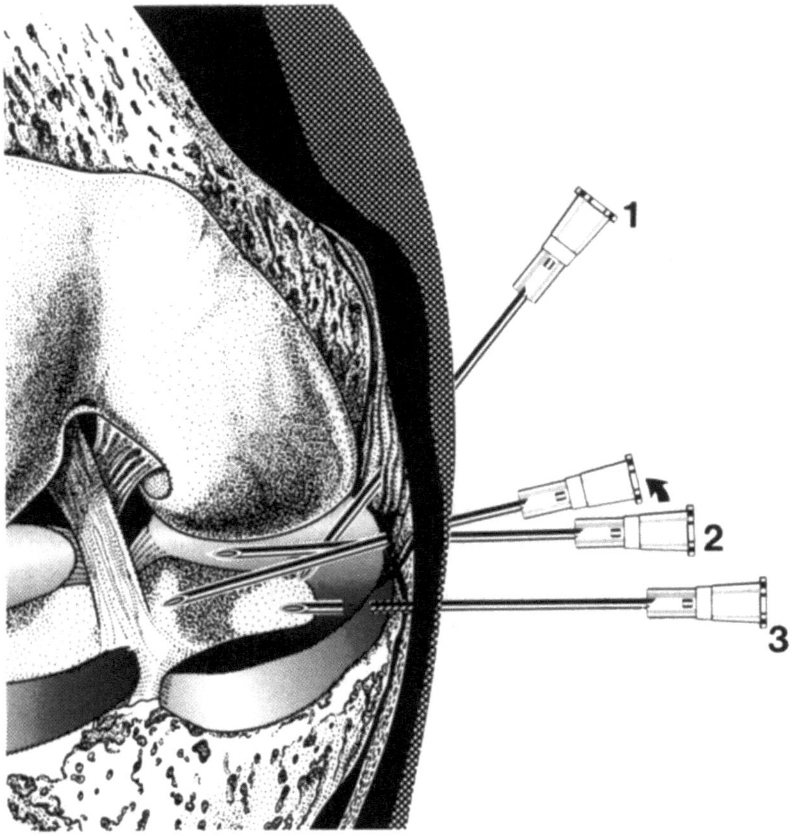

Fig. 6-18. Placement of the medial suprameniscal instrument portal using the cannula technique. If the portal is too high, the instrument will be deflected by the femoral condyle (1). Placing the portal just above the meniscal surface ensures adequate freedom of movement while giving access to the anterior cruciate ligament and the posterior part of the meniscus (2). If placed too low, the portal endangers the meniscal tissue (3)

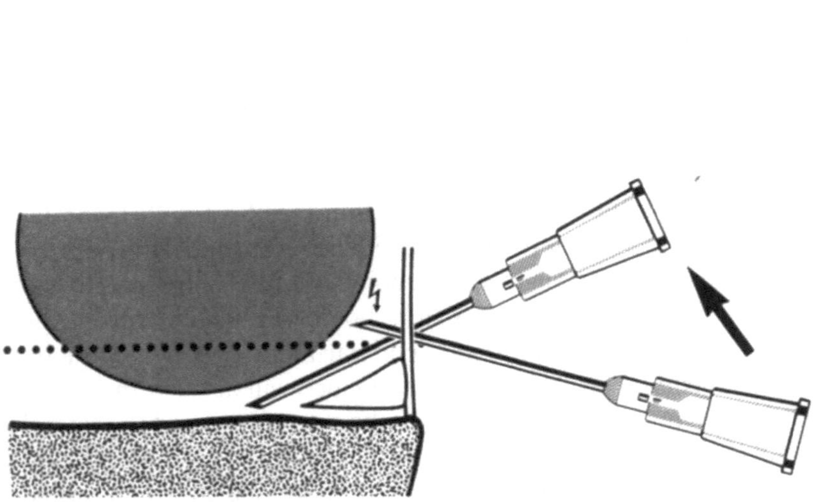

Fig. 6-19. "Pricking" of the medial femoral condyle should be avoided when determining the location of the suprameniscal portal

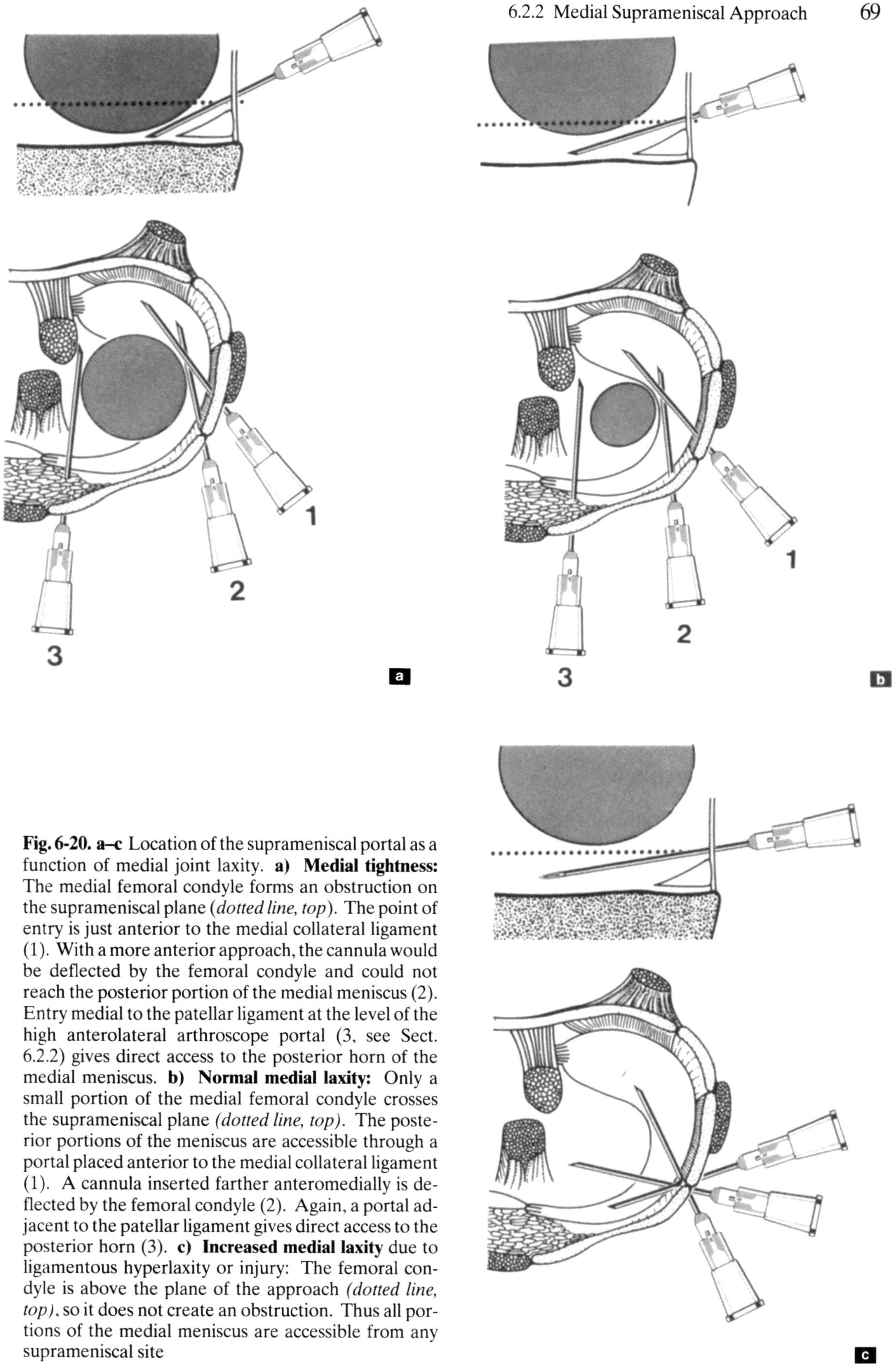

Fig. 6-20. a–c Location of the suprameniscal portal as a function of medial joint laxity. **a) Medial tightness:** The medial femoral condyle forms an obstruction on the suprameniscal plane (*dotted line, top*). The point of entry is just anterior to the medial collateral ligament (1). With a more anterior approach, the cannula would be deflected by the femoral condyle and could not reach the posterior portion of the medial meniscus (2). Entry medial to the patellar ligament at the level of the high anterolateral arthroscope portal (3, see Sect. 6.2.2) gives direct access to the posterior horn of the medial meniscus. **b) Normal medial laxity:** Only a small portion of the medial femoral condyle crosses the suprameniscal plane *(dotted line, top)*. The posterior portions of the meniscus are accessible through a portal placed anterior to the medial collateral ligament (1). A cannula inserted farther anteromedially is deflected by the femoral condyle (2). Again, a portal adjacent to the patellar ligament gives direct access to the posterior horn (3). **c) Increased medial laxity** due to ligamentous hyperlaxity or injury: The femoral condyle is above the plane of the approach *(dotted line, top)*, so it does not create an obstruction. Thus all portions of the medial meniscus are accessible from any suprameniscal site

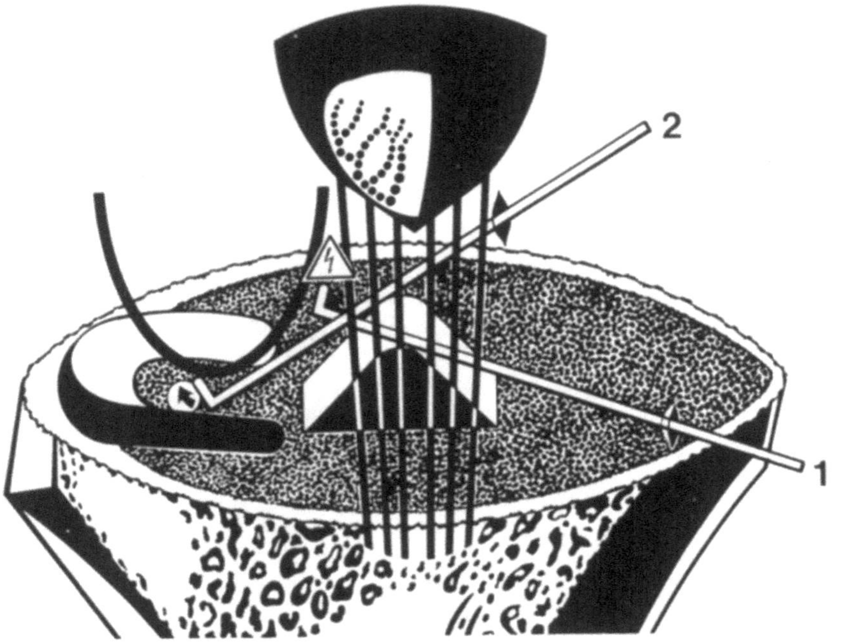

Fig. 6-21. Ramp effect. The lateral compartment cannot always be reached through a medial suprameniscal portal (1). Often the probe is deflected upward toward the lateral femoral condyle by the ramp-like medial intercondylar tubercle. A high medial portal directly adjacent to the patellar ligament gives unobstructed access for probing and other instrumentation of the lateral compartment (2)

6.2.3 High Medial Approach

In very tight joints, the posterior horn of the medial meniscus often cannot be probed or instrumented directly from the medial side. In these cases a high medial paraligamentous portal can be utilized to provide direct access to the posterior horn. As with other instrument portals, the optimum site for the high medial portal is determined by the use of a cannula (see above). The needle is inserted at the same level as the high anterolateral arthroscope portal, but on the anteromedial side. The puncture is made directly adjacent to the patellar ligament at the level of the patellar apex, affording direct access to the posterior horn of the medial meniscus between the medial femoral condyle and the posterior cruciate ligament (Fig. 6-22).

This approach can be difficult in osteoarthritic joints with large marginal osteophytes, and multiple punctures may be required to establish the optimum location for the portal.

The high medial paraligamentous portal also gives good access to the lateral joint compartment. Before this portal is created, the knee should be moved to the figure-four position and an effort made to reach the target structure in the lateral compartment with a cannula (Fig. 6-23). The knee remains in that position while probing and any necessary operative measures are performed. Returning the leg to the initial extended position causes a relative shifting of the tissue layers, and often this requires making a second capsular incision through the original skin incision before the portal can be used, say, for probing the posterior horn of the medial meniscus.

6.2.4 Suprapatellar Approaches

Some procedures, such as accurate probing or shaving of the retropatellar cartilage or separating intraarticular adhesions, may necessitate a suprapatellar approach if the inferior

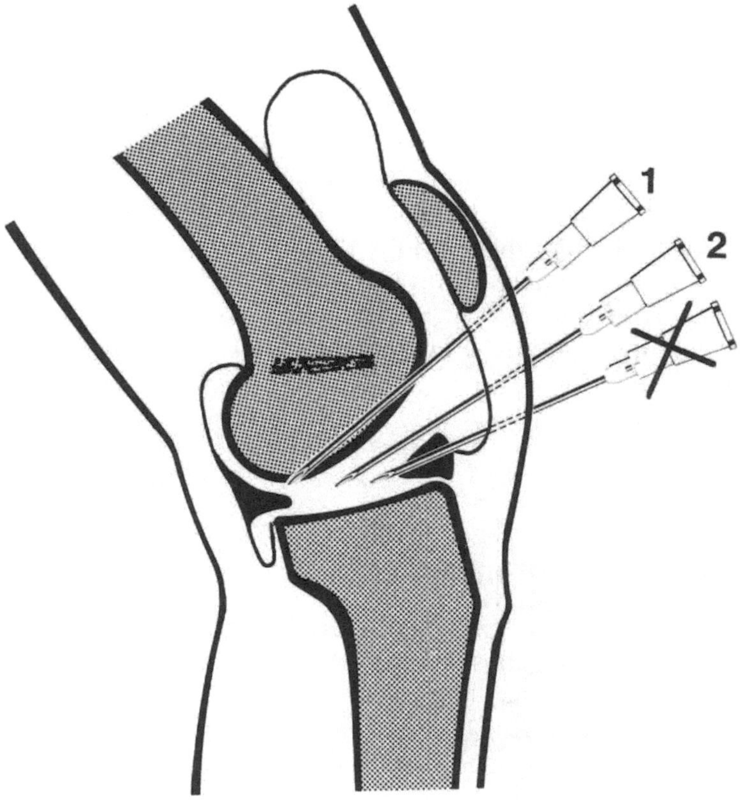

Fig. 6-22. A high medial paraligamentous portal gives direct access to the posterior horn of the medial meniscus. The optimum approach to the posterior horn is through the high medial portal (1). In joints with high valgus laxity, the posterior horn is also accessible through the suprameniscal portal (2). Perforation or incision of the anterior horn of the meniscus should be avoided (X)

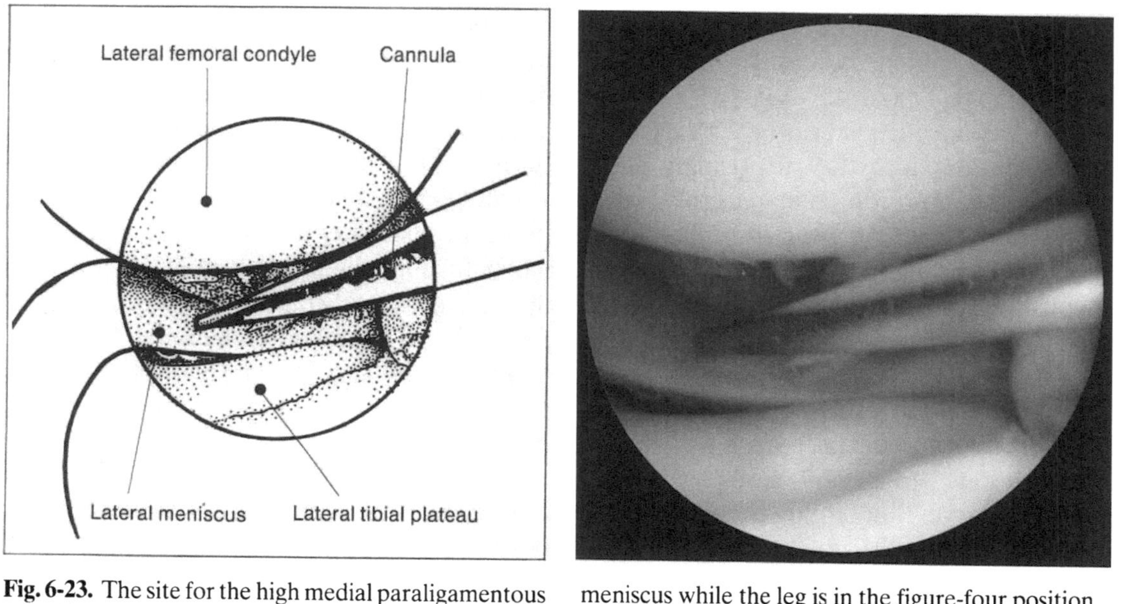

Fig. 6-23. The site for the high medial paraligamentous portal is determined by passing a cannula to the lateral meniscus while the leg is in the figure-four position

portals do not give satisfactory access. Suprapatellar portals are also indicated for the removal of large loose bodies from the suprapatellar pouch and for synovectomies.

A large-bore irrigation cannula can be passed into the joint through a suprapatellar portal. It is essential to preserve the vastus medialis obliquus muscle, so we prefer to go through the tendinous portion of the vastus medialis obliquus (see Sect. 3.5) (Fig. 3-28) or, preferably, to utilize a lateral suprapatellar approach.

6.2.5 Posterior Approaches

A posteromedial instrument portal is required for finding loose bodies or identifying a meniscal flap that has become displaced into the posteromedial recess. The posterior cruciate ligament can be directly inspected by introducing a second sheath under vision through a posteromedial portal (see Fig. 11-2) and switching the telescope to the posteromedial sheath.

The first step in making the posteromedial portal is to visualize the posteromedial recess by inserting the arthroscope from a high anterolateral portal and advancing it between the medial femoral condyle and anterior cruciate ligament. The route for traversing the intercondylar notch is easily recognized. With the knee flexed 45°–60°, the scope is carefully advanced posteriorly with a slight rotating motion into the surprisingly large cavity of the posteromedial recess, a brief "yellow-out" occurring just before the recess is entered. The light post is turned to the 8:00 position (4:00 in the left knee) to direct vision toward the posteromedial capsule (see Sect. 7).

The knee is now flexed 90° so that the posteromedial portal can be placed above the flexor tendons, great saphenous vein, and saphenous nerve. Fluid inflow is turned on to maximally distend the posteromedial recess; this is easily done owing to the lax condition of the posterior capsule in this position.

As with other instrument portals, the site for the posteromedial portal is determined by the cannula technique (Fig. 6-24). A probe, operating instrument, or even a second sheath with blunt obturator can be passed through this portal under arthroscopic vision. This permits an excellent evaluation of the posteromedial recess and the posterior suspension of the medial meniscus.

When proper technique is used to make the posteromedial portal, there is virtually no chance of injury to the neurovascular bundle in the popliteal fossa. When the initial puncture is made in the posteromedial corner, there is a danger that the tough posterior capsule may deflect the cannula posteriorly. This is avoided by inserting the cannula as well as the knife and other instruments (or sheath) perpendicular to the surface of the skin. Instruments that miss the capsular opening and deviate posteriorly will produce an arthroscopically visible bulge in the posterior capsule.

Technically demanding, the posteromedial portal should be reserved for seasoned arthroscopists. This portal is necessary for arthroscopic operations that involve a posterior synovectomy.

Relative shifting of the soft-tissue layers is particularly pronounced in the posteromedial region. Moreover, once an instrument has passed through the skin incision, it must traverse a considerable thickness of subcutaneous tissue. So it may take some probing to maneuver the instrument through the capsular incision and into the posteromedial corner of the joint. Thus, in arthroscopic operations via the posteromedial portal, we recommend using an instrument sheath with a one-way valve through which the operating instruments can be safely passed into and out of the joint. The constant interchanging of instruments without such guidance is not only difficult and time-consuming but also traumatizing.

Due to the proximity of the posterolateral portal to the peroneal nerve, the knee should be well flexed (approximately 110°) when the portal is created. After the leg is moved to the

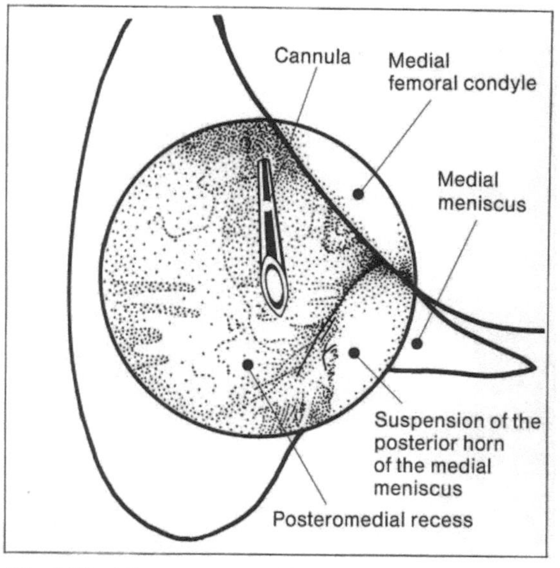

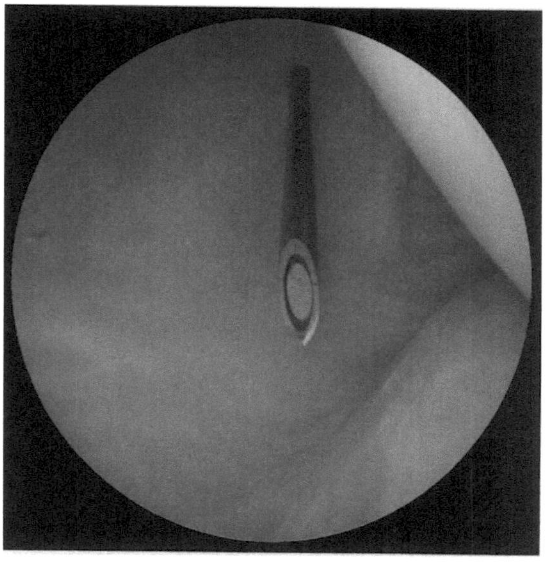

Fig. 6-24. The posteromedial portal is located using the cannula technique. The cannula is inserted into the posteromedial recess

figure-four position, the arthroscope is further advanced over the posterior horn of the lateral meniscus and into the posterolateral recess, which can be satisfactorily inspected when the light post is positioned at 5:00 (7:00 in the left knee). Utilization of the posterolateral portal is reserved for exceptional situations (arthroscopic synovectomy, suturing the posterior horn of the lateral meniscus).

6.2.6 Problems with the Instrument Portal

If the probing hook or operating instrument cannot be passed through the instrument portal, or passed only with difficulty, one of the following problems may exist:

- ***The portal is too small.*** The scalpel is reintroduced through the portal, making certain that the blade enters from the same direction as in the original incision. Reincision of the capsule is performed under arthroscopic control to ensure that the blade extends the original capsulotomy and does not make a second capsular incision.

- ***The joint position is altered.*** Any change in the joint position causes a relative shifting of the capsule, subcutaneous tissue, and skin. The incisions can be realigned by returning the knee to the position in which the instrument portal was made.

- ***Vision is obscured.*** Synovitis or osteophytes can interfere with arthroscopic visualization of the percutaneous needle and hamper instrument insertion.

7
Basic Principles of Arthroscopy

The secret of successful diagnostic and operative arthroscopy lies in a clear understanding of the physical principles of the optical system and how they apply to the compartmentalized interior of the knee joint. The goal is to inspect the entire joint cavity as efficiently as possible, without unnecessary movements of the arthroscope. Every movement of the scope that does not give added visual information needlessly aggravates the risk of cartilage damage.

The examiner has the option of moving the arthroscope and/or the knee joint to bring the various intraarticular structures into view. The examiner as well as any observers watching the monitor should feel as if they are taking a walk through the joint (Fig. 7-1). The experienced examiner, through his systematic, unhurried guidance of the arthroscope, can consistently achieve this sense of "taking a walk" as he visually explores the intraarticular compartments. This expertise contrasts with the jerky, uncoordinated maneuvers of the inexperienced arthroscopist.

The harmonious conduct of the arthroscopic examination and operation relies on a smooth, coordinated sequence of knee-joint and arthroscopic movements. Achieving this requires an understanding of the ways in which an arthroscope can be moved or maneuvered while inside the joint.

7.1 Movements of the Arthroscope

The factors that hamper or prevent free movement of the arthroscope consist of bony, cartilaginous, and ligamentous structures, as well as the portal selected for insertion of the scope. Because any contact at all with the cartilage can score or contuse the cartilage surface, and given the very poor regenerative capacity of the articular cartilage, any unnecessary contact between the arthroscope and cartilage should be scrupulously avoided.

While the examiner cannot directly influence the location of the intraarticular structures, he can and does select the site of arthroscope insertion. Thus, the placement of this portal has an essential bearing on the ability of the arthroscopist to conduct the examination smoothly.

Once the viewing portal has been created, there are three different ways in which the telescope can be maneuvered in the knee joint. It can be:

- advanced or retracted
- swept medially, laterally, upward, or downward
- rotated.

7.1.1 Advancing and Retracting the Scope

Moving the arthroscope in or out along the axis of its shaft alters the size of the visual field: advancing the scope makes the visual field smaller, while retracting the scope expands it (Fig. 7-2). The basic goal is to keep the distance between the scope tip and target structure (e.g., the medial meniscus) as large as possible so that a satisfactory overview is obtained (Figs. 7-3 and 7-4). If fine details are not appreciated, the arthroscope is readvanced toward the target.

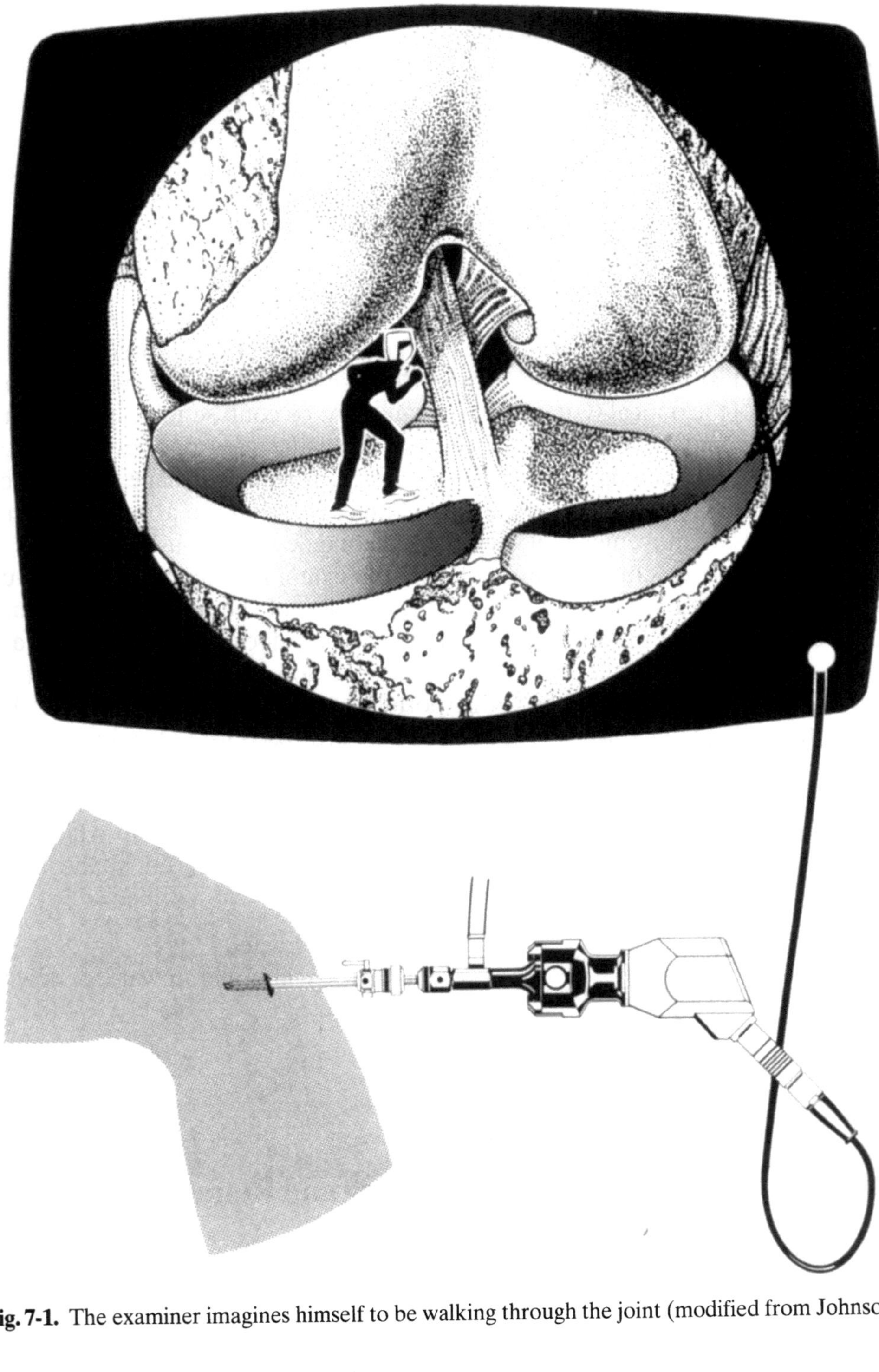

Fig. 7-1. The examiner imagines himself to be walking through the joint (modified from Johnson 1986)

Fig. 7-3 a, b. If the scope tip is brought very close to the target structure, orientation can be difficult (**a**). The location of the loose cartilage fragments is not apparent. As the scope is retracted, the structures of the lateral compartment come into view. The loose bodies are lodged beneath the lateral meniscus (**b**)

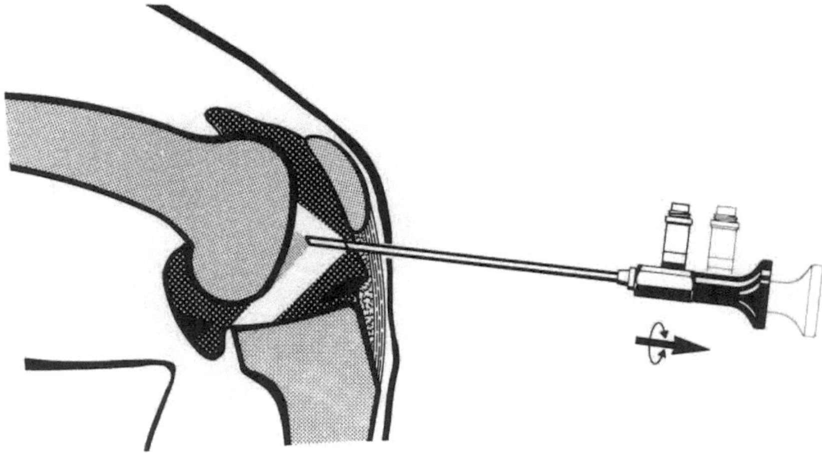

Fig. 7-2. The arthroscope is advanced and retracted with a slow rotating motion. As the scope is retracted, the visual field expands

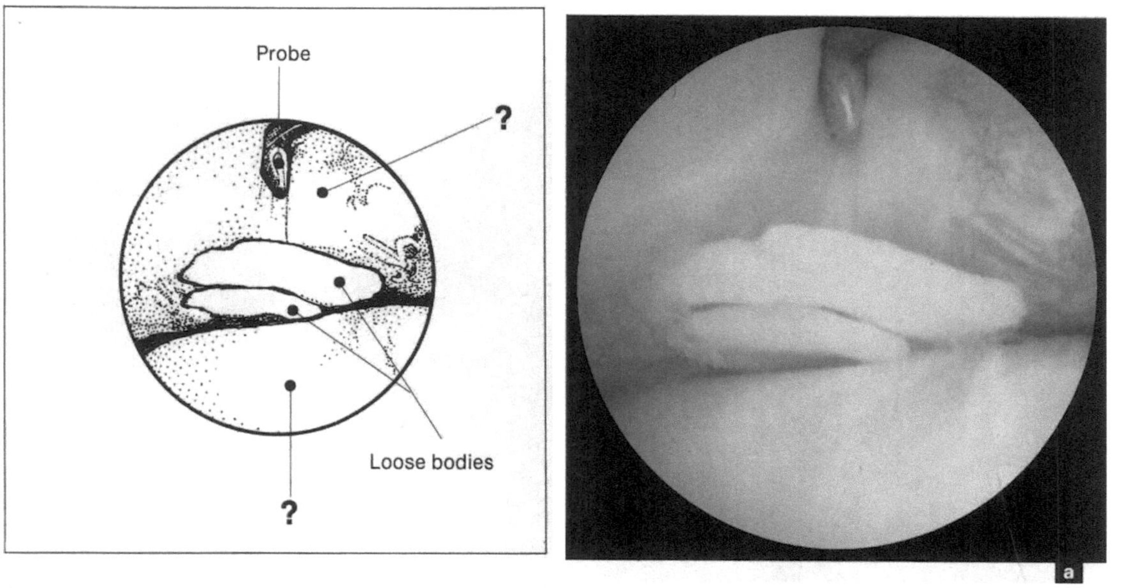

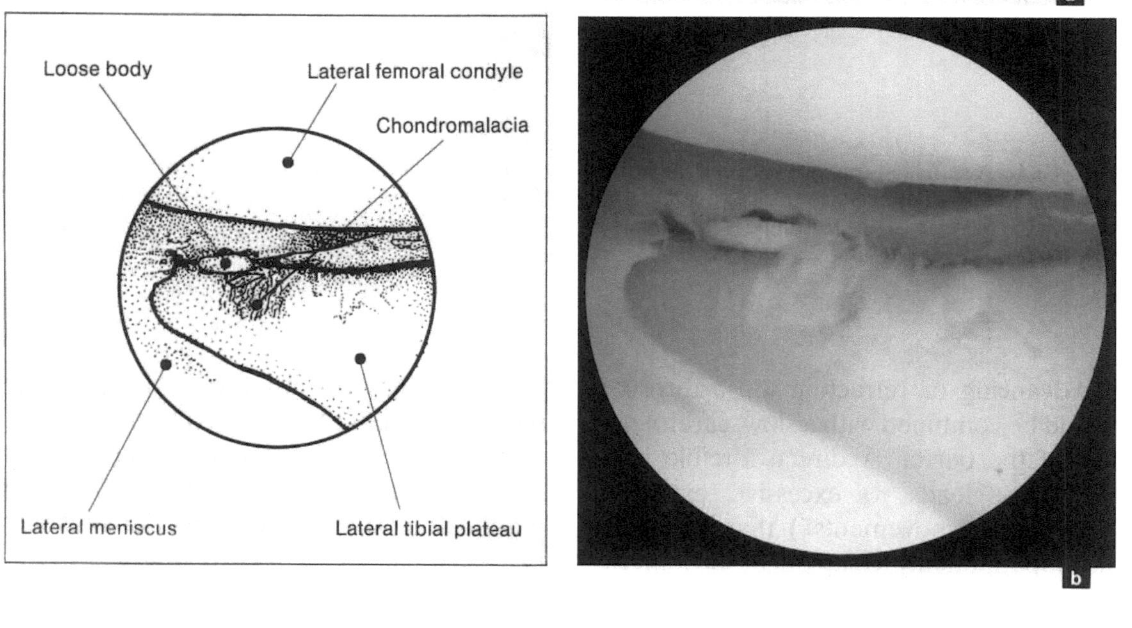

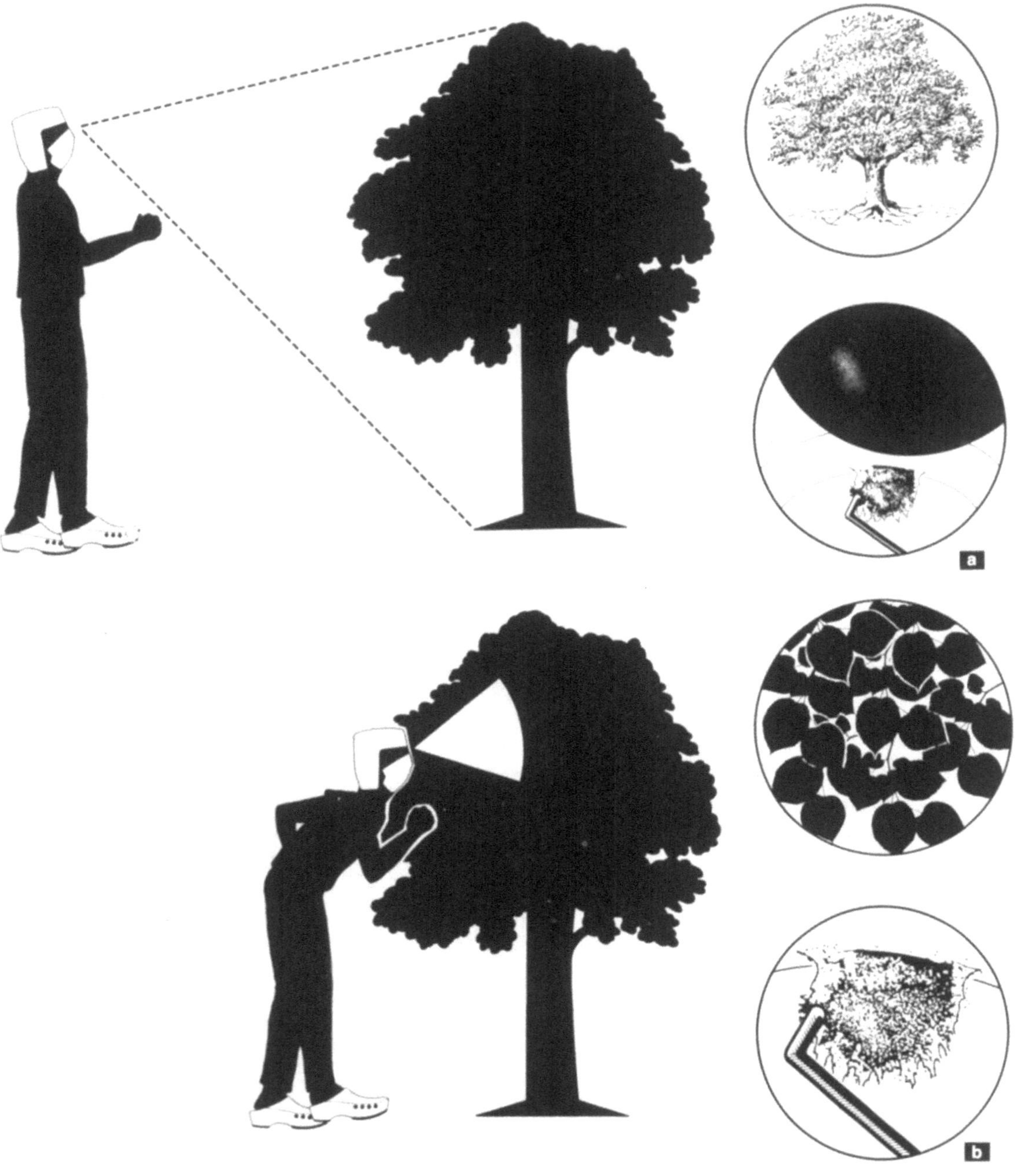

Fig. 7-4 a, b. A sufficient distance between the arthroscope and lesion is necessary for a clear overview and comfortable working (**a**). If the scope is too close, orientation and instrument guidance become much more difficult (**b**) (modified from Johnson 1986)

Advancing or retracting the arthroscope should be combined with a slow, careful rotation of the barrel. A direct, forcible in/out movement leads to excessive excursions ("centimeter movements") that may cause the scope suddenly to slip out of the joint cavity or impinge against the cartilage. If the scope slips from the joint cavity while the inflow is on, the subcutaneous tissue will become distended with irrigating fluid, making it difficult to reinsert the scope. Forceful contact between the arthroscope and articular cartilage can deeply score the cartilage or damage the telescope.

If the scope tip is closely apposed to the cartilage or capsule wall, a featureless yellow-white image will appear on the monitor (see Sect. 11.2). This "yellow-out" can usually be eliminated by retracting and rotating the scope slightly to expand the visual field and reestablish orientation *(note position of light post!)*.

7.1.2 Sweeping the Scope

The arthroscope can be swept upward, downward, to the right or to the left, the portal forming the pivot point for this motion (Fig. 7-5). The intraarticular portion of the scope moves precisely opposite to the extraarticular portion. "Sweeping the scope upward" means that the external part of the arthroscope is moved downward, causing the the intraarticular portion to pivot upward. Similarly, the scope is swept medially by moving its extraarticular portion laterally.

The arthroscope should never be swept with a fast or abrupt motion, and intraarticular structures should be constantly kept in view as if the examiner were visually scanning the interior of the joint. If a white or yellow wall suddenly comes into view, a more meaningful image can be obtained by retracting and/or rotating the scope.

As the arthroscope passes more deeply into the joint, sweeping becomes more difficult since the long portion of the scope is more likely to impinge on the articular cartilage. If the scope is inserted to a depth of only a few centimeters, considerable clearance is left between the scope tip and articular surface, and a much clearer overview is obtained. All movements of the arthroscope should be performed slowly and deliberately, for moving the scope even a millimeter can significantly alter the visual field.

Attention should be given to the long extraarticular lever arm of the arthroscope (Fig. 7-6). The lever arm is greatly extended if the examiner uses a tube camera and holds the system at the camera end rather than by the sheath at the level of the spigots. The long extraarticular lever (= high torque) can transmit powerful forces to the short intraarticular portion of the scope. Abrupt movements can cause bending of the telescope and sheath or produce deep cartilage lesions (Fig. 7-7).

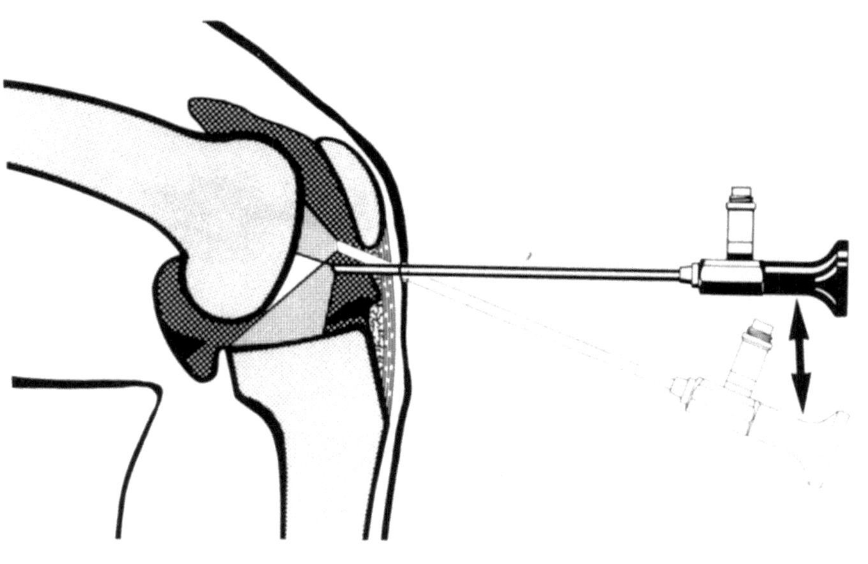

Fig. 7-5. Sweeping the arthroscope downward (to direct the visual field downward) requires a corresponding upward sweep of the extraarticular portion of the scope. If a constant distance is maintained between the scope tip and the target structure, the size of the visual field is not changed

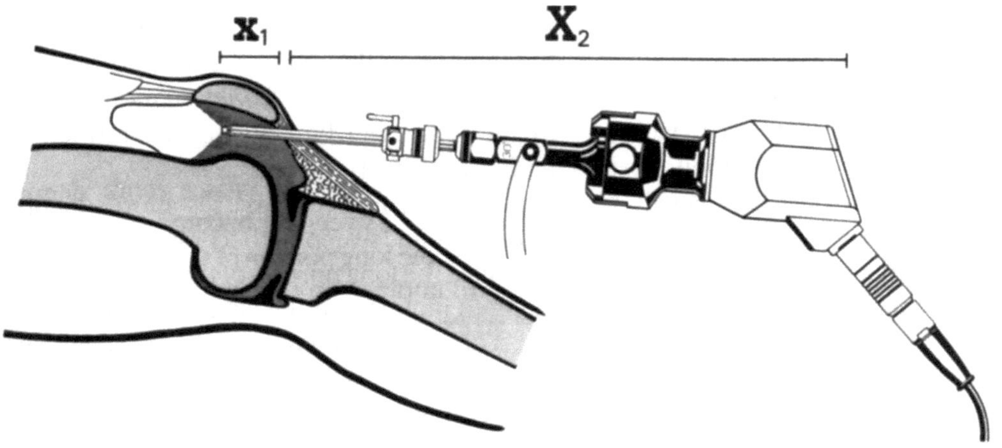

Fig. 7-6. A short intraarticular lever arm (X_1) and long extraarticular lever arm (X_2) are obtained in video arthroscopy if the examiner holds the arthroscope at the level of the video camera

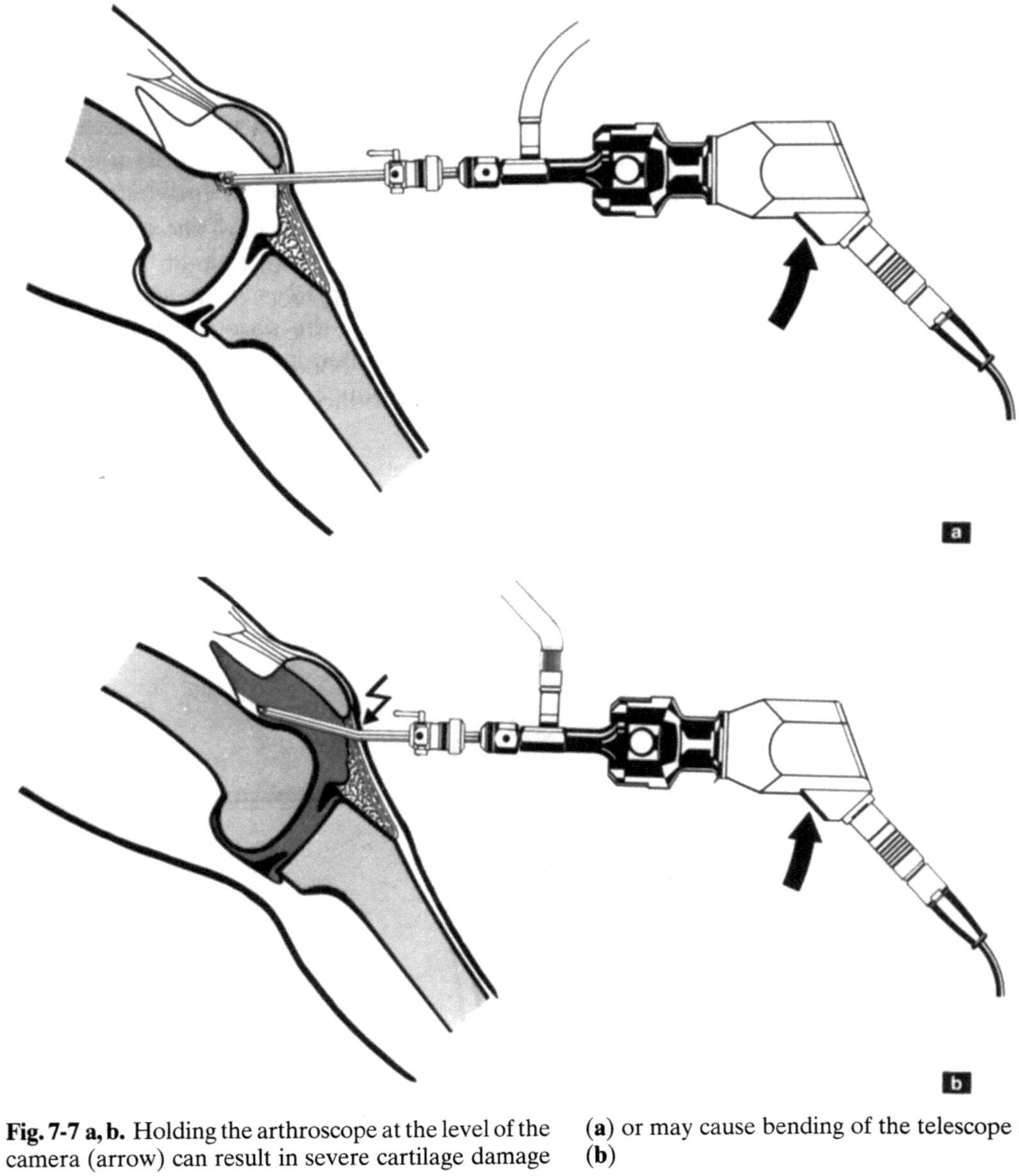

Fig. 7-7 a, b. Holding the arthroscope at the level of the camera (arrow) can result in severe cartilage damage (**a**) or may cause bending of the telescope and sheath (**b**)

The importance of moving the arthroscope slowly, carefully, and deliberately within the joint can scarcely be overstated. The examiner should never try to forcibly overcome a sudden resistance or obstruction to sweeping of the scope. Rather, the scope should be withdrawn slightly with a careful rotating motion to expand the visual field so that the obstruction can be identified and the scope maneuvered around it. Repositioning the knee (e.g., extending it) is sometimes helpful in getting past an obstruction.

An excessive external lever arm can be avoided by proper guidance of the arthroscope. The controlling hand (arthroscope hand) should hold the arthroscope by the sheath at the level of the spigots (see Fig. 3-3).

7.1.3 Rotating the Scope

As noted previously, the rotation of a 0° direct-viewing telescope does not alter its field of vision, much as rotating a flashlight does not change the area illuminated by its beam.

However, the rotation of a 30° wide-angle telescope has a very pronounced effect and can greatly extend the portion of the joint that can be visualized (see Fig. 3-12).

Rotation is accomplished by turning the telescope clockwise or counterclockwise within the sheath.

The visual field of an oblique scope is always directed away from the side carrying the light post.

Thus, if the light post points upward, the visual field is directed downward. If the light post is on the left, the visual field is directed to the right.

7.2 Position of the Light Post

For simplicity and clarity of understanding, we imagine the light post of the arthroscope to be projected onto a clock face that encircles the eyepiece of the scope (Fig. 7-8). The number 12 is always at the top, regardless of which direction the scope is pointing or what area of the joint is being viewed. The position of the light post can be described by saying "the light post is at 3 o'clock" or "light post at 5 o'clock" (Fig. 7-9).

When the 30° wide-angle telescope is used, its visual field covers a 90° sector directly opposite the light post (Fig. 7-9). Since the light post is extraarticular, its position provides the most useful guide to orientation.

The position of the light post is an important aid to orientation!

To illustrate the principles involved in the basic movements of the arthroscope (in/out, sweeping, rotation), we can imagine the tip of the scope to be at the center of the T-shaped intersection of two channels or spaces (Fig. 7-10). To inspect the interior of the channels with a 30° oblique telescope, precise maneuvering of the scope will be required.

The lower part of the vertical channel can be viewed by directing the visual field of the 30° scope straight downward. This is accomplished by rotating the light post to the 12:00 position (Fig. 7-10 a). Keeping the scope tip stationary while moving the light post to 9:00 directs vision toward the wall of the channel, and the visual field is greatly diminished (Fig. 7-10 b). The field could be expanded by sweeping the scope to the left so that its tip enters the horizontal channel.

Moving the light post to 5:00 affords partial views of the upper and horizontal channels (Fig. 7-10 c). Neither channel can be inspected completely, but the entrance to the horizontal channel is seen. Further rotation to 3:00 directs vision into the horizontal space (Fig. 7-10 d). The scope must be swept into the horizontal channel to inspect its interior. An optimum view of the entrance to the horizontal channel is obtained only when the light post is at 3:00 (Fig. 7-10 d).

The horizontal space can be inspected only if the scope tip is level with the space. If the scope is correctly rotated (to the 3:00 position) but is not level with the channel, the vis-

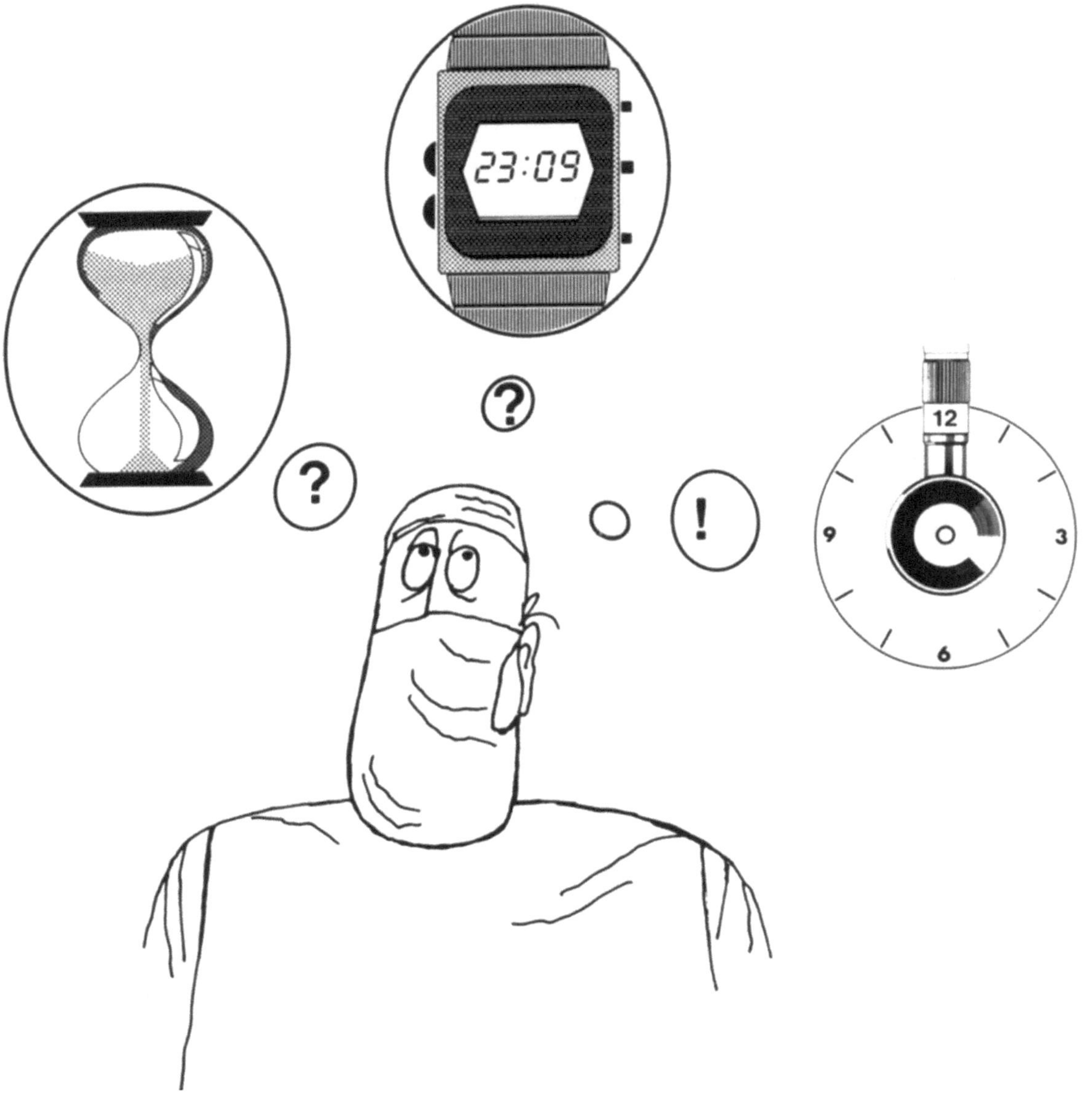

Fig. 7-8. The rotational position of the light post is projected onto an imaginary clock

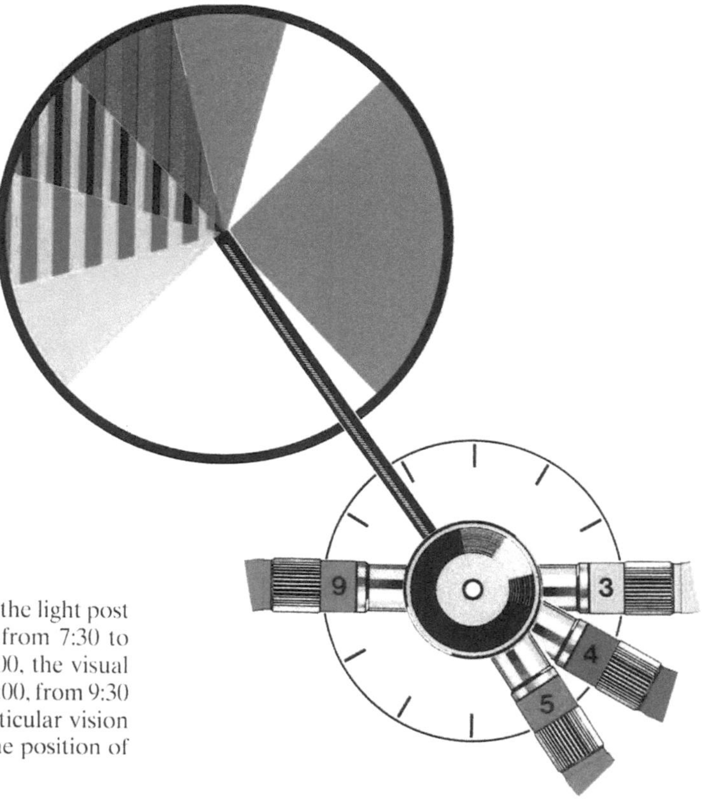

Fig. 7-9. Rotation of the light post. With the light post at 3:00, the visual field covers the area from 7:30 to 10:30 (*yellow*). With the light post at 4:00, the visual field extends from 8:30 to 11:30 (*red*); at 5:00, from 9:30 to 12:30 (*blue*). The direction of intraarticular vision can be precisely determined by noting the position of the light cable

ual field is greatly restricted (Fig. 7-10 e), and the entrance to the space is poorly demonstrated.

If the scope is level with the space and the light post is at 3:00 (Fig. 7-10 d), the scope tip can be swept into the interior of the horizontal space. The scope may shift from the 3:00 position during this maneuver, directing the lens toward the wall of the space. This creates a yellow-out situation with a marked reduction of the visual field (Fig. 7-11 a). The narrower the space, the more careful the operator must be to keep the light post in the optimum position. The yellow-out is corrected, and the interior of the space visualized, by returning the light post to its "optimum" 3:00 position (Fig. 7-11 b).

The caudal portion of the vertical space is visualized by sweeping the arthroscope downward with the light post at 12:00 (Fig. 7-12).

The narrower the space to be inspected, the more accurately the light post and arthroscope must be positioned.

This theoretical example in a geometric system of intersecting channels can be applied to the tissue spaces of the knee joint. To inspect the interior of larger channels, corresponding to the suprapatellar pouch and the lateral and medial recesses of the knee, the light post of the arthroscope should be positioned so that it is parallel to the axis of the channel. For viewing into the lateral recess from above, the light post should be positioned at 12:00. For viewing into the suprapatellar pouch from the medial side, the light post should be at 3:00 in the right knee and 9:00 in the left knee.

The principles of inspecting a narrow space (Fig. 7-11 a,b) are also applicable to the knee joint. This means that the light post of the arthroscope must be directed parallel to the joint space being examined. To inspect the joint space of the right knee from the medial side, the light post is positioned at 3:00 (9:00 in the left knee). Deviations from this optimum position lead to reduction of the visual field.

Accurate positioning of the light post is even more important during the inspection of

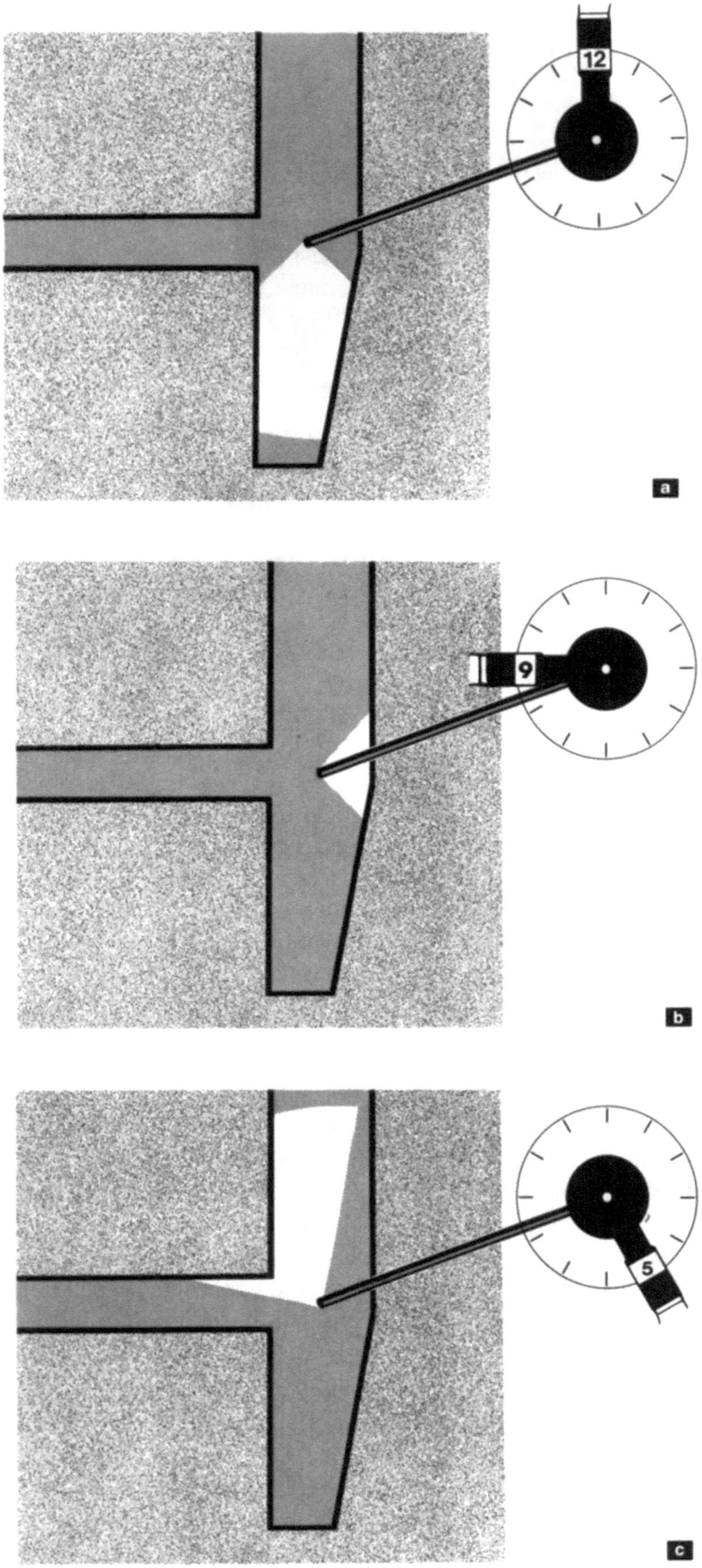

Fig. 7-10 a–e. Inspection of intersecting channels with the 30° oblique scope. **a)** The lower part of the vertical channel is inspected by moving the light post to 12:00. **b)** The 9:00 position gives a very limited view of the channel wall. **c)** Portions of both channels can be viewed by moving the light post to 5:00.

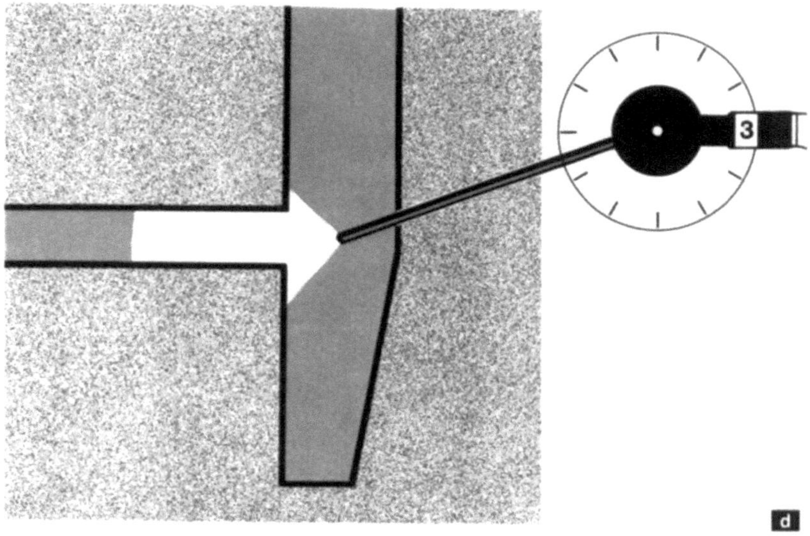

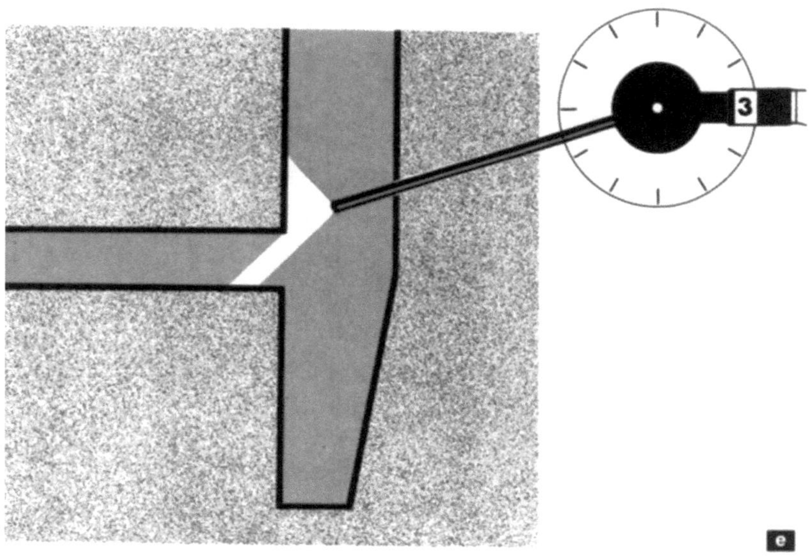

Fig. 7-10 a–e (continued) **d)** The entrance to the horizontal channel is inspected with the light post at 3:00. **e)** If the scope is not at the level of the horizontal space despite a correct rotational position (3:00), only a small portion of the space is visualized

a narrow joint space. The slightest change in the rotational position of the scope will significantly reduce the visual field (Fig. 7-11 a,b). Optimum visualization is obtained only at the 3:00 position in the right knee and at 9:00 in the left knee.

Thus we can see how arthroscopic exploration of the compartments of the knee joint consists of a combination of maneuvers in which the scope is rotated, advanced/retracted, and swept to the right, left, up or down (Fig. 7-13).

The arthroscopist should have a clear appreciation of the individual components of arthroscope movements. It is recommended that the beginner limit scope maneuvers to one type of movement at a time, i.e., he should sweep the scope to the right or left, advance or retract it, or rotate the scope while holding the video camera stationary. Combined movements, such as sweeping the scope while simultaneously advancing or retracting it and rotating the light post, come naturally to the seasoned arthroscopist, but the less experienced examiner cannot expect to achieve this fine coordination right away.

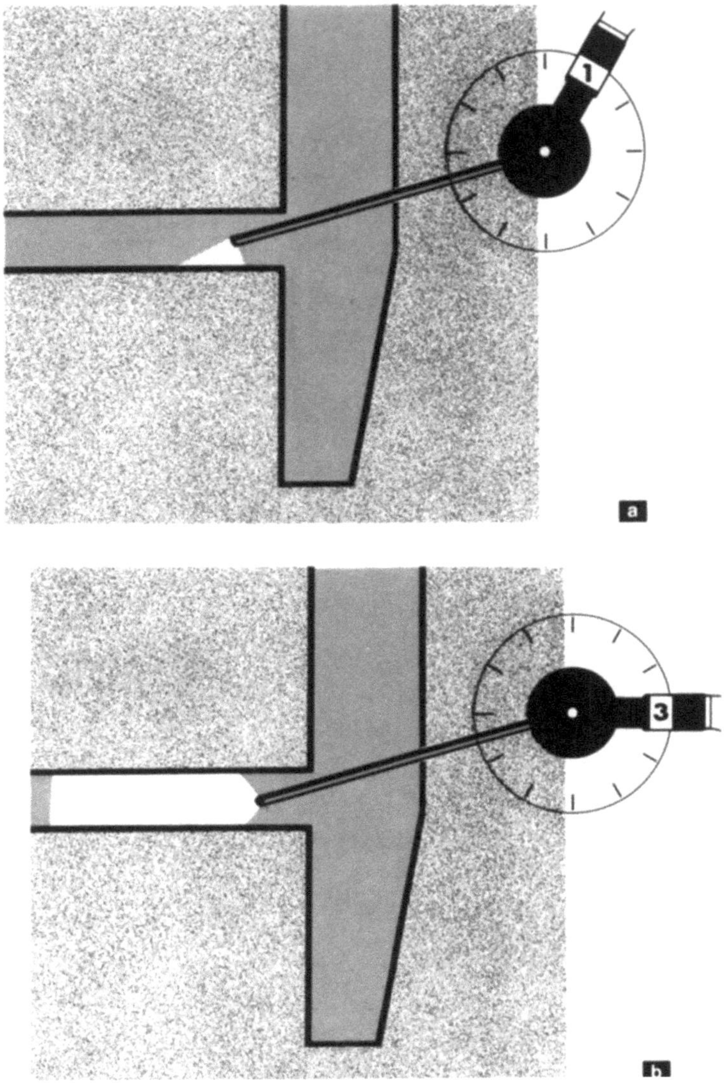

Fig. 7-11 a, b. Inspection of the horizontal space with the 30° scope. **a)** Deviations from the optimum rotational position (e.g., shifting the light post to 1:00) greatly restricts the field of view. **b)** Returning the light post to 3:00 redirects vision into the horizontal space

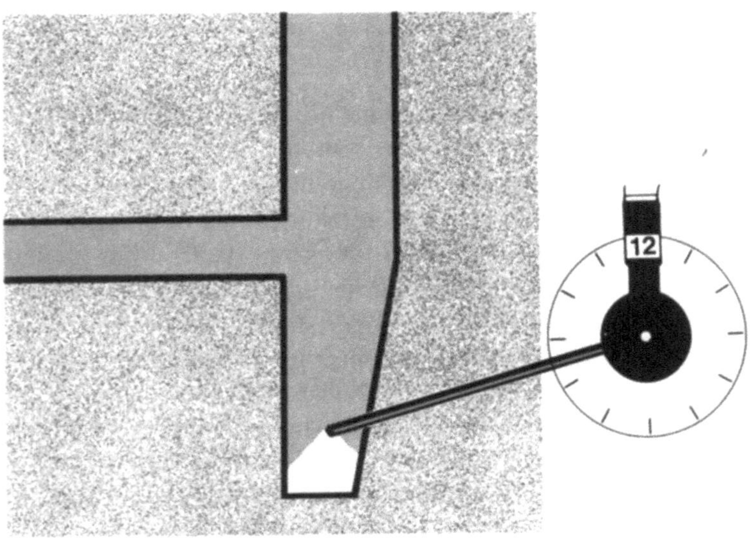

Fig. 7-12. To visualize the floor of the vertical channel, the scope is swept downward while keeping the light post at 12:00

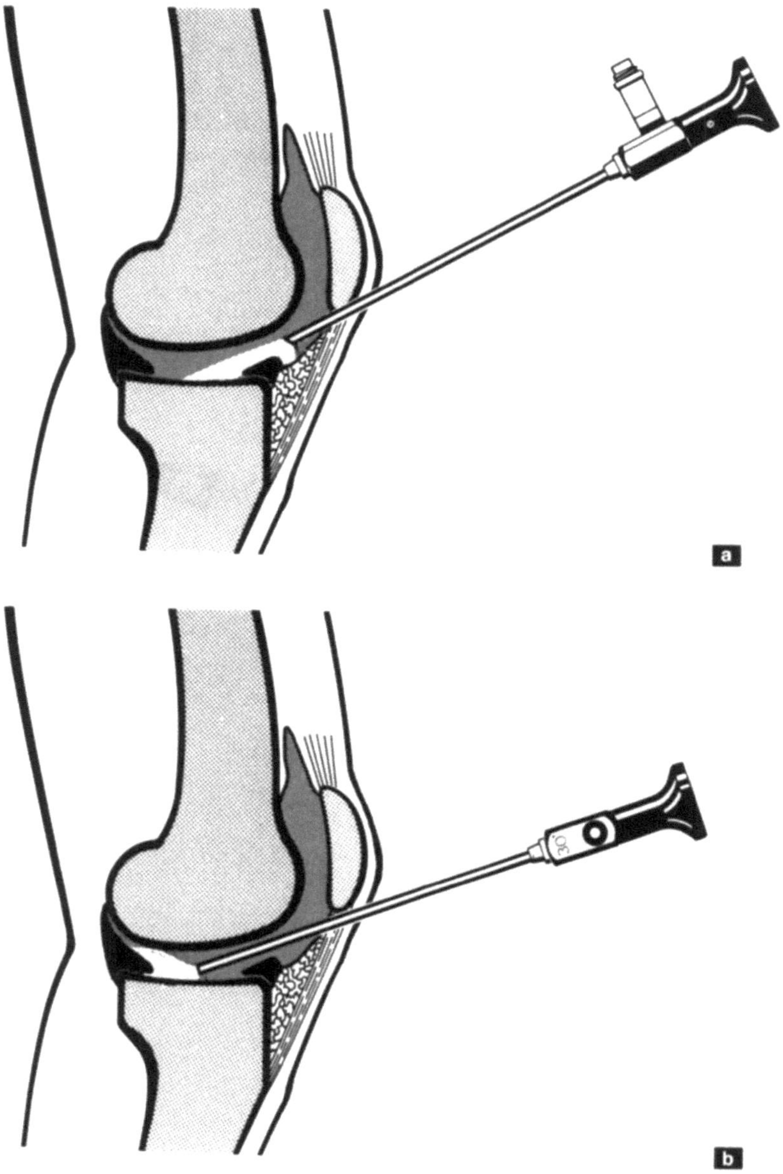

Fig. 7-13 a, b. Exploration of the joint space. **a)** If the scope tip is cranial to the joint space, the anterior portions of the joint space are visualized (light post at 12:00). **b)** By advancing the scope tip, thus bringing it to the level of the joint space, and moving the light post to 3:00 (9:00 in the left knee), the joint space and the posterior horn of the meniscus are visualized

7.3 Movements of the Knee

Besides movements of the arthroscope, movements of the knee joint itself provide a second means for obtaining optimum views of intraarticular structures. The following types of knee movement are available:

- flexion and extension
- internal and external rotation
- medial and lateral opening
- anterior and posterior drawer motion.

These movements not only are utilized for optimum arthroscopic visualization but also convey an impression of the functional condition and stability of the knee.

7.3.1 Flexion and Extension

Flexion and extension of the knee joint are a necessary part of the arthroscopic examination. They permit the examiner to evaluate contact between the patella and femoral trochlea in the femoropatellar joint. The relation of the patella to the femoral groove is evaluated in maximum extension and in various degrees of flexion.

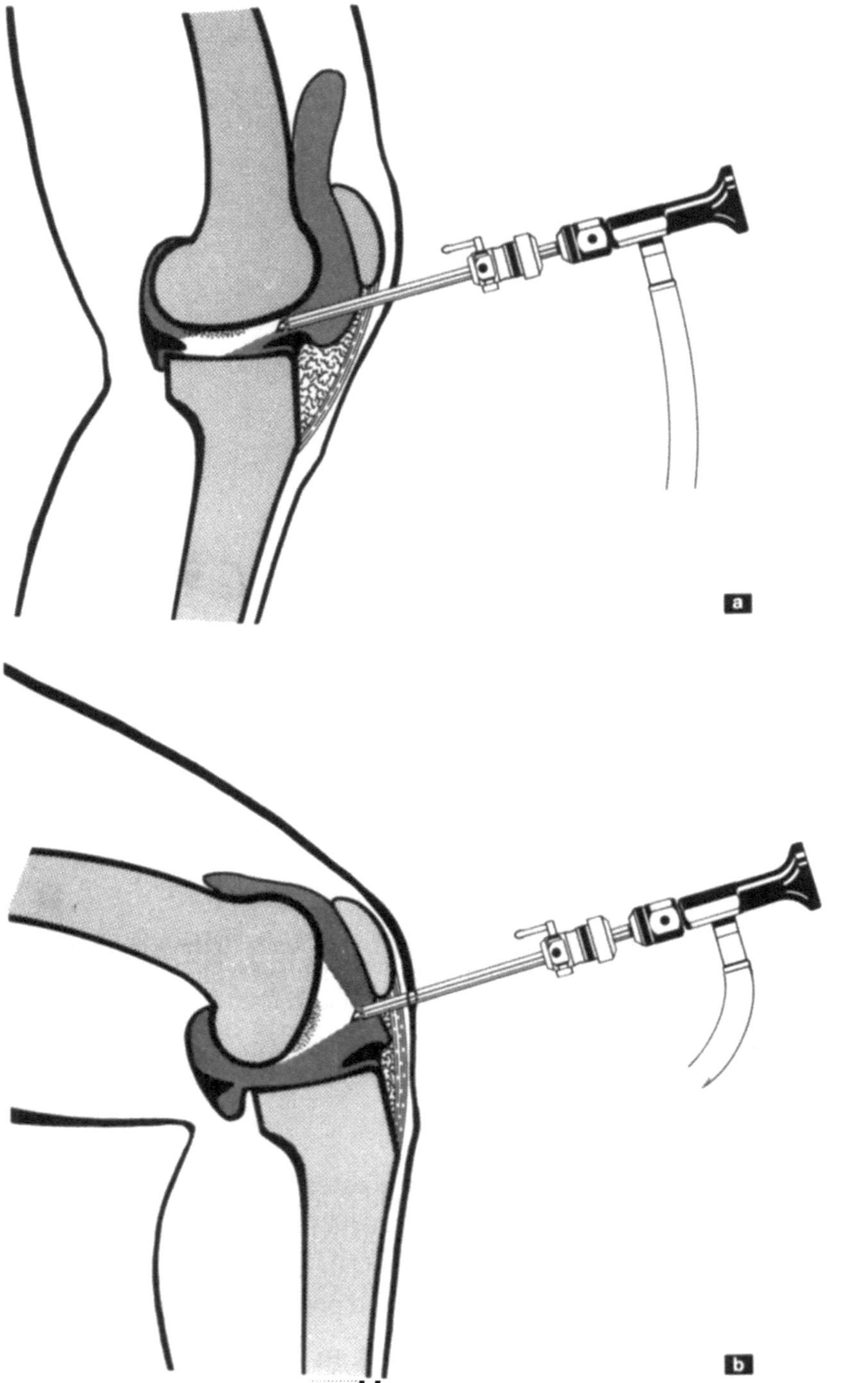

Fig. 7-14 a, b. Inspection of a cartilage lesion on the femoral condyle. With the knee extended, only a portion of the cartilage lesion can be discerned (**a**). When the knee is flexed, the true extent of the cartilage damage can be appreciated (**b**)

As the knee is flexed and extended during arthroscopy, different sites on the cartilaginous surfaces of the femoral condyles pass through the field of view. As the flexion angle increases, posterior cartilage areas can be evaluated (Fig. 7-14).

Increasing flexion is also accompanied by a posterior excursion of the menisci. While posterior gliding of the femoral condyle on the tibial plateau dominates in the initial phase of flexion, the condyle mainly rolls upon the tibia as flexion proceeds. Thus, the menisci recede disproportionately during initial flexion (see Sect. 12.6.1), so the knee should not be sharply flexed for inspecting the posterior horn of the medial meniscus; approximately 10° of flexion is sufficient.

7.3.2 Internal and External Rotation

The visual field of the arthroscope can be modified by internal and external rotation of the tibia. In joints with tight ligaments, it is necessary to combine external rotation of the knee with a valgus stress to visualize the posterior portions of the medial meniscus. External rotation untwists the cruciate ligaments, reducing the axial pressure across the joint and allowing greater opening of the medial joint space.

7.3.3 Medial and Lateral Opening

The narrow joint space must be opened up so that the arthroscopist can look into it and evaluate the condition of the menisci and tibial articular cartilage. The joint space is opened by applying a valgus or varus stress, and for this the thigh must be supported or stabilized on the medial and lateral sides. When the leg is flexed over the edge of the table, this support is provided by the leg holder (see Sect. 4.2.2, Fig. 4-3).

When the leg is extended on the table, the padded lateral post adjacent to the distal third of the thigh serves as a fulcrum for stressing open the joint (see Fig. 4-1). A massive, abrupt valgus force should be avoided as it might cause a capsuloligamentous injury or a femoral fracture, especially in older patients. It might also convert a partial ligament rupture into a complete rupture. Often the medial joint space can be opened sufficiently by abducting the lower leg off the side of the table. A varus stress for opening the lateral joint space is created by moving the leg to the figure-four position (see Sect. 8.8).

In most cases the medial meniscus can be adequately visualized by flexing the knee slightly (not past 10°) while externally rotating the tibia and applying a valgus stress. Inspection of the posterior horn also requires a correctly placed portal and correct positioning of the arthroscope, i.e., with the scope tip in the joint space and the light post at 3:00 (9:00 in the left knee) (see Sect. 11.8 for further details).

7.3.4 Anterior and Posterior Drawer

As in the clinical examination, the anterior and posterior drawer tests and the Lachman test (anterior drawer test in slight flexion) can be performed intraoperatively under arthroscopic vision. In many cases pathologic mobility can be demonstrated and its morphologic basis (e.g., anterior cruciate deficiency) identified. The examiner can also detect the pathomechanical sequelae of the underlying lesion, such as damage to the articular cartilage or to the posterior horn of the medial meniscus.

During arthroscopy the Lachman test can be administered under arthroscopic control while the anterior cruciate ligament (or its remnant) is simultaneously examined (Fig. 7-15). The drawer stress is applied by an assistant who stabilizes the femur with one hand while pulling the proximal tibia anteriorly with the other.

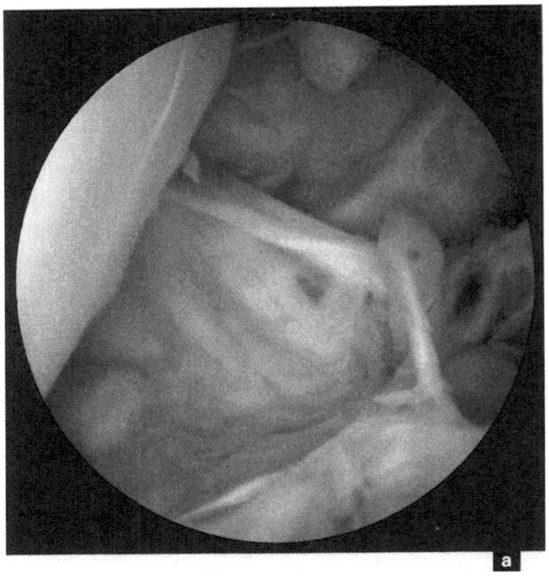

Fig. 7-15 a, b. Arthroscopic Lachman test.
History: Man 27 years of age sustained a rotational knee injury with subsequent hemarthrosis while playing soccer. Arthroscopy revealed a proximal tear of the anterior cruciate ligament, which was repaired with transcondylar sutures 2 years before. For 4 months the patient has experienced an increasing feeling of instability. He has a positive Lachman test with a soft endpoint; the pivot shift test is positive only under anesthesia.
Arthroscopic findings: The anterior cruciate ligament appears intact (**a**), but arthroscopic Lachman testing demonstrates marked elongation signifying functional deficiency of the ligament (**b**).
Procedure: Anterior cruciate ligament reconstruction is indicated

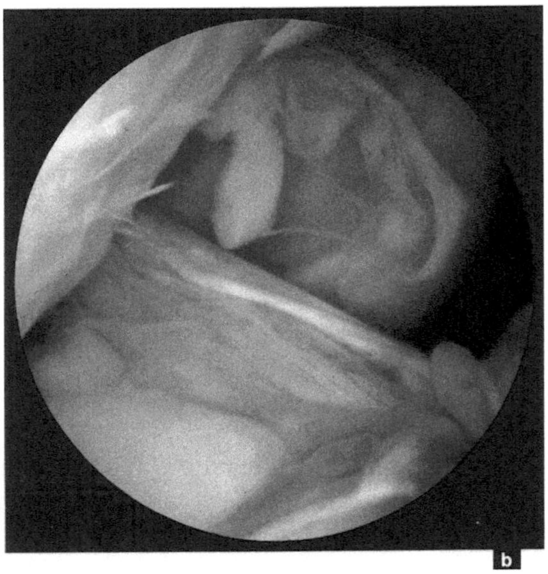

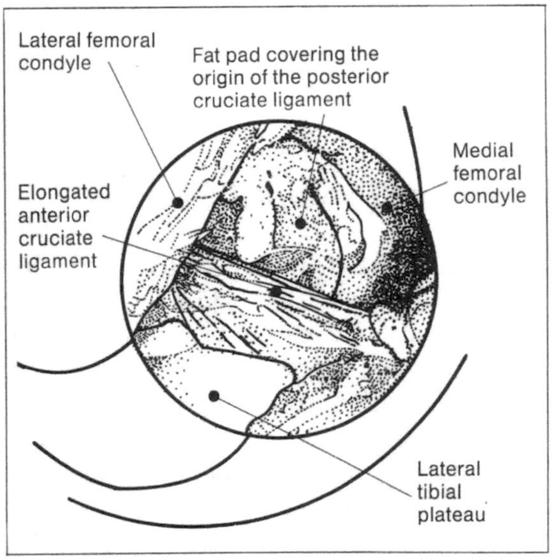

7.4 Direct Manual Maneuvers

These are maneuvers in which the examiner applies a direct pressure to the anatomic structures of the knee joint for the purpose of localizing them, examining them, or becoming oriented on the monitor (see Sect. 7.5 for further details).

A simple direct maneuver is to press on the patella with the finger while observing the motion of the patella on the monitor, i.e., the movement of the retropatellar cartilage toward the opposing femoral cartilage (see Fig. 7-17). Before an instrument portal to the medial or lateral recess is created, it can be helpful to apply external pressure to the capsule to differentiate the capsular wall from the condylar surface (see Fig. 6-11). Indentation of the capsule by digital pressure is visible on the monitor. The spatial relationship of the indentation to the monitor image can be used to adjust the position of the camera or confirm that it is correctly positioned.

Finally, visualization of the medial meniscus can be enhanced by applying direct manual pressure to the meniscus in the popliteal fossa at the level of the joint line. This tends to push the meniscus anteriorly in the direction of the joint cavity (see Fig. 11-10).

7.5 Orientation

7.5.1 Basic Rules

It is always fascinating to watch an experienced arthroscopist at work-to note the thoroughness and apparent ease with which he explores the joint interior and displays the structures of interest on the monitor. This seems remarkable indeed to one who is taking his first "arthroscopic steps" and encountering problems at every turn. Often neither the arthroscopist nor other observers know just what part of the joint is being viewed. Everything appears yellowish-white, inverted, or turned on its side-a most frustrating situation.

It is useful, therefore, to review some basic rules of orientation. The monitor image serves as the ultimate reference point for the arthroscopist, assistant, and nurse, as well as for the patient and any others observing the procedure.

Basic rule. *The joint is displayed on the monitor as if the observer were looking into the knee from the anterior side.*

Specific structures are displayed as follows:

1 Joint space horizontal
2 Patella above, femur below
3 Medial and lateral recesses vertical
4.1 Right knee: medial structures on the right side of the monitor, lateral structures on the left
4.2 Left knee: medial structures on the left side of the monitor, lateral structures on the right.

The medial meniscus in the right knee is displayed on the right side of the screen and appears horizontal, following the course of the joint line. While the content of the monitor image is determined by the position of the arthroscope, the orientation of the image is determined by the position of the video camera in relation to the telescope (Fig. 7-16).

The basic rules of monitor orientation are *independent* of the position of the knee or arthroscope. A few arthroscopists prefer to display the joint space on the monitor in a vertical or diagonal orientation. This practice, dating back to a time before video systems were available, is not recommended because it can confuse orientation and even lead to cervical spine problems since the examiner must tilt his head to view the image.

The joint space should always be horizontal!

The video camera should be positioned so that its top surface, which usually bears the manufacturer name plate, is uppermost. Image orientation is then fine-adjusted as needed by rotating the camera a few degrees relative to the arthroscope (Fig. 7-16).

7.5.2 Intraarticular Orientation

Once inside the joint, the tip of the arthroscope is advanced into the medial suprapatellar recess. The light post is moved to the 6:00 position, and the arthroscope is slowly retracted with a careful rotating motion. The first feature to appear on the monitor is a whitish, homogeneous structure representing the retropatellar cartilage. It may appear on the right or left side of the screen. To display it at the top of the screen, the video camera is rotated relative to the arthroscope (see Fig. 7-16).

To confirm that the whitish feature is indeed the retropatellar cartilage, the examiner applies external manual pressure to the patella while watching the monitor for a corresponding movement of the cartilage surface (Fig. 7-17).

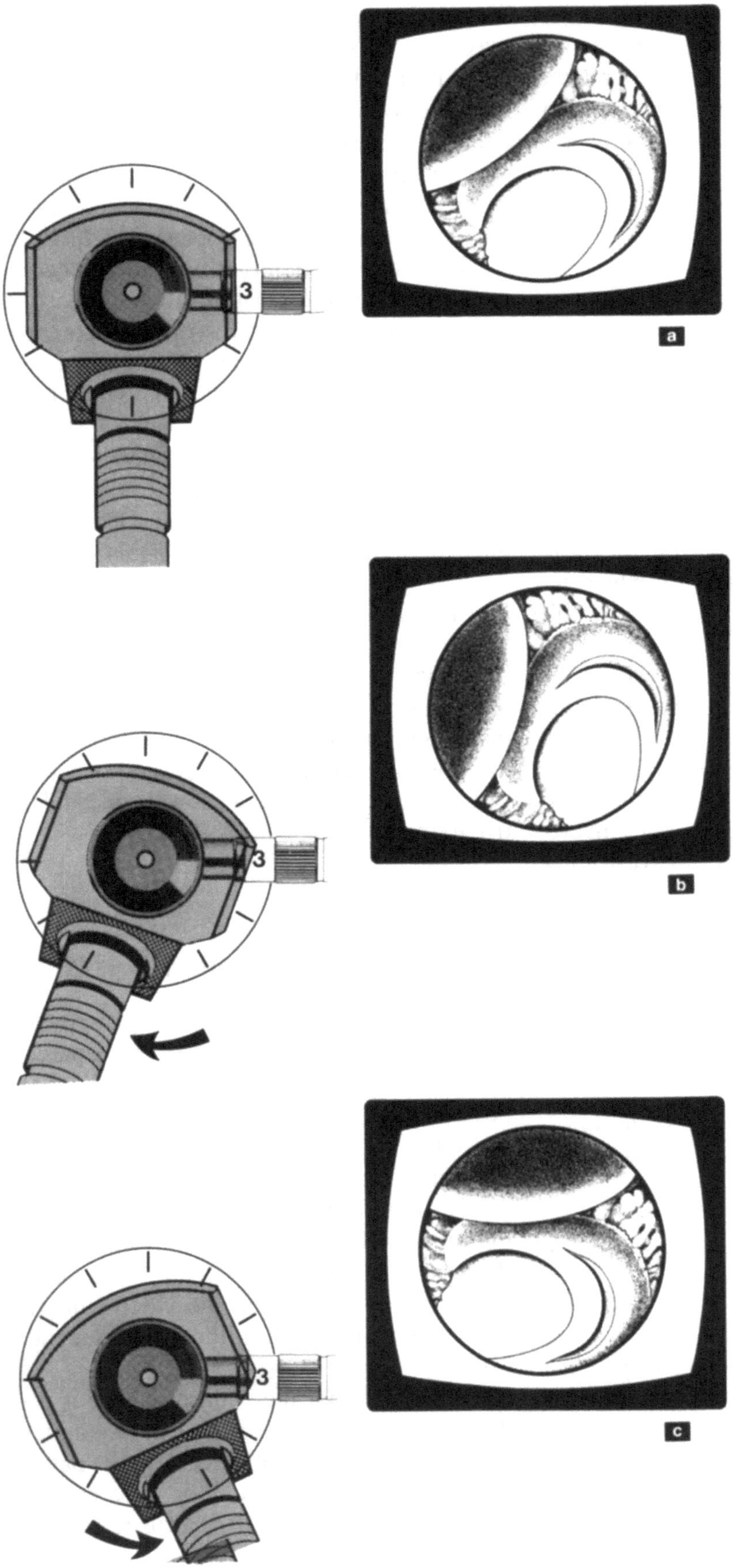

Fig. 7-16 a–c. Visualization of the medial joint space (right knee). **a)** Despite correct positioning of the light post (at 3:00), the joint space appears diagonal on the monitor. **b)** If rotating the camera relative to the arthroscope causes the joint space to appear more vertical, the camera is being turned in the wrong direction. **c)** Correct camera rotation produces the desired horizontal joint-space orientation

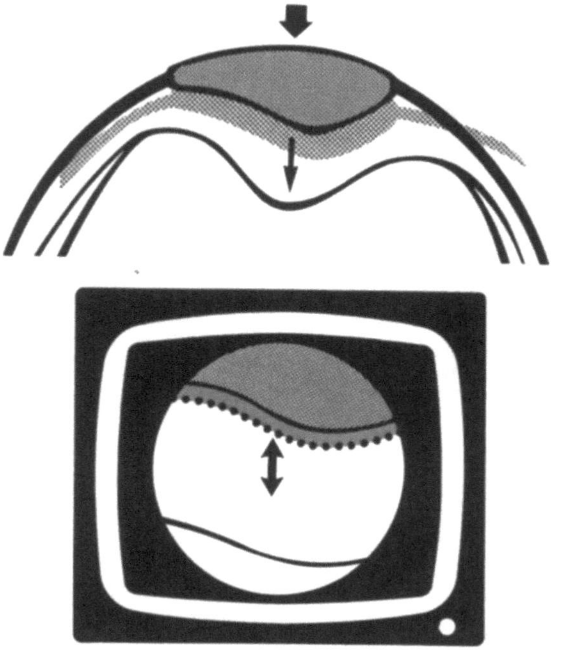

Fig. 7-17. Manual compression of the patella (top) elicits movement of the retropatellar surface that is visible on the monitor (bottom)

Table 7-1. Procedure for establishing orientation in the knee joint

1. With the knee extended, advance the arthroscope into the suprapatellar pouch.
2. Position the light post at 6:00.
3. Place the top of the camera at 12:00.
4. Carefully retract the scope with a rotating motion (knee is still extended).
5. Locate a whitish or yellowish area (= retropatellar cartilage).
6. Display the retropatellar cartilage at the top of the monitor by rotating the camera relative to the scope.
7. Confirm by manual pressure that the whitish area is the retropatellar cartilage.

As the examination proceeds, it will be necessary to make repeated fine adjustments of the monitor image by rotating the video camera relative to the scope.

The examiner should see to it that once the monitor image has been calibrated, orientation is not lost. Since the image changes constantly in response to movements of the arthroscope and knee, an effort must be made to keep the video camera in a constant position. Especially when the arthroscope is rotated, the camera should be held stationary so that it does not turn with the scope. With some cameras this requires temporarily loosening the connection between the camera and telescope while the scope is turned.

If, for whatever reason, orientation is lost, it can be reacquired by identifying one or more major landmark features. Attempting to examine a joint without proper orientation not only increases the risk of iatrogenic cartilage damage but is also unsatisfying for the examiner and observers. Reorientation can always begin in the suprapatellar pouch. Initial orientation and reorientation are established by following a standard sequence of steps (Table 7-1).

When arthroscopy is performed without a video system, the foregoing calibration procedure is simplified since the examiner is looking directly through the scope. Thus, the position of the arthroscope correlates directly with the arthroscopic image.

Other useful landmarks besides the retropatellar cartilage are (1) the *lateral triangle,* bounded by the lateral tibial plateau, the lateral femoral condyle, and the anterior cruciate ligament and (2) the *medial triangle,* bounded by the medial femoral condyle, the medial tibial plateau, and the medial meniscus.

7.6 Principle of Triangulation

Once the instrument portal has been created, it is often difficult to bring the probe into the visual field of the arthroscope. This may result from:

- a small field of view,
- monocular vision,
- lack of experience.

It is helpful to imagine that the probe and arthroscope form two sides of an equilateral triangle. A common error is to cross the tips of

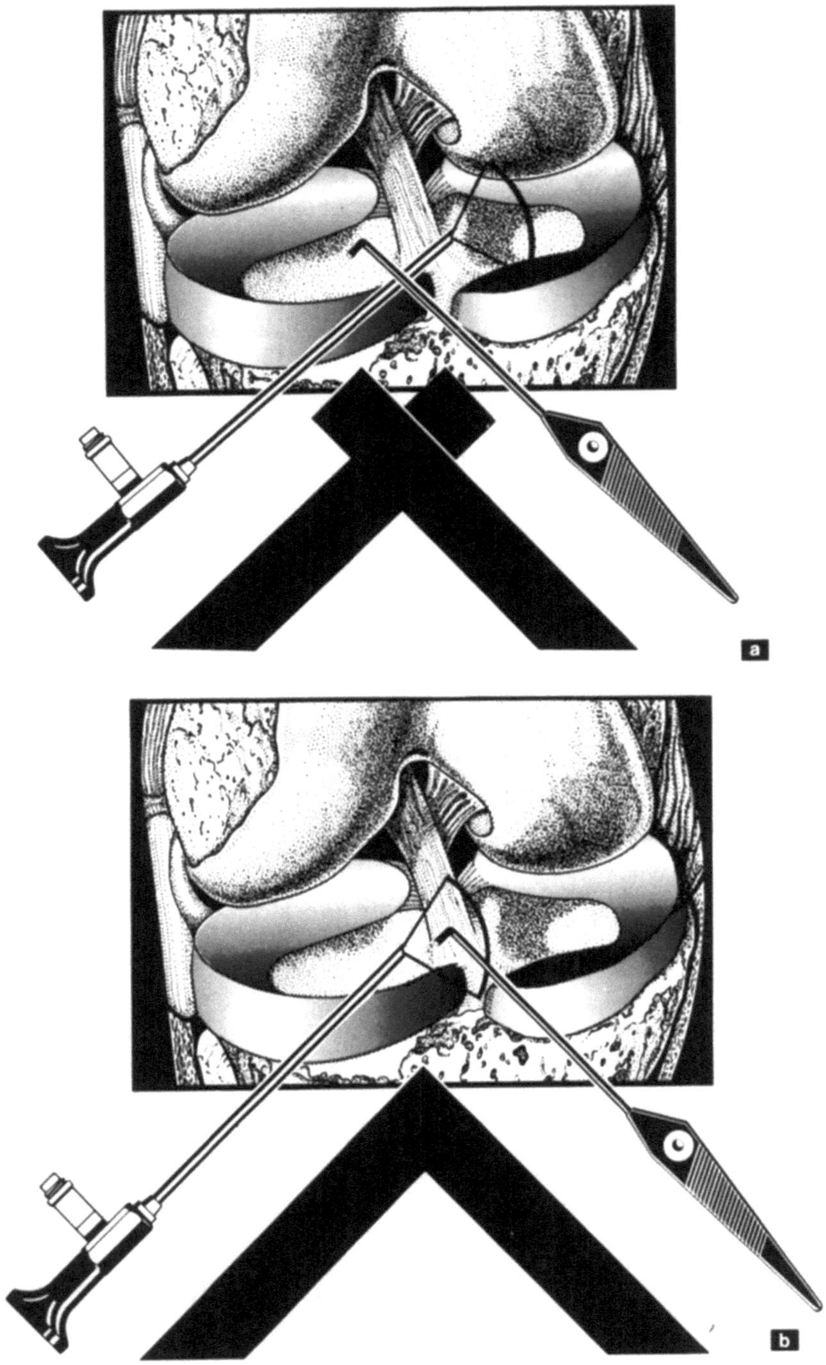

Fig. 7-18 a, b. Principle of triangulation. If the probe crosses the arthroscope in the joint, it will be outside the visual field of the scope (**a**). The probe is visualized only if the tips of the probe and arthroscope converge at the apex of an equilateral triangle (**b**)

the probe and arthroscope. Although a triangle is formed, the probe is not within the optical field of the scope (Fig. 7-18).

As the probe is moved into the field, the examiner should control both the arthroscope and probe so that the two objects can be more easily brought together. Handling of the arthroscope and probe is comparable to eating with a knife and fork. The diner does not look alternately at the knife and fork but at the point where the "instruments" meet, the plate. Similarly, the arthroscopist does not look at the arthroscope and probe but watches the monitor with the idea of bringing the tips of his "knife and fork" together "on the plate," i.e., within the joint.

It should be emphasized that the true sense of "triangulation" is achieved only when the examiner holds the arthroscope in one hand while simultaneously holding the probe or operating instrument in the other.

7.7 Rendezvous Technique

The "rendezvous technique" is recommended for cases where a desired portion of the joint cannot be reached with the probe or other instrument. In this technique the examiner makes a "rendezvous" with the probe (instrument) in a portion of the joint where such a meeting is easily arranged, e.g., in front of the anterior cruciate ligament or at the undersurface of the patella. From that meeting point, the probe can then be directed under vision to sites that are more difficult to reach. Often it will be found that the instrument portal has not been optimally positioned. It is better in these cases to make a new portal than bend the probe in an attempt to reach the target structure from an unsatisfactory portal.

The rendezvous technique is used when the joint position is changed frequently but the examiner does not want to keep adding portals. Given the relative shifting tendency of the capsule, subcutaneous tissue, and skin, the probe is introduced in the initial joint position and visualized on the monitor. It is kept in sight as the knee is moved to the desired position.

8
Examination Procedure – Normal and Pathologic Findings

The arthroscopic examination should follow a predetermined routine to ensure that nothing is overlooked (Table 8-1). The sequence of the examination depends in large part on the position of the extremity. When the knee is extended for arthroscopy, the examination begins with inspection of the retropatellar cartilage. While it may seem more appropriate to start with the suprapatellar recess, since that is where the sheath is first introduced, the retropatellar cartilage is the first feature used to orient the monitor image by rotation of the camera, so it is convenient to begin the examination there (see Sect. 7.5).

When the knee is examined in the flexed position, the sheath is first directed into the anteromedial part of the joint at the level of the joint space, in front of the medial femoral condyle. In that position the inflow and outflow lines can be connected to the sheath and the telescope inserted. The examination then commences in the medial joint compartment.

The particular examination sequence or routine that is followed is immaterial as long as all portions of the joint are covered by the examination.

Table 8-1. Systematic arthroscopic exploration

1. Retropatellar cartilage
2. Suprapatellar recess
3. Lateral recess
4. Patellofemoral joint
5. Medial capsule
6. Medial compartment
7. Intercondylar notch
8. Move leg to figure-4 position
9. Lateral compartment

If pathology is found, the arthroscopist should not discontinue the examination and proceed at once to arthroscopic or open treatment. Frequently the pathology will coexist with other lesions requiring treatment or other conditions that will influence the prognosis of the underlying disease.

The portal for the probing hook is made only after the interior of the joint has been thoroughly inspected. Only then can the examiner determine whether the suspicious structures can be probed and treated through one favorably placed portal or whether multiple punctures will be needed-bearing in mind that one portal may give sufficient access for the treatment of two or three different lesions.

After the arthroscope has been inserted through a high anterolateral portal, the retropatellar cartilage identified, and the video horizon established (with the light post at 6:00 and the top of the camera at 12:00), the arthroscopic examination may begin (see Sect. 7.5).

The examination procedure is described below in detail. If the arthroscopist is to conduct the examination smoothly, he should know something of the basic rules for positioning the leg and arthroscope (light post) as well as the potential obstacles and problems that may arise. The normal findings and the most common pathologic findings will be described for every portion of the joint and every anatomic structure. Because the evaluation of normal and pathologic changes in the cartilage and synovial membrane are particularly complex, separate chapters (9 and 10) are devoted to the *articular cartilage* and *synovium.*

Every compartment in the knee joint can be reproducibly described in terms of five parameters:

Position
This pertains essentially to the angle of knee flexion and the rotational position of the tibia.

Visualization
The position of the light post is stated using clock-face notation (see Fig. 7-8) so that the arthroscope position and the structures visualized can be reproducibly described. The position of the light post is independent of the location of the arthroscope, i.e., it does not matter whether the scope is in the suprapatellar pouch or in the lateral or medial compartment.

All photographs, drawings, and data on arthroscope position pertain to the **right** knee. The position of the light post for the left knee is stated in parentheses.

Besides the position of the light post, necessary movements of the arthroscope (in/out, sweeping, rotation) are also indicated. External movements of the joint (flexion, extension, rotation, drawer tests) are used to evaluate for functional abnormalities, as in the clinical examination.

Normal Findings
Normal findings and their variants are not always easy to differentiate from pathologic conditions.

Pathologic Findings
Clinically relevant pathologic findings, which may be present in varying degrees, are described. It is often difficult for the novice to correlate clinical and arthroscopic findings, so numerous arthroscopic photographs and correlative drawings are presented along with illustrative case reports giving essential facts about the patient's history, the result of the clinical examination, and a suggested therapeutic approach.

Problems
Errors in positioning the arthroscope, anatomic variants, and pathologic changes can hamper the conduct of the examination and operation. If the cause of a problem is known, it should be fairly easy to correct. Thus, the examiner should be familiar with the potential problems and errors that can occur in the various joint regions. Several possible solutions are offered for each problem situation that may arise.

8.1 Retropatellar Space

Position
The knee is fully extended. Even slight flexion will narrow the retropatellar space.

Visualization
The light post of the arthroscope is at 6:00 (Fig. 8-1).

The arthroscope is swept from side to side (medially and laterally) while it is slowly retracted so that both patellar facets can be visualized. Inspection of the larger lateral facet is made easier by manually pushing and tilting the patella medially with the light post at 4:00 (Fig. 8-2). The junction between the lateral patellar facet and retinaculum can also be evaluated from this position.

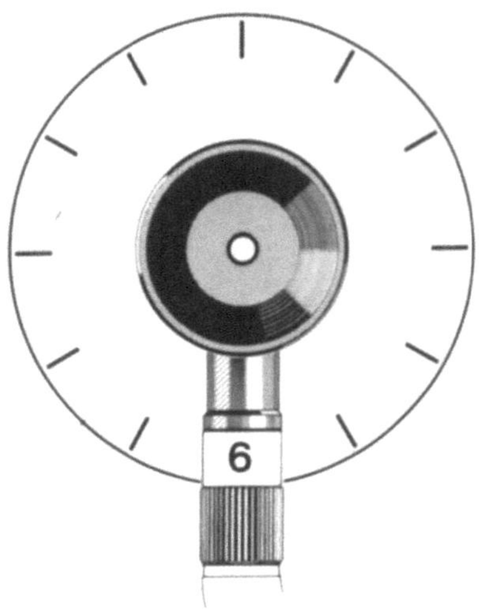

Fig. 8-1. Light post at 6:00 for examination of the retropatellar cartilage

Normal Findings

Healthy retropatellar cartilage is smooth, yellowish-white, and resilient. The cartilage is usually probed from a suprameniscal portal.

The cartilage of the femoral portion of the femoropatellar joint should not be overlooked. It is examined during the evaluation of femoropatellar contact (see Sect. 8.4).

Pathologic Findings

Lesions of the retropatellar cartilage are among the most common pathologic changes detectable by arthroscopy (Fig. 8-3). It should be noted that arthroscopically diagnosed retropatellar cartilage lesions frequently do not correlate with clinical findings. Thus, it is common to find extensive cartilage lesions in clinically asymptomatic patients, or to find no evidence of chondropathy in patients experiencing severe retropatellar pain. Such cases should not be lumped under the heading of "chondromalacia" for lack of a better diagnosis (see Sect. 9.2.1). While areas of softening (grade I chondromalacia) are frequently detected on probing the retropatellar surface, especially in young patients, one should not assume that they are responsible for the patient's overall complaints.

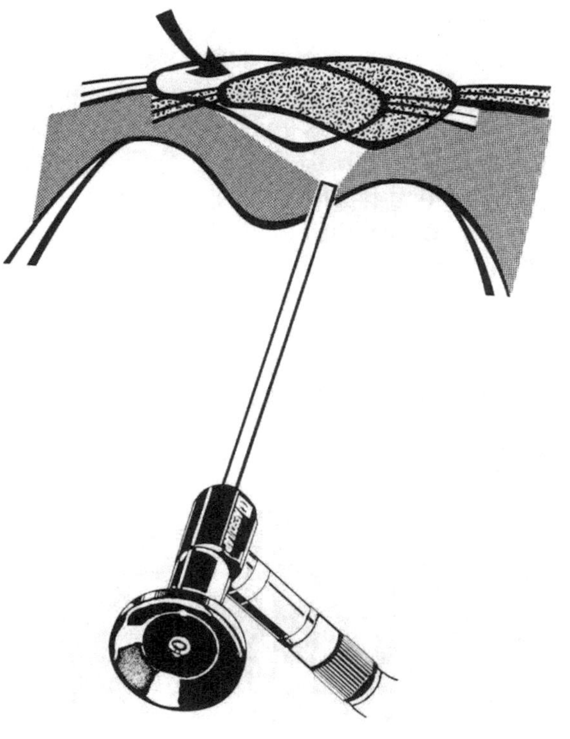

Fig. 8-2. Manual medialization of the patella to improve visualization of the lateral patellar facet. The light post is at 4:00 (8:00 in the left knee)

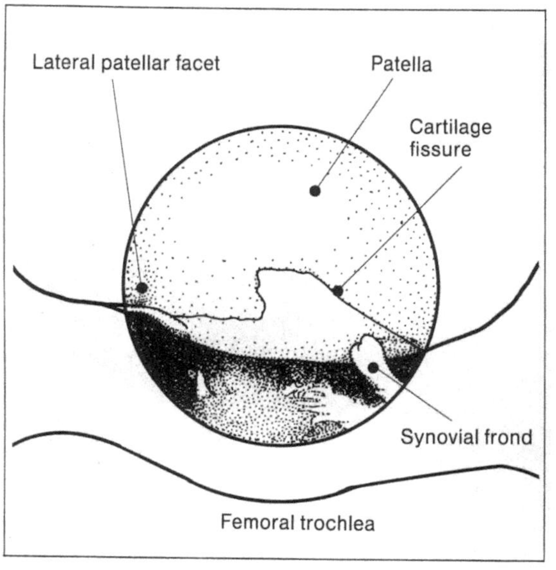

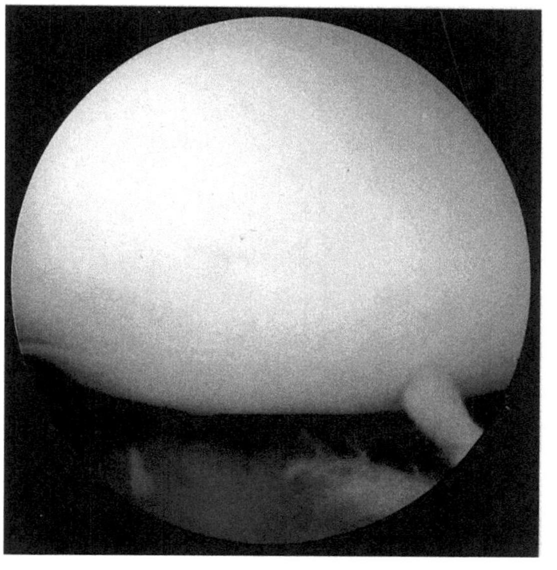

Fig. 8-3. Inspection reveals fine fissuring of the retropatellar cartilage. Probing is necessary for a more accurate evaluation

It should be noted, moreover, that various grades of traumatic or degenerative retropatellar cartilage pathology can be found in virtually all patients over 50 years of age (Fig. 8-4, see Chap. 9).

The medial facet of the patella may demonstrate contusional marks, sites of bloody imbibition, or chondral or osteochondral fractures as sequelae to a patellar dislocation. Rarely the fracture may involve the entire medial facet and portions of the patellar ridge. The detached osteochondral fragments may enter the suprapatellar pouch or the lateral recess. The mediodistal retinaculum usually shows tearing or hemorrhagic change following a patellar dislocation (Fig. 8-5) and should be inspected during the evaluation of femoropatellar contact (see Sect. 8.4).

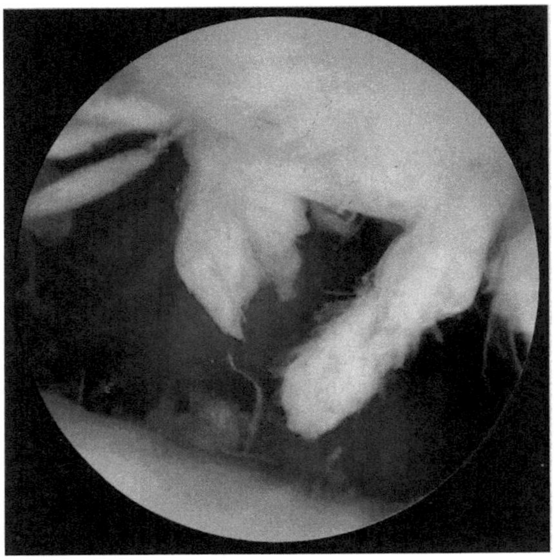

Fig. 8-4. Fraying of the retropatellar cartilage. Probing is necessary to determine whether the lesions extend to the subchondral bone

Problems

Inspection and probing of the retropatellar cartilage are difficult when the patellofemoral space is narrowed. This may result from:

- *Incomplete extension of the knee.* Any degree of flexion significantly reduces the femoropatellar distance. In a knee that cannot fully extend due, say, to an entrapped meniscus or loose body, a contracture of the joint capsule, or a bone deformity, the retropatellar space can be reexpanded only by eliminating the cause of the extension deficit. With an entrapped loose body, extension should not be forced due to the risk of iatrogenic cartilage damage. If necessary, the patella can be examined through a lateral or medial suprapatellar portal.

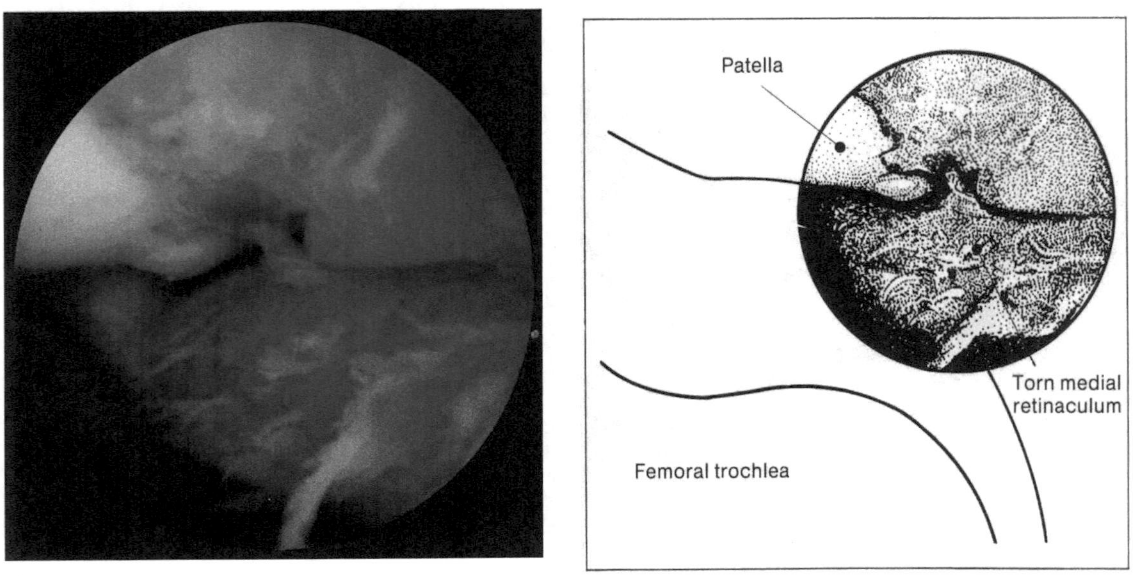

Fig. 8-5. Tearing and hemorrhage in the medial retinaculum following patellar dislocation

- *Insufficient distention with irrigating fluid.* The supply of irrigating fluid may be exhausted, the fluid pressure may be too low, or the inflow may be obstructed (tubing clogged or kinked, spigot turned off, faulty placement of inflow needle). After the inflow path is checked for patency, one can attempt to distend the joint by raising the fluid pressure (elevating the fluid bag to a higher level).
- *Adhesions.* When adhesions are present in the superior portion of the joint, they must be divided before the femoropatellar space can distend.
- *Failure of expansion* of the suprapatellar pouch due to a suprapatellar septum (see under "Adhesions" above).
- *Yellow-out* due to proximity of the scope tip to the cartilage or synovial membrane. First the position of the light post is checked (6:00?). Then the arthroscope is carefully retracted and swept downward toward the anterior surface of the femur (floor of the suprapatellar pouch) to increase its distance from the patella.

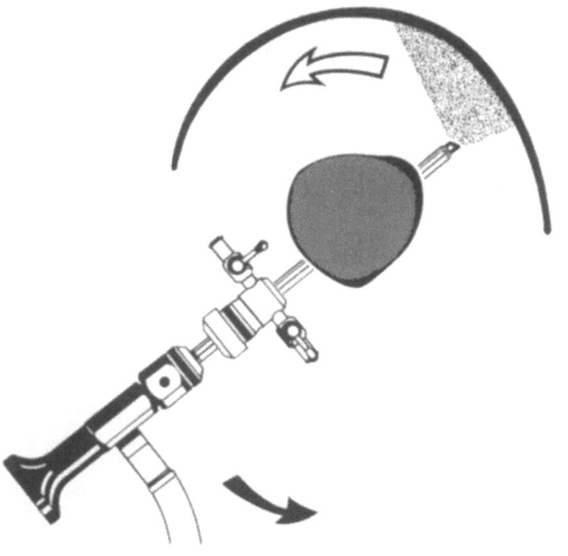

Fig. 8-6. Inspection of the suprapatellar pouch. The light post is at 3:00 (9:00 in the left knee). The arthroscope is swept from the medial to the lateral side

8.2 Suprapatellar Pouch

Position

The knee is maximally extended.

Visualization

The light post is at 3:00 (9:00 in the left knee).

Starting from the retropatellar cartilage, the arthroscope is advanced proximally and medially into the joint. The suprapatellar pouch is inspected by sweeping the scope from medially to laterally (Fig. 8-6).

Normal Findings

The suprapatellar pouch appears as a proximal saclike extension of the joint cavity. The tendon and muscle fibers of the quadriceps femoris muscle form the whitish roof of pouch. Fiber tracts frequently appear in the medial and lateral portions of the pouch, and dark red muscle tissue showing through the pouch lining should not be mistaken for residual hematoma or hemarthrosis. The floor of the pouch is formed by the anterior aspect of the femur, whose marked convexity is evened out medially and laterally by fat and connective tissue. The floor of the pouch is studded with fat-laden synovial villi, which tend to undergo hypertrophy in response to a chronic intraarticular irritation such as a meniscal tear (see Chap. 10).

The entrance to the suprapatellar pouch is bounded medially and laterally by variants of the suprapatellar plica.

Pathologic Findings

The contents and extent of the suprapatellar pouch are clinically significant. The pouch may contain loose bodies-osteochondral fragments from a patellar dislocation or other trauma, meniscal fragments, cartilage flakes-that should be removed or, if possible, reattached. If there is a loose body in the suprapatellar pouch, it can be transfixed with a percutaneous needle. (Further movement of the loose body would necessitate an additional, time-consuming search!) With the fragment immobilized, the instrument portal can be placed at an optimum site for inserting a grasping instrument to retrieve the loose body. Following hemarthrosis, the suprapatellar pouch will contain blood clots in acute cases or fibrin clots in cases of longer standing (Fig. 8-7).

With synovitis, hypertrophied synovial fronds can hamper inspection of the pouch. Blood and fibrin clots can be aspirated through a large-bore needle, but this can be done more rapidly and effectively with a motorized synovial or Rosenberg resector. Large fibrin clumps are extracted with a grasping forceps.

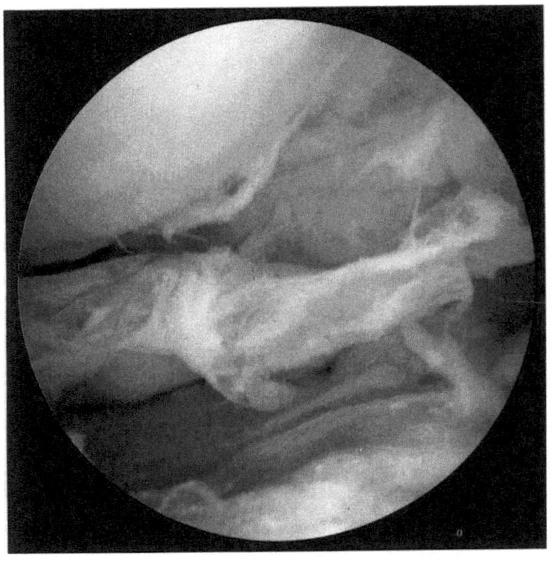

Fig. 8-7. Fibrin clots fill the suprapatellar pouch following hemarthrosis

The joint cavity may appear to terminate just proximal to the base of the patella, signifying either the presence of a suprapatellar septum (see Sect. 8.2.1) or obliteration of the suprapatellar pouch by adhesions (Fig. 8-8).

Following hemarthrosis or a knee operation with subsequent prolonged immobilization, it is common to find individual or multiple adhesive bands within the suprapatellar pouch. They become clinically significant when they cause mechanical interference of patellofemoral tracking.

Many patients with adhesions in the suprapatellar pouch complain of a feeling of pressure or tenseness in the anterior part of the knee or in the knee joint as a whole. The range of knee motion is frequently restricted. The treatment of choice is arthroscopic division and removal of the adhesions followed by intensive therapeutic exercise (indwelling peridural catheter, continuous passive motion).

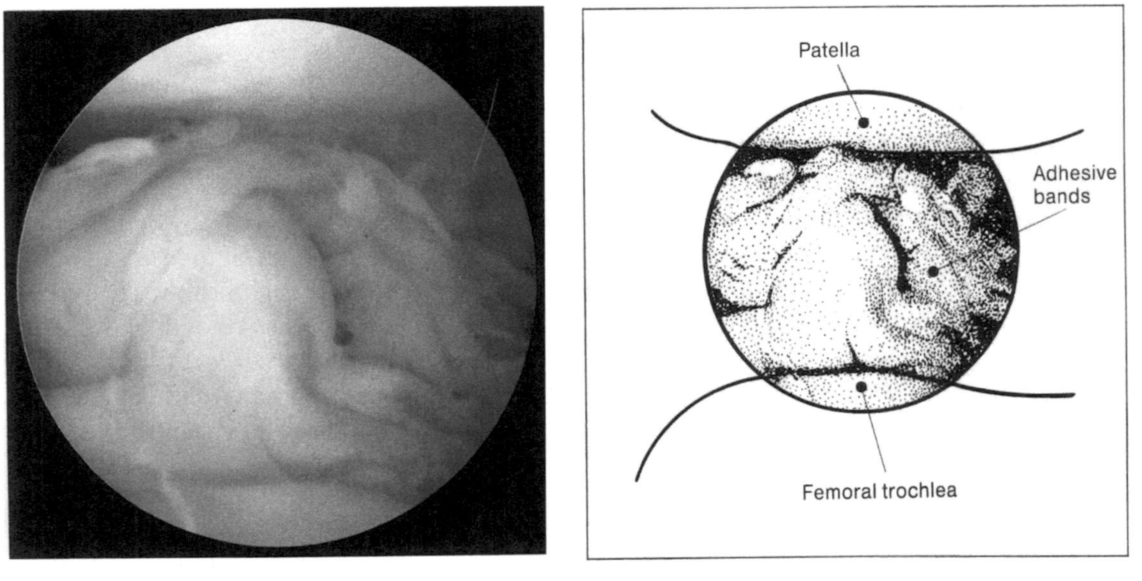

Fig. 8-8. Adhesions in the suprapatellar pouch

Problems

- *Dark monitor image.* Since the suprapatellar pouch contains no reflective cartilage surfaces, illumination of the pouch requires a high-power light source (set to maximum intensity). The telescope and light cable should be in good operating condition. The arthroscope is advanced into the suprapatellar pouch until its proximal boundary is identified. With hemarthrosis, residual blood coating the synovium will cause it to appear darker than usual. This residue is removed by copious irrigation.
- *Absent suprapatellar pouch.* Adhesions or a suprapatellar septum can cause the joint cavity to terminate just above the base of the patella. Division of the adhesions, which often form almost a transverse wall, will restore vision into the residual pouch.
- *Incomplete knee extension.* The suprapatellar pouch, like the retropatellar cartilage, cannot be inspected in the presence of an extension deficit or adhesions.

8.2.1 Suprapatellar Plica

The suprapatellar plica, known also as the superior synovial plica, runs transversely from the proximal rim of the femoral trochlea at the floor of the suprapatellar recess to the base of the patella. Though consistently present, the suprapatellar plica is highly variable in its development. It may present as small folds flanking the entrance to the superior pouch or as a complete suprapatellar septum. As early as 1928, Kenji described three basic types of suprapatellar plica, while Hempfling (1987), drawing on Watanabe, recognized five types (Table 8-2, Figs. 8-9 to 8-11).

More differentiated classifications have been proposed (e.g., the 9 types recognized by Watanabe) but are of little value due to their lack of clinical significance.

Table 8-2. Classification of suprapatellar plicae, after Hempfling (1987)

Type I:	Suprapatellar septum is completely preserved, separating the suprapatellar bursa from the femoropatellar joint.
Type II: other	Central perforation (porta) with no septum in the suprapatellar bursa (most common form).
Type III:	Lateral perforation in the suprapatellar septum.
Type IV:	Medial and lateral perforation.
Type V:	Rudimentary, consisting only of a medial rim of plica or synovial fold of variable prominence.

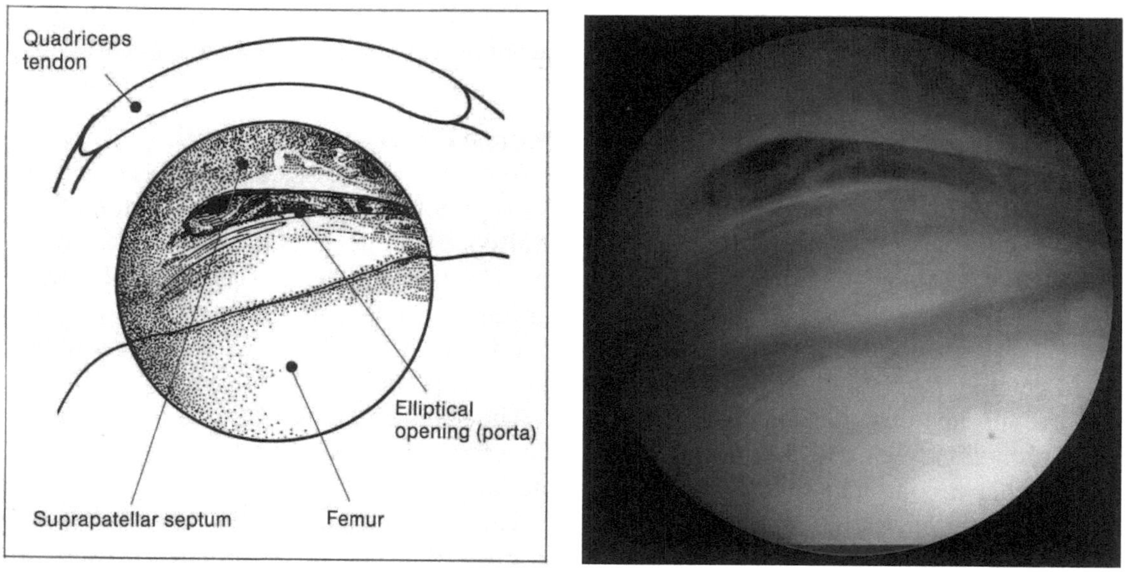

Fig. 8-9. Suprapatellar septum with a transverse elliptical opening (porta) (type II)

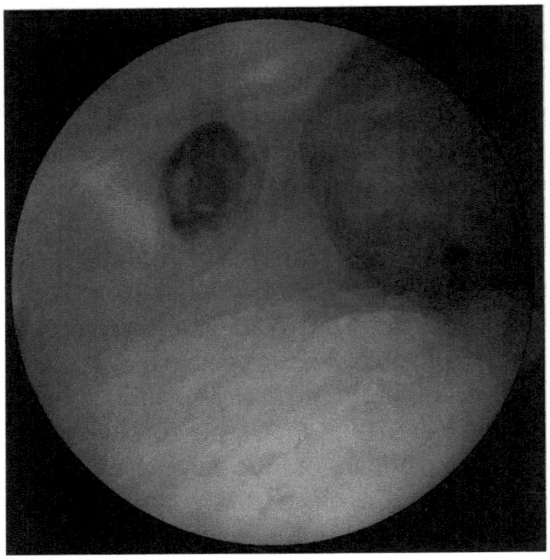

Fig. 8-10. Suprapatellar septum with 2 openings. The type IV septum can be difficult to distinguish from adhesive bands

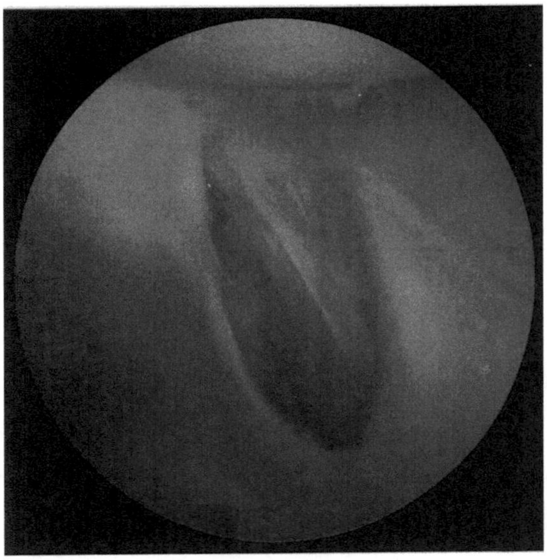

Fig. 8-11. Suprapatellar plica (type III)

Unlike the mediopatellar plica (see below), the suprapatellar plica is not subject to typical pathologic changes, although it is conceivable that a complete suprapatellar septum or fibrotic plica, by restricting patellar mobility, could adversely affect patellofemoral tracking. Shelflike septa occurring medially and laterally form an excellent hiding place for loose bodies. Thus, if loose bodies are suspected, the arthroscope should be advanced far into the suprapatellar pouch and the light post moved to 9:00 (3:00 in the left knee) to inspect the back surface of the medial portion of the plica, or to 3:00 (9:00 in the left knee) to inspect the lateral portion.

In some joints the medial portion of the suprapatellar plica or septum is perforated by a small, round or oval foramen (Figs. 8-9 and 8-10). This is a physiologic variant and should not be confused with a puncture made by overvigorous insertion of the arthroscopic sheath.

8.3 Lateral Recess

Position
The knee is slightly flexed, and a mild valgus stress is applied to relax the lateral capsule.

Visualization
The light post is at 12:00.

Just before the scope tip reaches the lateral capsule wall following inspection of the suprapatellar pouch, the light post is moved to 12:00, and the arthroscope is slowly retracted and brought to an upright position as the tip is swept downward (Figs. 8-12 and 8-13).

Normal Findings
To enter the lateral recess, the tip of the scope is swept downward. Between the lateral femoral condyle and lateral capsule, the scope must be maneuvered past a *synovial fold* of variable prominence which is usually duplicated (Fig. 8-14). This fold is not known to have any pathologic significance.

The synovial lining of the lateral recess is smooth and translucent with fine vascular markings.

The lateral aspect of the lateral femoral condyle (the "cheek" of the condyle) and the lateral capsule are inspected. At this point the

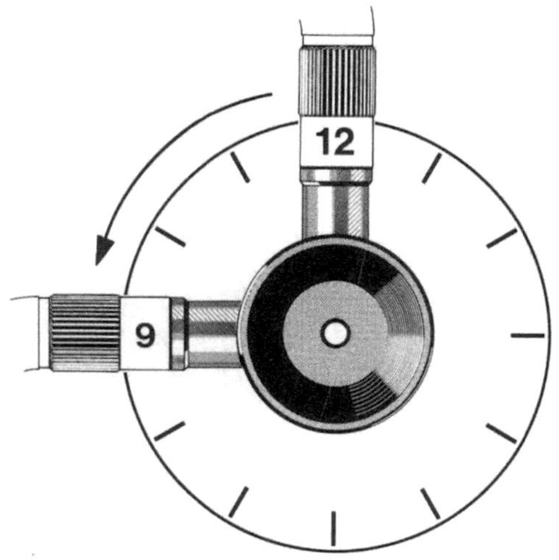

Fig. 8-12. The light post is at 12:00 for inspecting the lateral recess. From there it is rotated past 11:00 to 9:00 (past 1:00 to 3:00 in the left knee) to visualize the popliteal hiatus

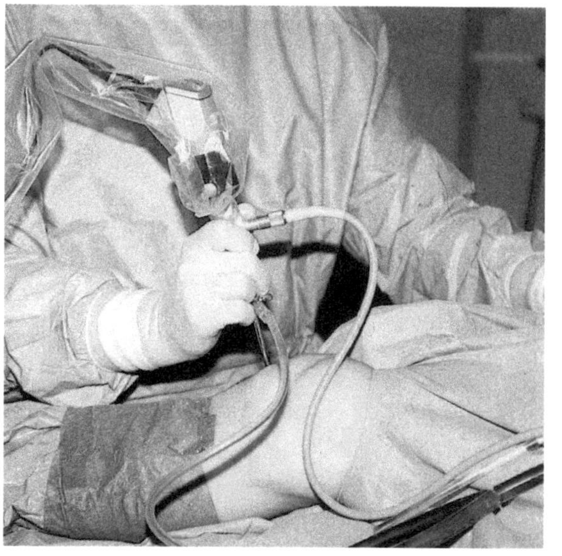

Fig. 8-13. Arthroscope position for viewing the lateral recess (light post at 12:00)

examiner may indent the lateral capsule externally with his finger to assist orientation.

Pathologic Findings

Blood clots, fibrin clots, loose bodies (fixed or detached), hypertrophied synovial villi, and osteophytes are the most common pathologic findings encountered in the lateral recess or on the lateral femoral condyle (Figs. 8-15 to 8-18).

Problems

- *Yellow-out.* If the arthroscope is advanced too far, it may hang up on the transverse synovial plica (Fig. 8-14) and cannot be swept downward, creating a yellow-out on the monitor. This is remedied by carefully retracting the scope while slowly rotating it.
- *Extraarticular position of the arthroscope.* Abrupt withdrawal of the arthroscope may retract the tip into the subcutaneous tissue

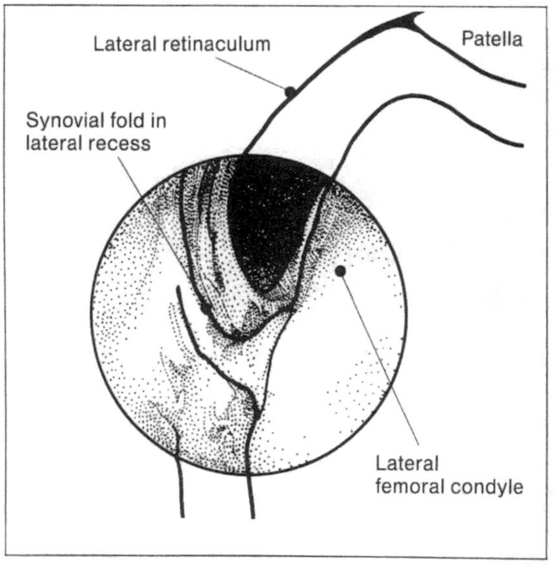

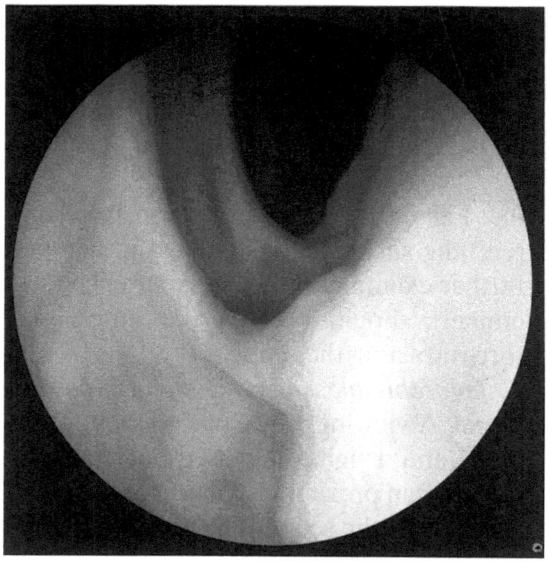

Fig. 8-14. Transverse, usually two-part synovial fold in the lateral recess

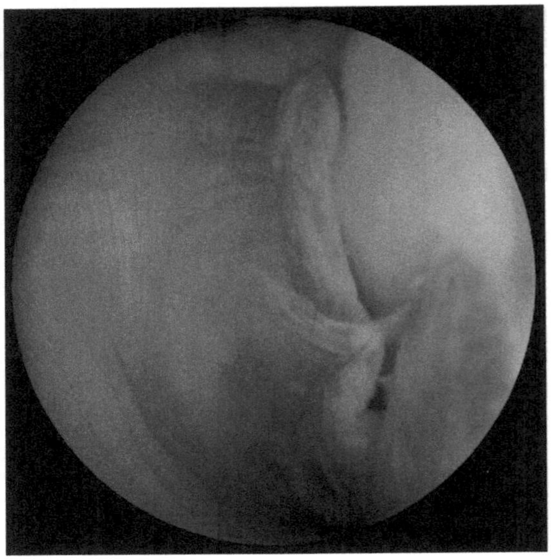

Fig. 8-15. Fibrin clots in the lateral recess following hemarthrosis
◀

Fig. 8-16. Loose body (osteochondral fragment from the medial patellar facet following patellar dislocation) that has become loosely attached to the wall of the lateral recess
▼

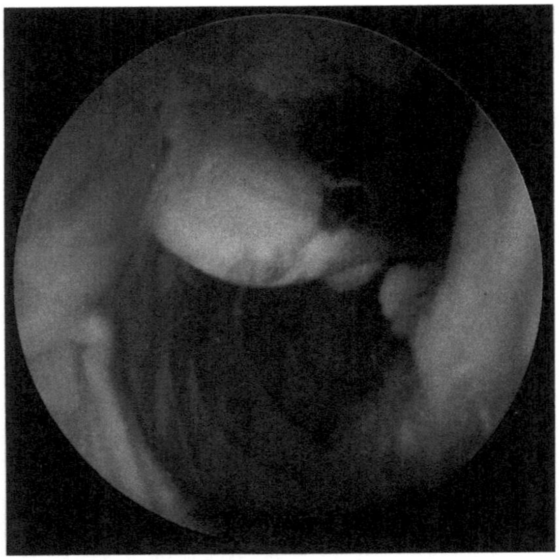

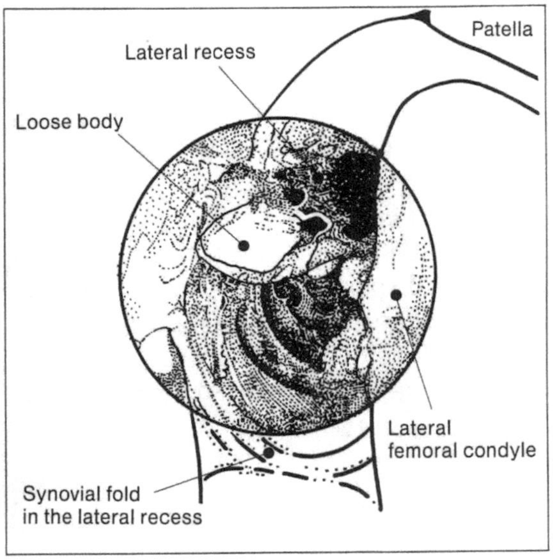

(see Fig. 6-9 b). If the inflow is on, it will distend the subcutaneous tissue and hamper further examination. Less experienced examiners should occlude the inflow before retracting the scope.

- *Unfavorable placement of the arthroscope portal.* A viewing portal placed too far medially and a tight, unincised anterolateral capsule can prevent inspection of the lateral recess. If the scope is forced into the recess, the monitor image will become out of round and blurred at the edges.

8.3.1 Lateral Aspect of the Lateral Meniscus

The arthroscope is swept farther downward, and the light post is rotated to 11:00 (Fig. 8-13).

Caudal to the lateral femoral condyle, a white structure comes into view that is easily mistaken for the lateral tibial plateau. This is the lateral aspect of the lateral meniscus. When a mild valgus stress is applied to the

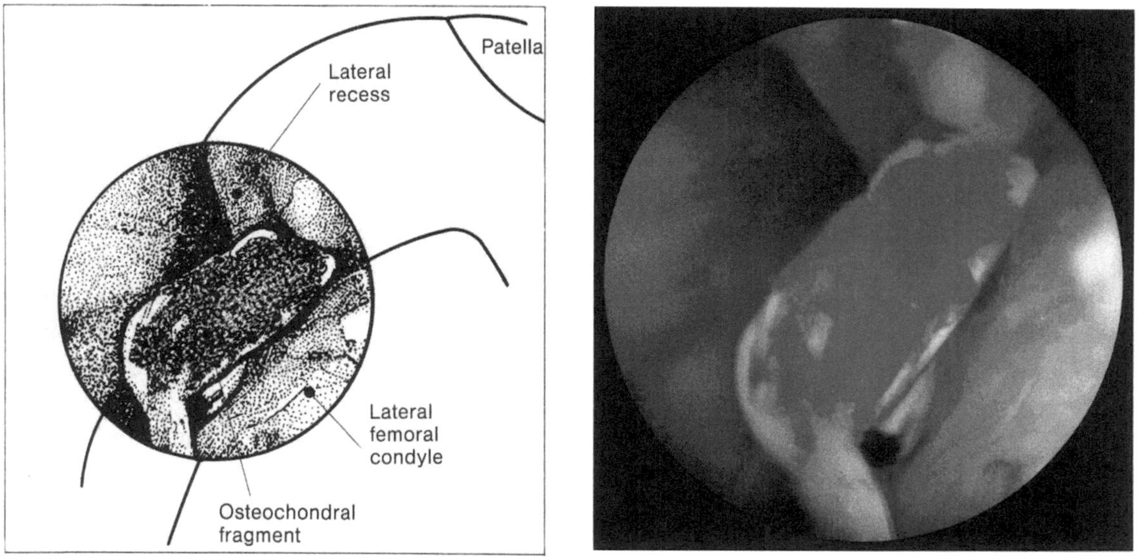

Fig. 8-17. Large, fresh osteochondral fragment in the lateral recess following patellar dislocation. Site of origin: lateral femoral condyle or medial patellar facet

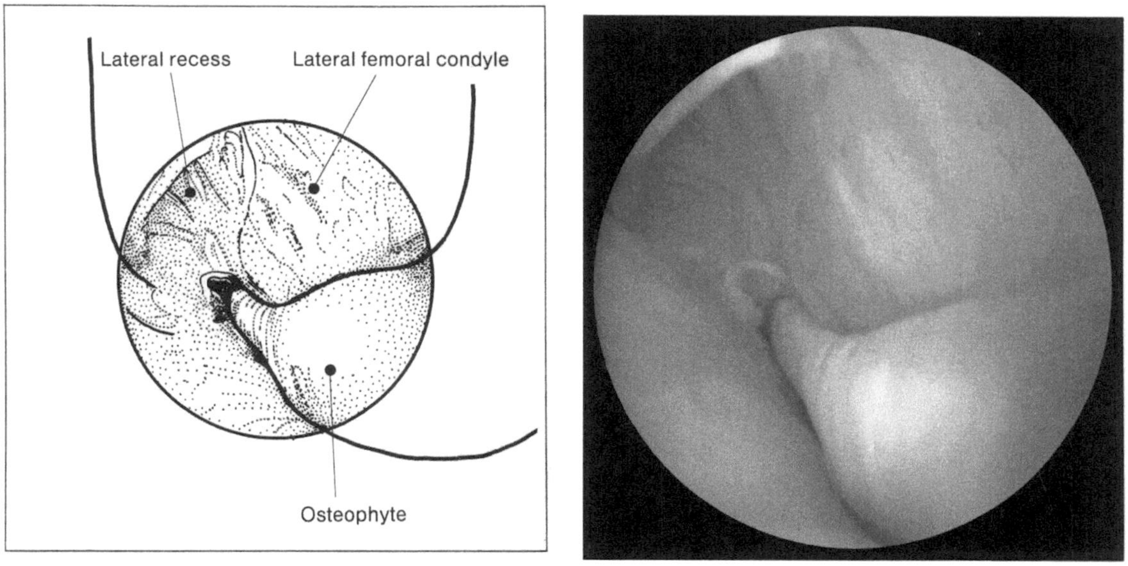

Fig. 8-18. Large osteophyte on the lateral femoral condyle

knee, the scope can be positioned to view into the lateral joint space from the lateral side (light post at 10:00). When degenerative changes are present, vision may be obscured by osteophytes or villous hypertrophy (Fig. 8-18).

8.3.2 Popliteus Tendon, Popliteal Hiatus

Inspection of the distal, posterior portion of the lateral recess reveals the synovium-covered bulge of the popliteus tendon. This tendon, which has no attachment with the lateral meniscus, arises from the distal part of the lateral femoral condyle just anterior to the origin of the lateral collateral ligament. Its course can be traced arthroscopically as far as the posterior aspect of the tibia. As the light post is moved from 11:00 past 10:00 to 9:00 (Fig. 8-12), the synovial attachment between the tibia and lateral meniscus and the course of the popliteus tendon are visualized (Figs. 8-19 and 8-20). Farther posteriorly the tendon disappears in the caudal portion of the popliteal hiatus, whose boundaries can be inspected (Fig. 8-21).

Hypertrophied synovial villi and loose bodies are the most common pathologic findings. Small loose bodies lodged in the popliteal hiatus can be aspirated through the arthroscopic sheath (see Fig. 3-6). Manual percussion and distal-to-proximal "milking" are helpful in uncovering loose bodies. Isolated tearing or hemorrhage in the popliteus tendon are uncommon.

8.3.3 Outerbridge Ridge

Before the femoropatellar joint is examined, the lateral aspect of the lateral femoral condyle and the Outerbridge ridge (junction of bone and cartilage on the lateral femoral condyle) are inspected. For this the arthroscope is swept upward and rotated to the 10:00 position. Osteophytic outgrowths are commonly found there when degenerative disease is present (Fig. 8-22).

Following dislocation of the patella, inspection of the Outerbridge ridge may show areas of subchondral hemorrhage, cartilage flakes, or even extensive chondral and osteochondral fractures (Fig. 8-23). Because the patella always dislocates laterally and generally reduces spontaneously to a normal position, many cases of patellar dislocation can be diagnosed only by clinical testing (positive Fairbank's apprehension test) or arthroscopic examination.

Arthroscopic signs suggestive of a prior patellar dislocation are:

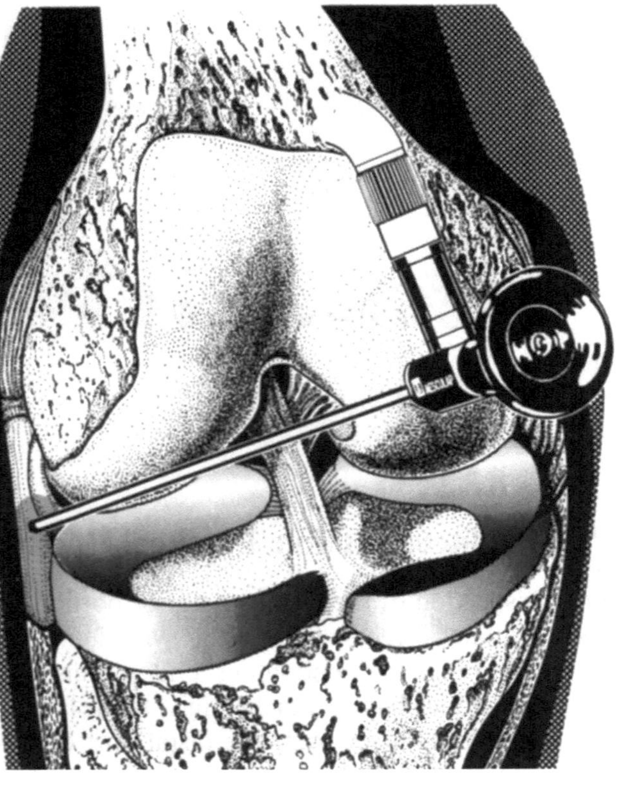

Fig. 8-19. Visualization of the lateral aspect of the lateral meniscus and popliteal hiatus. The light post is positioned at 11:00 and 10:00 (1:00 and 2:00 in the left knee)

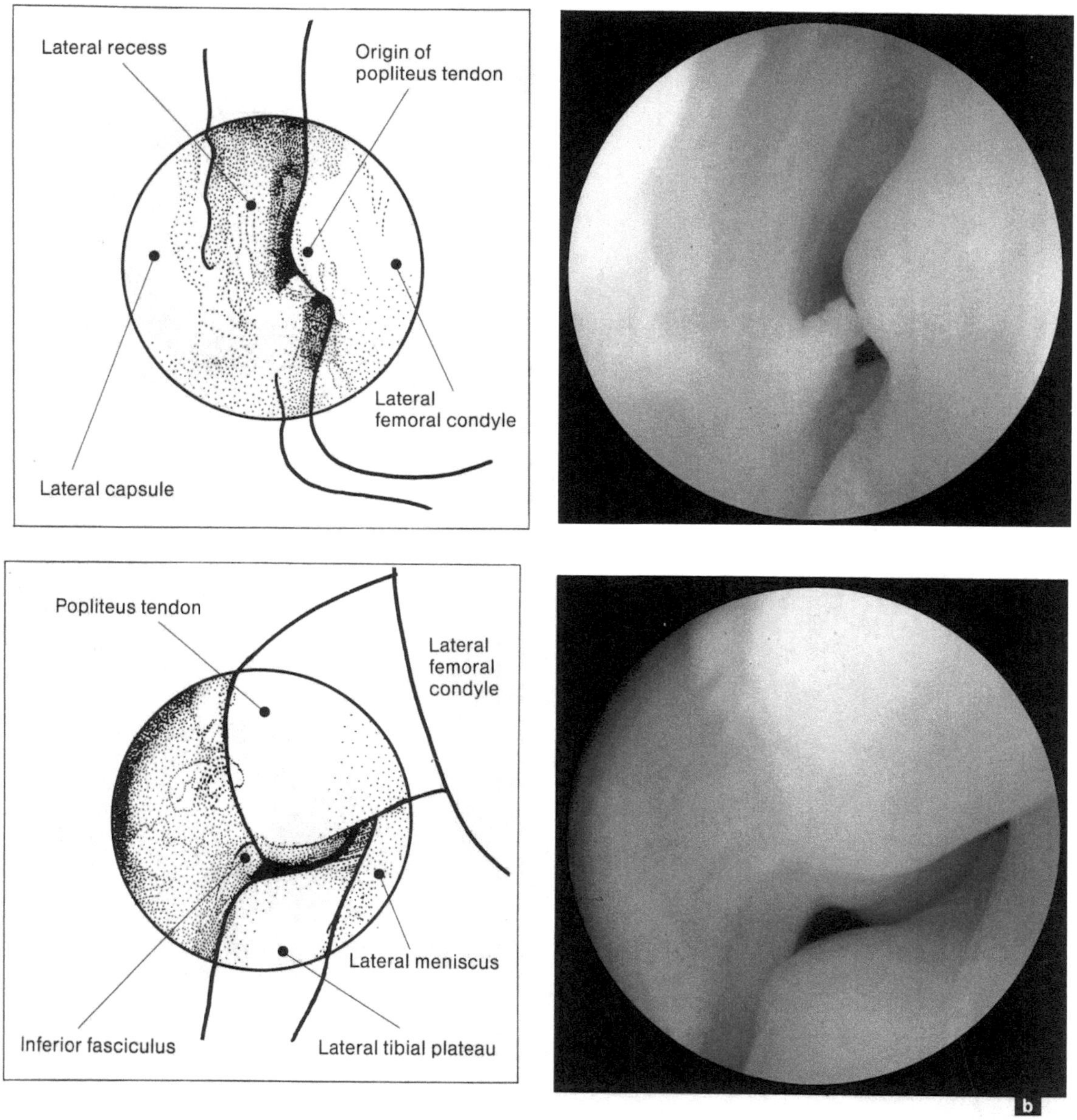

Fig. 8-20 a, b. Site of origin of the popliteus tendon on the lateral femoral condyle (**a**) and the posterior segment descending lateral to the tibial plateau (**b**)

- Hemorrhagic changes in the lateral surface of the lateral femoral condyle
- Chondral or osteochondral fractures involving the Outerbridge ridge
- Cartilage fragments detached from the medial patellar facet or contused areas on the facet
- Tears and/or hemorrhage in the medial retinaculum or synovial membrane

8.4 Femoropatellar Joint

Position

The knee is extended. The joint is alternately flexed and extended to evaluate patellar tracking on the femur.

8-21

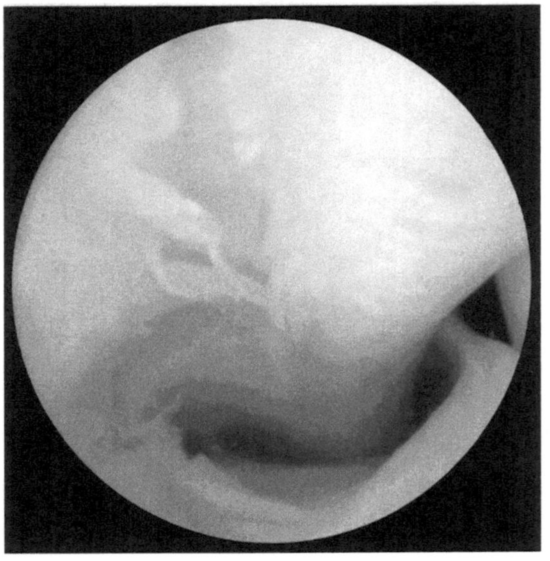

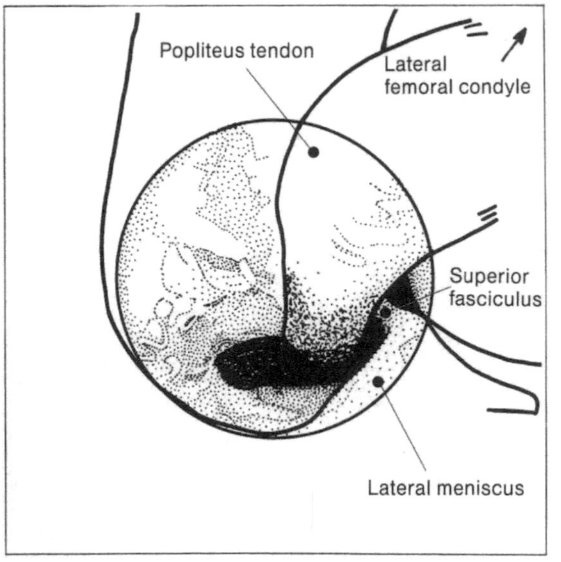

8-22

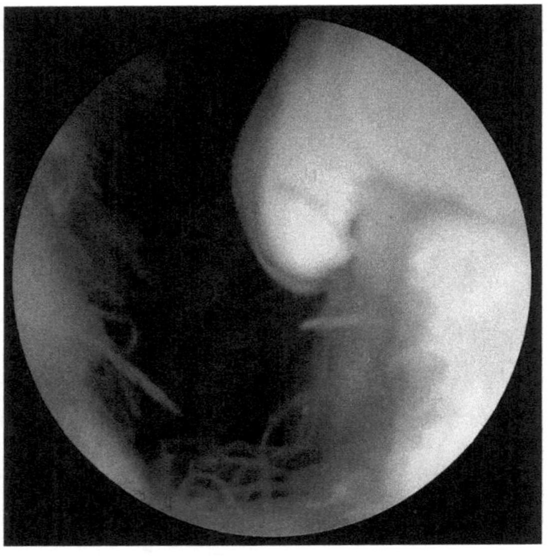

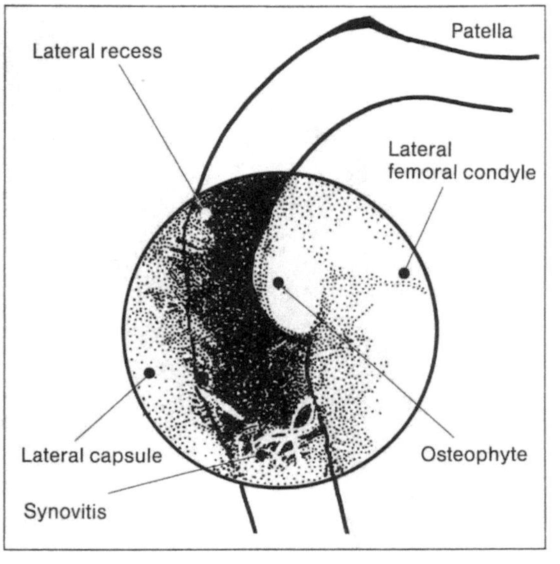

8-23

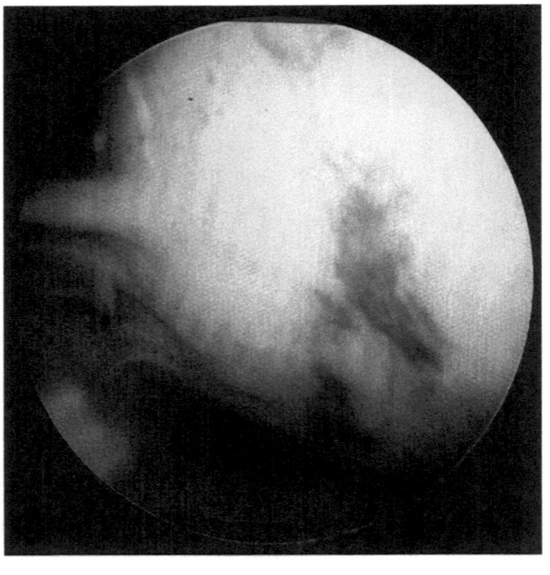

Fig. 8-21. The course of the popliteus tendon can be traced far posteriorly with the 30° scope (light post at 10:00 and 9:00)

Fig. 8-22. Osteophyte on the lateral femoral condyle (Outerbridge ridge)

Fig. 8-23. Contused areas on the lateral aspect of the femoral condyle following patellar dislocation (monitor image)

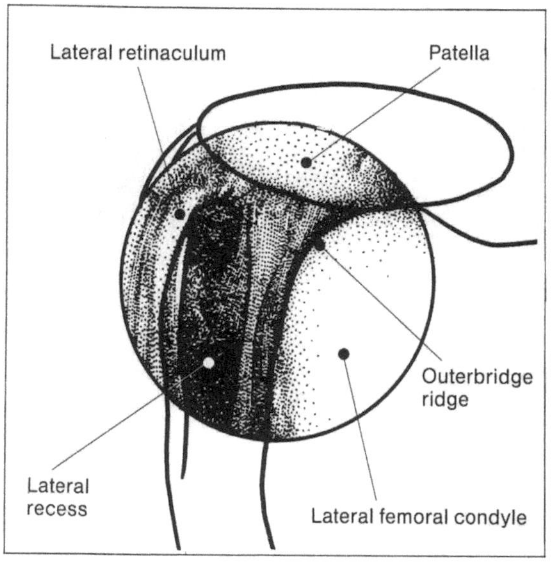

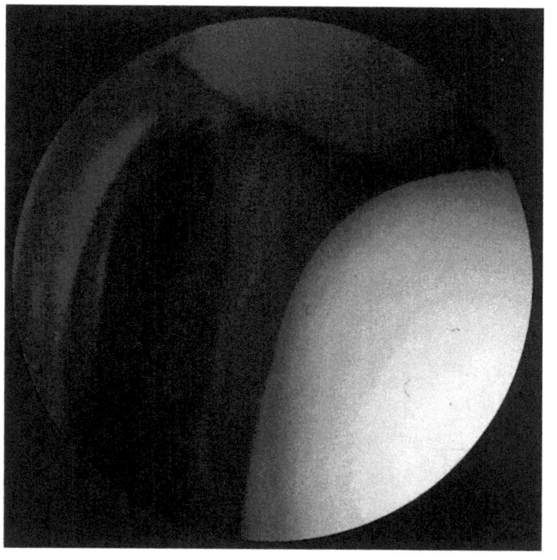

Fig. 8-24. The arthroscope enters the femoropatellar joint from the lateral side. The patella always appears slightly lateralized in the extended knee

Visualization

The lateral portion of the femoropatellar joint is inspected with the light post at 10:00. The arthroscope is directed parallel to the leg axis, as for inspection of the lateral recess, and the tip of the scope is in the area of the lateral recess (Fig. 8-24).

To evaluate centering of the patella in the femoral trochlea, the arthroscope is swept medially over the lateral femoral condyle and positioned anterior to the infrapatellar fat pad. The light post is rotated to 5:00 (left knee 7:00). The lateral portion of the femoropatellar joint appears first (Figs. 8-25 and 8-26); the rest of the joint is evaluated by advancing the scope toward the medial capsule.

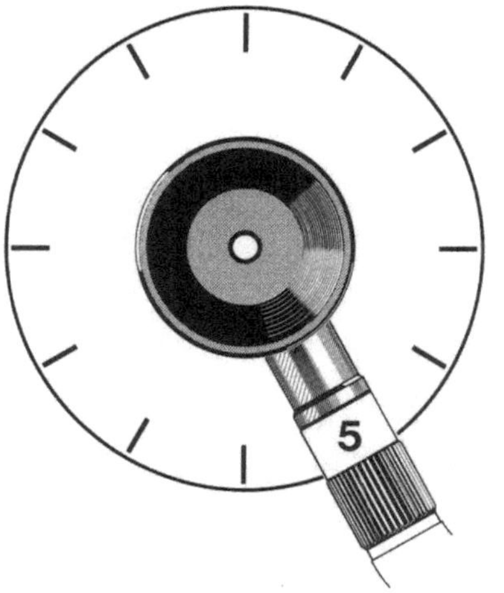

Fig. 8-25. The light post is at 5:00 (7:00 in the left knee) for examination of the femoropatellar joint

8.4.1 Centering and Lateralization of the Patella

Arthroscopy is the most accurate method available for the diagnosis of functional and morphologic changes in the femoropatellar joint. The condition of the cartilaginous surfaces can be assessed (see Chap. 9), and patellar tracking can be evaluated.

With the femoropatellar joint space in the field of view, the knee is alternately flexed and extended. The deepest point of the femoral trochlea should be at the center of the monitor, and both articular surfaces should be visible—the patella at the top of the screen and the femur at the bottom. Any malalignment or tilting of the patella is noted as the knee is alternately flexed and extended (Fig. 8-26).

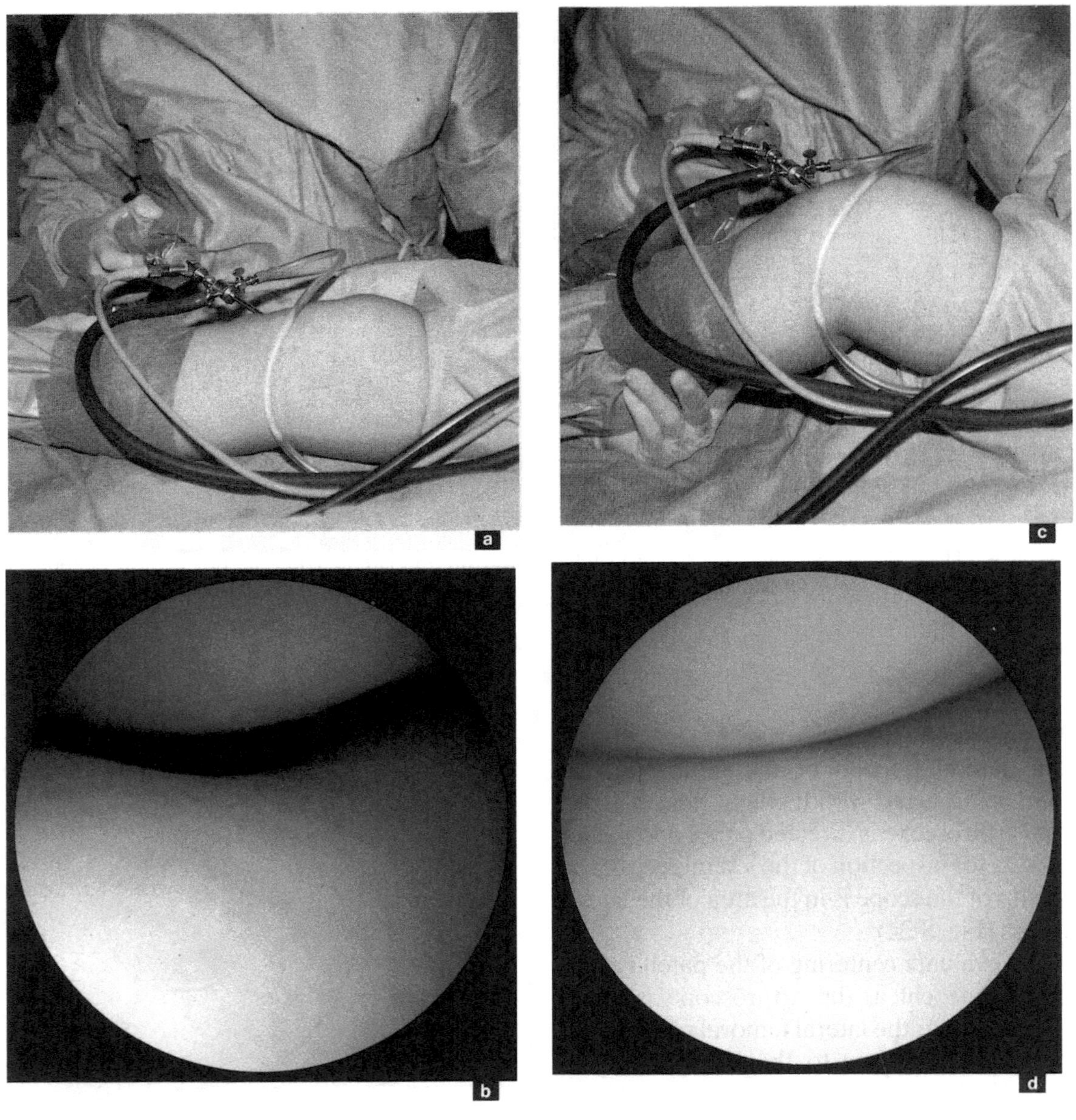

Fig. 8-26 a–d. Evaluation of patellofemoral tracking. With the knee extended or slightly flexed, an interspace is visible between the patella and femur (**a, b**). When the knee is flexed to 45°, the patella seats in the center of the femoral trochlea (**c, d**)

Normal Findings

The portion of the patella (midpatellar ridge, medial or lateral facet) that initiates contact with the femur (the patellar contact point) and the flexion angle at which the contact occurs are determined. The normal patellar position in the extended knee is slightly lateral to the lateral femoral condyle, the patella moving medially and distally with increasing flexion. Initial contact occurs between the lateral patellar facet and the lateral femoral condyle. At about 45° of flexion the patella seats in the center of the trochlea.

Pathologic Findings

Vague anterior knee complaints with giving-way episodes are common clinical manifestations of patellar subluxation. Arthroscopy shows that centering of the patella does not occur until the knee is flexed well past 45°. In

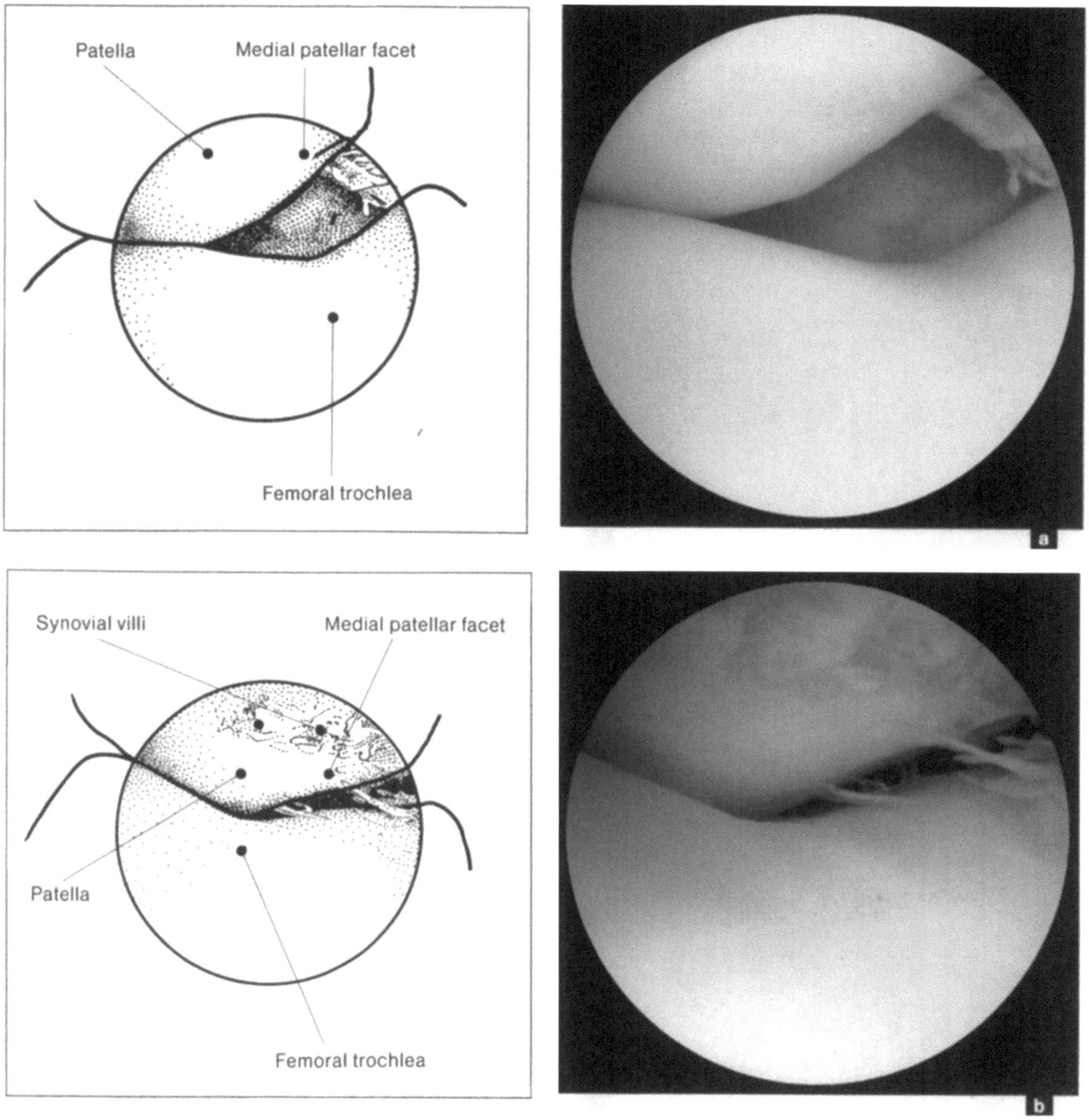

Fig. 8-27 a, b. Patellar subluxation. The patella does not seat in the center of the femoral trochlea at 45° (**a**). Centering does not occur until 80° of flexion is reached (**b**)

some cases this delay of centering is associated with marked lateralization and lateral tilting of the patella (Figs. 8-27 and 8-28).

When evaluating patellofemoral tracking, the examiner should watch for the entrapment of enlarged fat-pad villi or the mediopatellar plica. If a structure protrudes into the femoropatellar interspace, a high fluid pressure in the distended joint may keep the structure from becoming caught between the articular surfaces. If entrapment is suspected, it can be reproduced by lowering the intraarticular pressure (i.e., by turning off the inflow or by aspirating fluid) and repeating the flexion/extension maneuver (Figs. 8-29 and 8-30).

The lateral portion of the femoropatellar joint is visualized by sweeping the arthroscope laterally, the medial portion by sweeping the scope medially. From that position the junction of the medial patellar facet with the medial retinaculum is easily assessed.

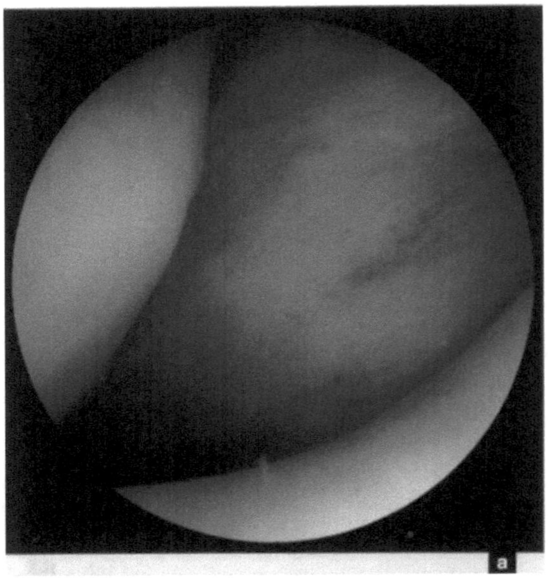

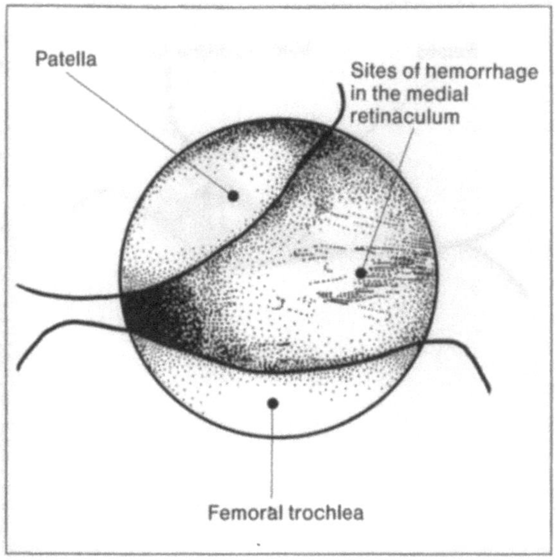
Patella
Sites of hemorrhage in the medial retinaculum
Femoral trochlea

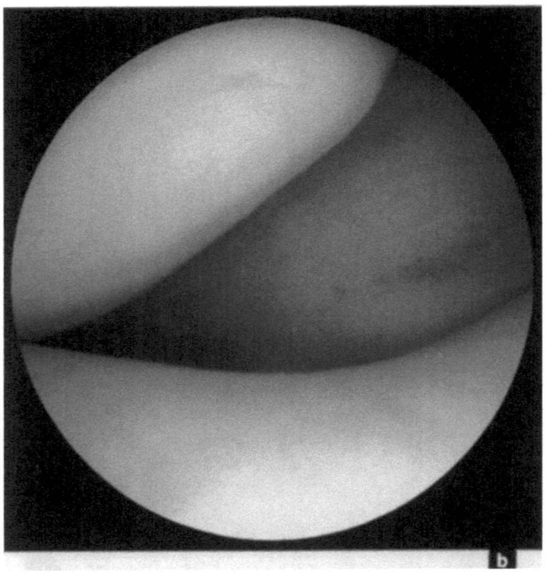

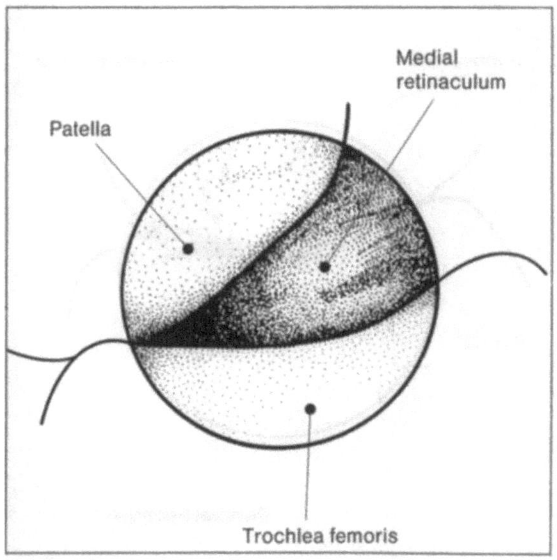
Medial retinaculum
Patella
Trochlea femoris

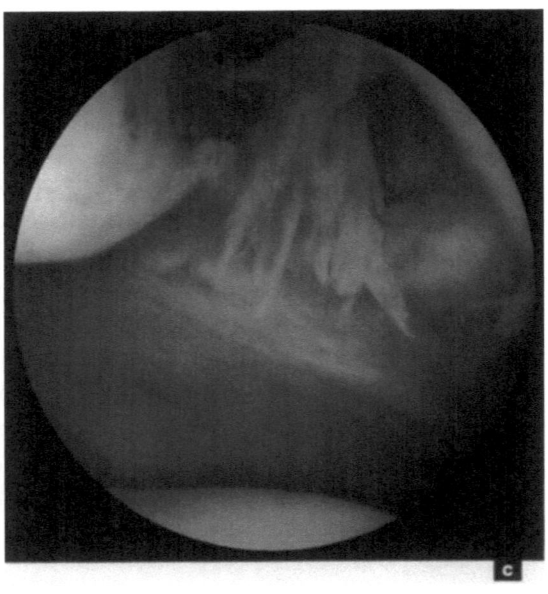

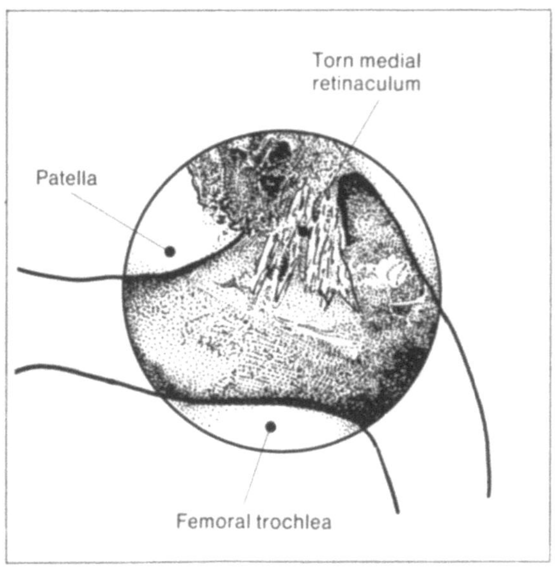
Torn medial retinaculum
Patella
Femoral trochlea

◀ **Fig. 8-28 a–c.** Patellar dislocation.
History: 15-year-old girl experienced 4 episodes of patellar dislocation in the left knee, the most recent 4 days ago. The knee was immobilized in a cast brace. During ambulation with forearm crutches, the patient experienced an initial dislocation of the right patella with a tense hemarthrosis. She had an Insall-Salvati index of 0.8 (low normal) and marked bilateral genu valgum.
Arthroscopic findings: Dysplastic medial patellar facet, the lateral facet forming most of the patellar surface. Marked tendency toward lateralization and tilting in extension (**a**) and 45° flexion (**b**). Tearing of the medial retinaculum with subjacent hemorrhage (**c**).
Procedure: Arthroscopic repair of the medial retinaculum, possibly combined with a lateral release. Another option would be to limit arthroscopic treatment to lavage and immobilize the leg for 5 weeks following postoperative mobilization to 90° (to prevent intra-articular adhesions). An arthroscopic lateral release could then be performed in a second sitting

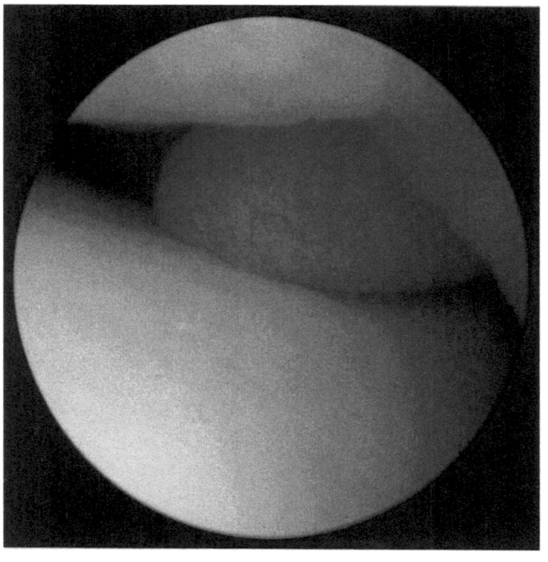

Fig. 8-29. Hypertrophied fat-pad villus entrapped in the femoropatellar joint. Synovitis is conspicuous even in the exsanguinated limb

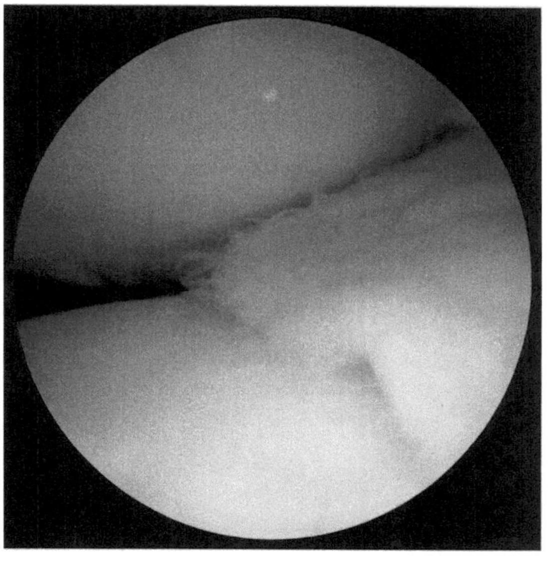

Fig. 8-30. Impingement of a hypertrophied fat-pad villus in the femoropatellar joint

Arthroscopy performed after a recent patellar dislocation will demonstrate tears and/or hemorrhage in this junctional area or in the medial retinaculum (Fig. 8-5 and 8-28 c).

8.4.2 Femoral Trochlea

The femoral trochlea is too often the neglected "stepchild" of the arthroscopic examination. Yet it forms an important site of predilection for pathologic change. Although the femoral trochlea articulates with the patella, lesions of the trochlear cartilage do not necessarily correlate with retropatellar findings. Lesions may be confined to the retropatellar cartilage or may involve both articular surfaces (Figs. 8-31 and 8-32).

In other cases the femoral trochlea is affected in isolation and is solely responsible for femoropatellar complaints. The extent of the lesions is ascertained by probing the cartilage from a medial suprameniscal or high medial portal (Figs. 8-33 and 8-34). Assessment is aided by flexion and extension to make the proximal and distal cartilage areas accessible to probing. A fat-pad villus that obstructs vision can be held aside with the probe or removed with a grasping instrument.

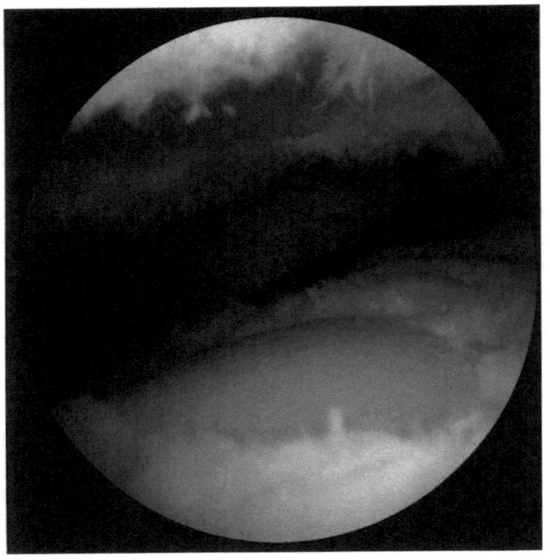

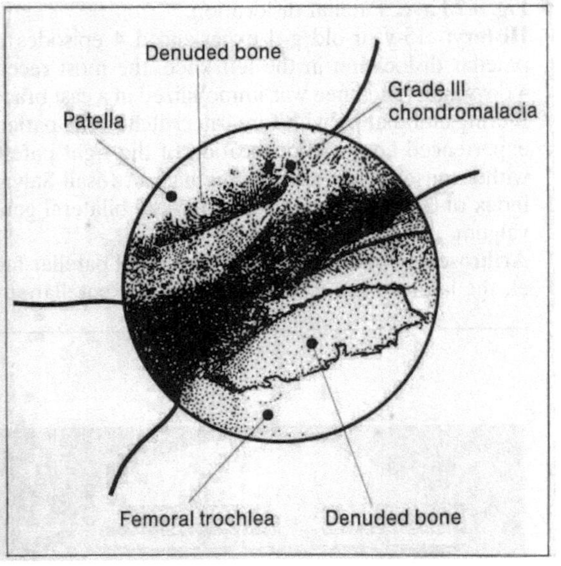

Fig. 8-31. Advanced femoropatellar osteoarthritis.
History: Woman 38 years of age had a history of bilateral knee pain for several years. Recently her complaints increased with no antecedent trauma and no effusion or instability. Clinical examination showed bilateral patellar subluxation with retropatellar crepitus.
Radiographic findings: Tangential films show massive lateralization of both patellae with osteophytosis in the femoropatellar joint and bilateral foci of chondromatosis.
Arthroscopic findings: Sites of bone denudation on both articular surfaces.
Procedure: Arthroscopic debridement of the cartilage. Lateral retinacular release is indicated to stabilize the patella

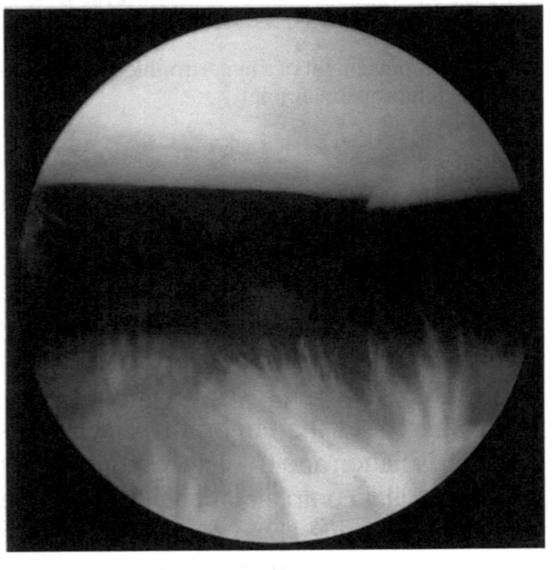

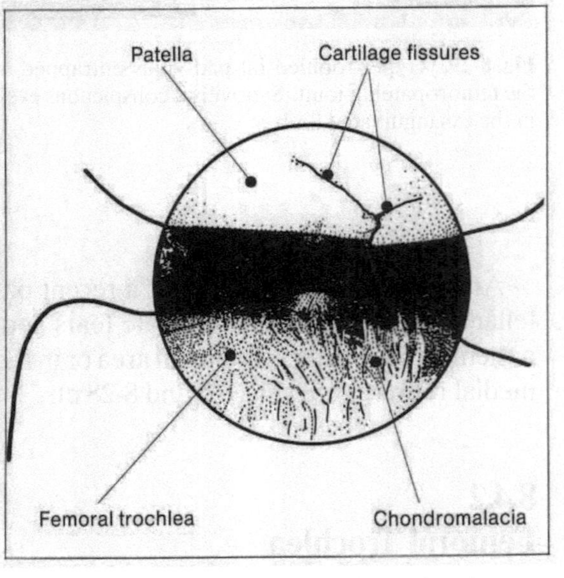

Fig. 8-32. Grade II and III chondromalacia of the femoral trochlea. Fissuring is apparent in the retropatellar cartilage. Probing is necessary to determine the presence and degree of cartilage separation

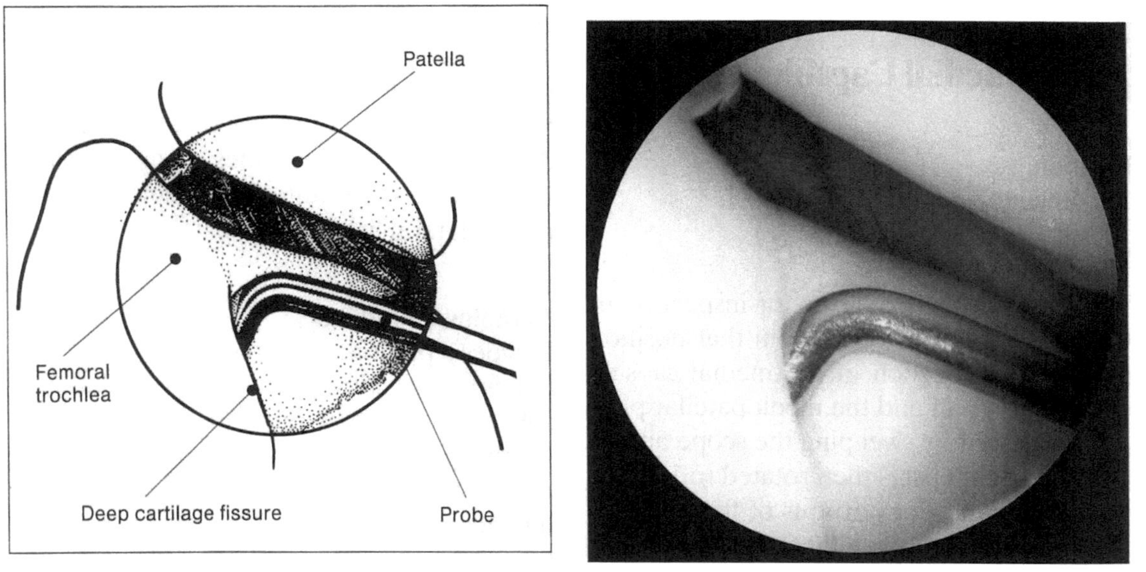

Fig. 8-33. Grade II chondromalacia in the central portion of the femoral trochlea. Selective palpation with the probing hook can establish whether the cartilage lesions extend to the bone

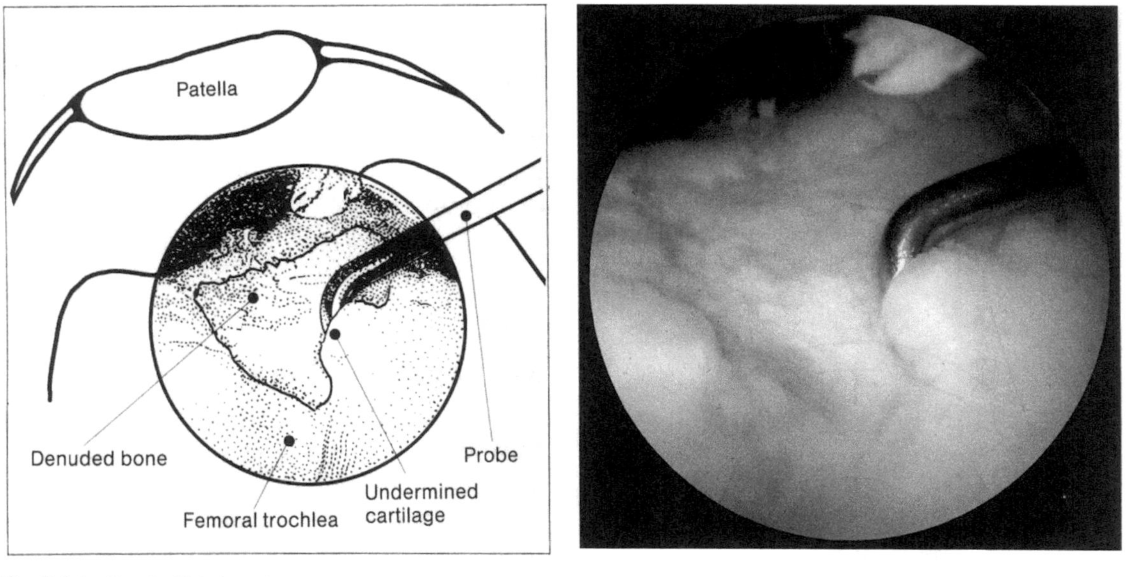

Fig. 8-34. Grade IV chondromalacia of the femoral trochlea. The probe is used to determine the extent of the undermined and separated cartilage areas

8.5 Anteromedial Capsule

Position

The knee is extended.

Visualization

The light post is at 5:00, as for inspection of the femoropatellar joint. From that position the proximal portion of the medial capsule can be surveyed, and the mediopatellar plica can be viewed by sweeping the scope anteriorly. The light post is then rotated to 10:00 to inspect the anterior portions of the plica extending to the infrapatellar fat pad.

Next the arthroscope is advanced and swept into the medial recess. At this stage the tip of the scope must be maneuvered past the medial portion of the femoral trochlea. This is most easily done by carefully sweeping the scope upward in the extended knee; abrupt or forceful movements might damage the cartilage on the femoral trochlea. The light post is rotated from 10:00 past 12:00 to 2:00; as this is done, the medial recess is inspected (Figs. 8-35 and 8-36).

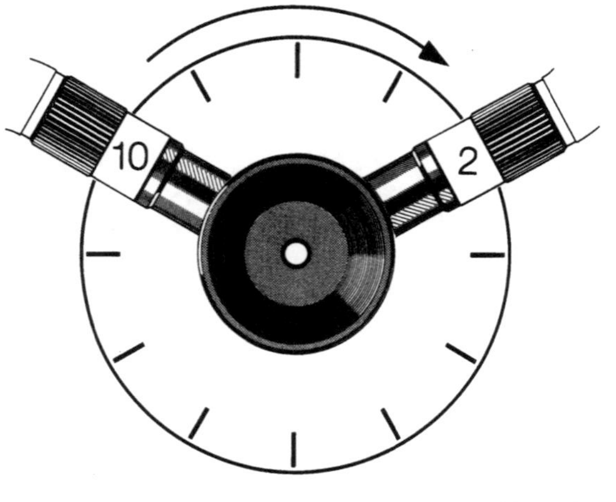

Fig. 8-35. The light post is positioned at 10:00 for inspecting the anteromedial capsule (2:00 in the left knee). It is then moved to 2:00 (10:00 in the left knee) and swept downward to view the central portion of the medial meniscus

Normal Findings

The medial recess is bounded medially by the medial capsule and ligaments and laterally by the medial aspect of the medial femoral condyle (Fig. 8-36). Sometimes a slight protrusion is noted in the anterior border of the medial collateral ligament.

Pathologic Findings

Besides a pathologic mediopatellar plica (see below), inspection of the anteromedial capsule wall may show areas of synovial hypertrophy, posttraumatic hemorrhage, or partial or complete tears of the medial capsule and ligaments (Fig. 8-36).

If strands of ligamentous tissue are seen floating in the joint, the arthroscopy should be performed as swiftly as possible to limit fluid drainage into the subcutaneous tissues. In some cases the torn ligament tissues may become displaced into the medial joint space (see Fig. 8-44). The medial aspect of the medial femoral condyle is inspected by sweeping the scope in the direction of the medial joint space and rotating the light post to the 1:00 and 2:00 position until the meniscosynovial junction is seen (Fig. 8-36 b). Osteophytes may obstruct arthroscopic access to the medial compartment.

8.5.1 Mediopatellar Plica

Position

The knee is extended. The joint is repeatedly flexed to check for impingement of the mediopatellar plica on the medial femoral condyle or patella.

Visualization

The medial portion of the mediopatellar plica is first inspected from the arthroscope position used to evaluate patellar tracking. The scope is advanced in the direction of the medial capsule. The light post is moved to 10:00 to demonstrate the anterior part of the plica that inserts on the infrapatellar fat pad.

Fig. 8-36 a, b. Medial recess with streaklike hemorrhagic areas in the medial capsule consistent with acute medial capsuloligamentous injury (**a**). Hemorrhagic areas are also commonly seen in the distal portion of the medial recess. The meniscosynovial junction is also inspected (**b**)

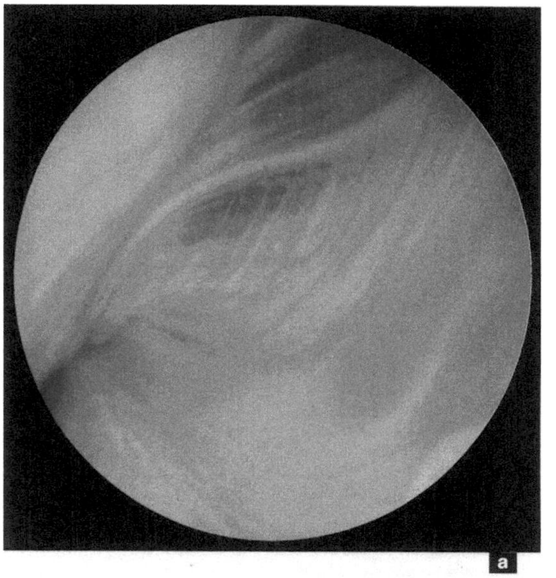
a

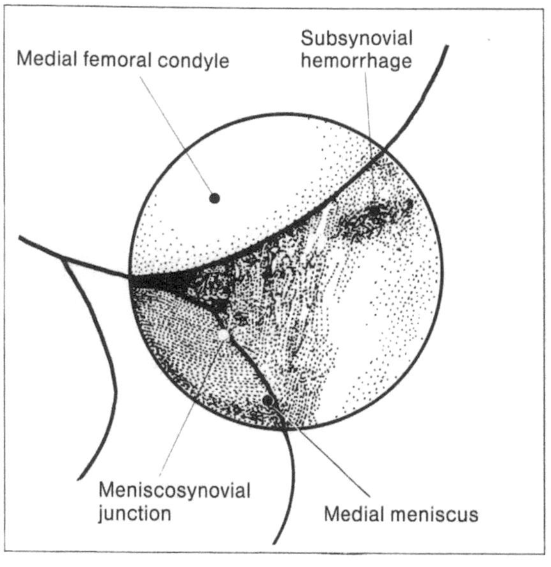

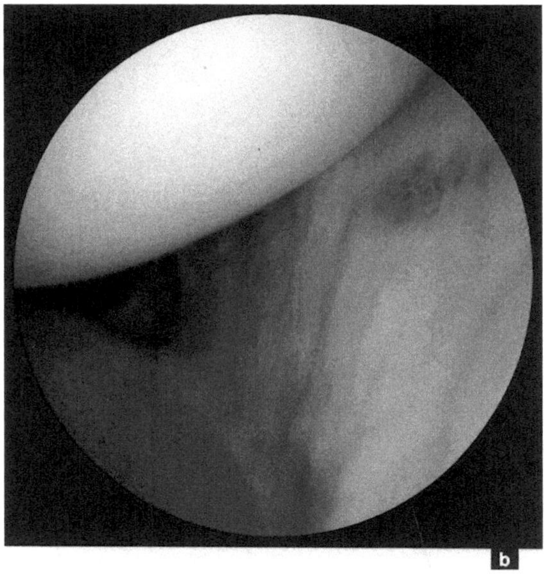
b

Normal Findings

The mediopatellar plica is known variously as the medial shelf, medial plica, intraarticular medial band, Iinos' band, and synovial chorda. Reports on its incidence range from 19% to 60%. It courses along the medial capsule wall between the infrapatellar fat pad and the medial capsule. Shaped somewhat like a shelf or sail, it divides the medial capsule wall into a superior and inferior portion. It is variable in its development, and duplicated forms are known. Three main types have been identified:

Type I: A rudimentary streaklike elevation on the anteromedial capsule wall.

Type II: A bandlike or cordlike structure that does not impinge on the medial femoral condyle or medial patellar facet during flexion.

Type III: A bandlike or shelflike structure that impinges on the medial femoral condyle or patella during flexion.

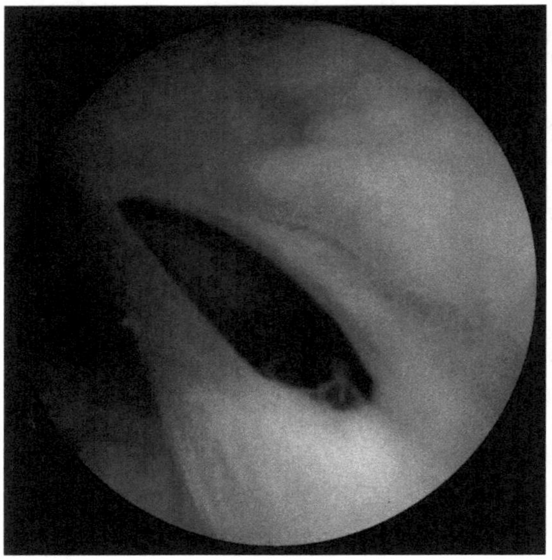

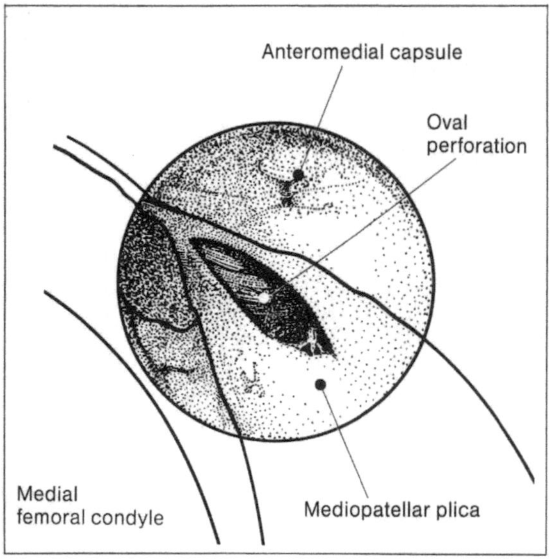

Fig. 8-37. Mediopatellar plica with a large, central oval perforation

This classification is not influenced by the presence or absence of a perforation in the plica (Fig. 8-37). The determining factor is whether or not the plica impinges on the medial femoral condyle during flexion, and whether the cartilage has become damaged at the site of contact.

We therefore check to see whether the mediopatellar plica comes in contact with the medial femoral condyle and/or the patella when the knee is flexed (Fig. 8-38), noting whether impingement occurs when the joint is distended by a high fluid pressure. In a minimally distended joint, almost every bandlike plica is likely to come in contact with the medial femoral condyle. If similar contact occurs in the well-distended joint, it must be decided whether the plica might be responsible for the patient's symptoms (Fig. 8-39).

Pathologic Findings

Unlike the other plicae in the knee joint—the suprapatellar, infrapatellar, and lateral (rare)—the mediopatellar plica can assume true pathologic significance. The symptoms produced by a pathologic mediopatellar plica are referred to as *plica syndrome* or *medial shelf syndrome*. During arthroscopy, it is often difficult to determine whether the plica is pathologic and whether it might be causing the patient's complaints. Diagnostic uncertainties result from the nonspecific symptoms of plica syndrome, which include anteromedial joint pain, irritative effusion, a palpable cord on the anteromedial capsule, a feeling of instability, retropatellar pain, as well as medial snapping, locking, and pseudolocking. The main disorders requiring differentiation from plica syndrome are retropatellar cartilage damage, femoropatellar pain syndrome, and meniscal injuries.

In patients with a type III plica, symptoms are easily explained. The plica may become caught in the femoropatellar joint or subluxate over the condyle. This subluxation can be reproduced with the probing hook and can account for the meniscus-like locking symptoms with pain projecting to the medial capsule. The cartilage lesions result from continual impingement of the plica upon the articular cartilage, especially during flexion (Fig. 8-40). A hypertrophied plica tends to hang up on the medial femoral condyle when the knee is flexed (pressure-induced chondromalacia) and then release when the knee is extended, causing the patient to report knee pain upon standing after prolonged sitting. A snapping sensation may also be perceived.

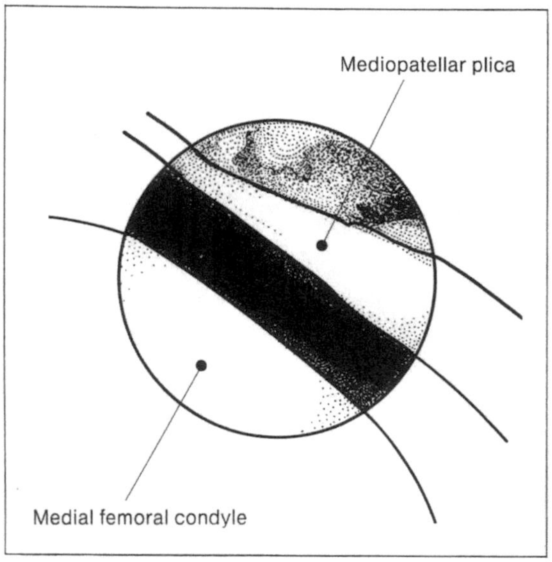

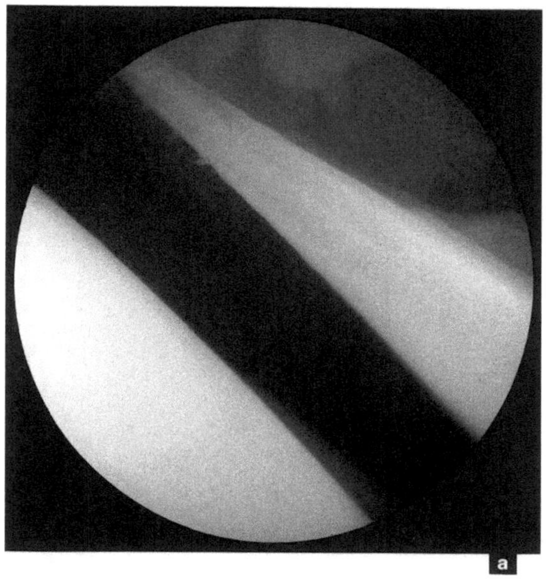

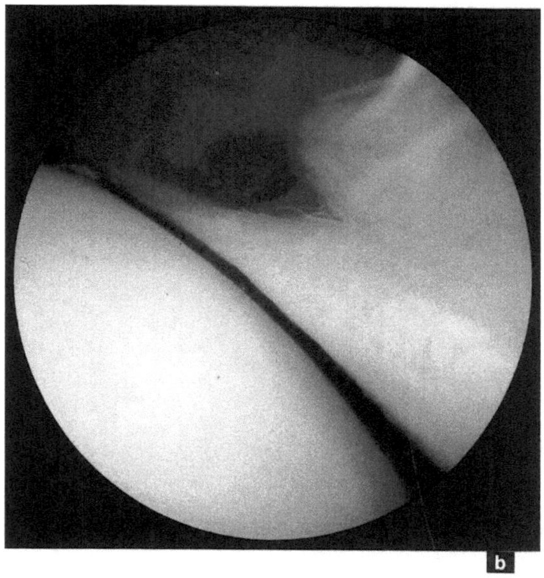

Fig. 8-38 a, b. Type II mediopatellar plica. Function testing shows no impingement on the medial femoral condyle in extension (**a**) or flexion (**b**). There are no visible cartilage changes on the condylar surface

When fraying of the free border of a type III mediopatellar plica coexists with erosive cartilage lesions at the site of contact with the medial femoral condyle, the pathologic significance of the plica cannot be questioned, and arthroscopic resection of the plica is indicated.

Plica syndrome should be considered in cases where the clinical and arthroscopic examinations show no morphologic causes for nonspecific complaints such as locking or vague medial joint pain. When a type III plica is identified in an otherwise normal-appearing joint but the patient is experiencing anteromedial joint symptoms, resection of the plica is appropriate even if the medial femoral condyle does not yet exhibit significant cartilage change.

Incision of the mediopatellar plica is not sufficient to relieve impingement, since scarring and contracture of the plica can cause symptoms to reappear. Total resection of the plica is advised. The resection is performed using the "bucket handle" technique. An instrument portal is placed over the medial portion of the plica, and the plica is divided very close to the capsule, leaving an intact bridge of connective tissue medially and also anteri-

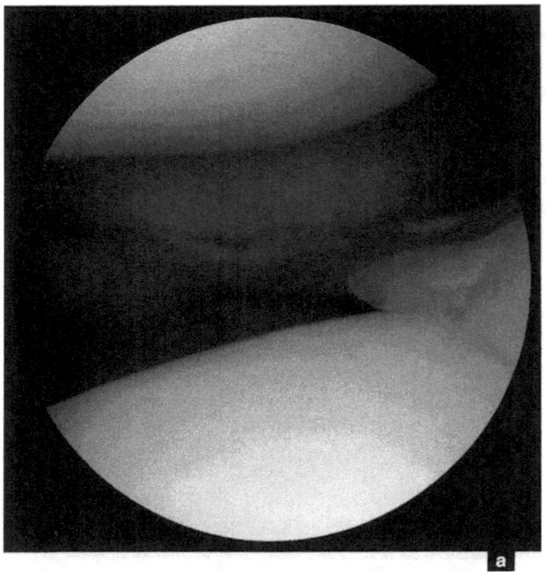

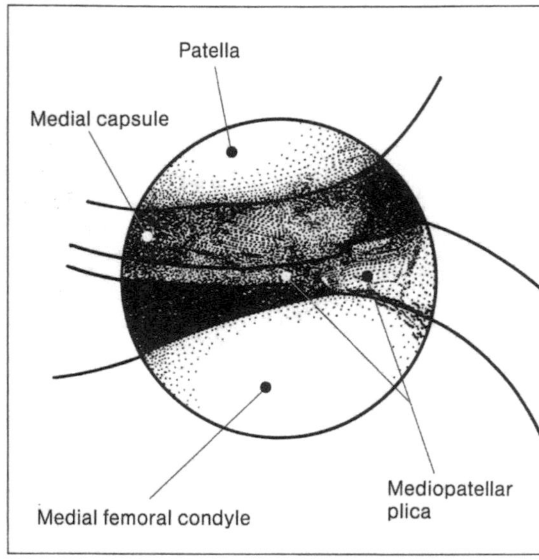

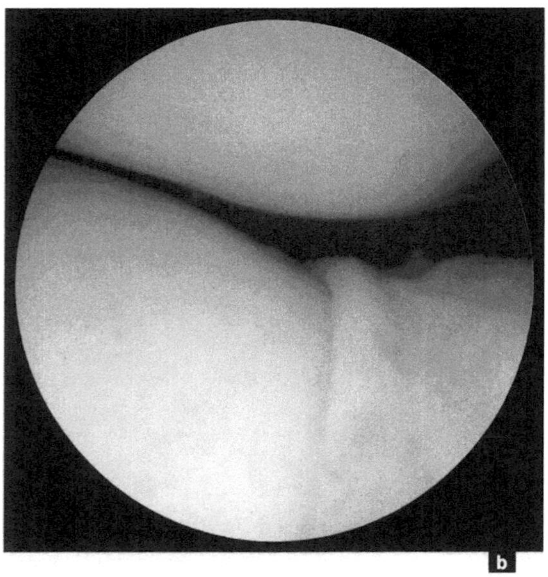

Fig. 8-39 a, b. Type III mediopatellar plica. Even in extension, the plica is in contact with the medial femoral condyle (**a**). As the knee is flexed, the free edge of the plica rolls upon the medial femoral condyle to escape entrapment between the femur and patella (**b**). The cartilage surfaces still show no pathologic changes

orly. When the plica is tethered only by the medial and anterior attachments, like a bucket handle, the anterior attachment is divided first. The plica falls into the medial recess, where it is easily grasped with a forceps and extracted, rupturing the medial bridge of connective tissue. This technique is advantageous in that it facilitates division of the plica close to the capsule. Completely resecting the plica in one step from a medial or anterior approach allows the detached portion of the plica to float within the joint, obstructing vision and hampering the rest of the resection.

Problems

- *The plica is not seen.* If the arthroscope is passed into the medial recess in the fully extended knee, even a large plica may be missed. So the examiner should make a specific search for the medial plica before entering the medial recess. If the plica is still not seen, the knee joint is briefly flexed. Often this will cause a large plica to snap downward into view. Care is taken that the scope is not advanced too far toward the medial capsule, as it may displace the plica upward and out of the visual field (requiring slight retraction of the scope).

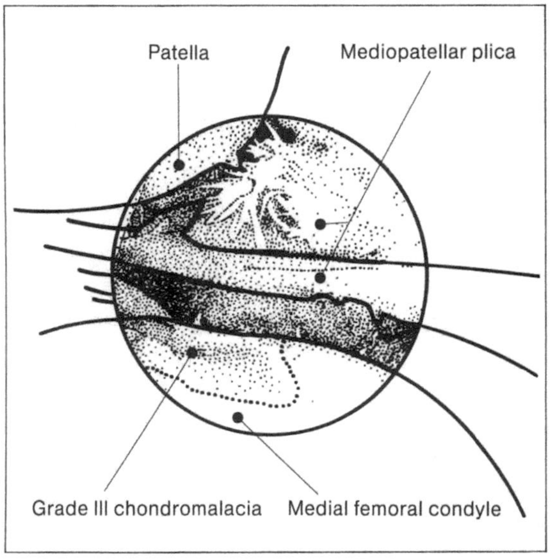

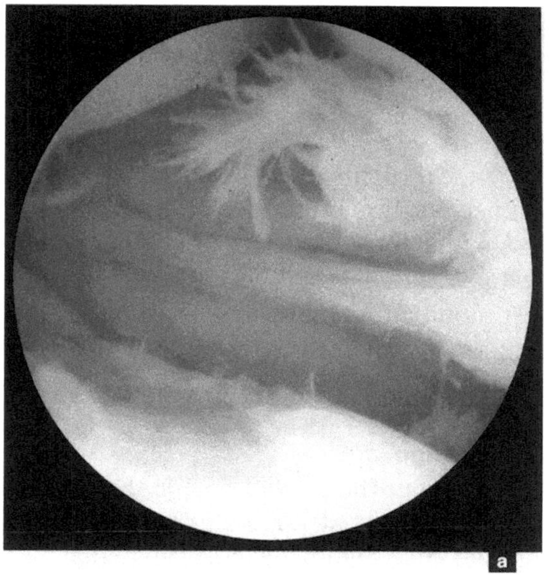
a

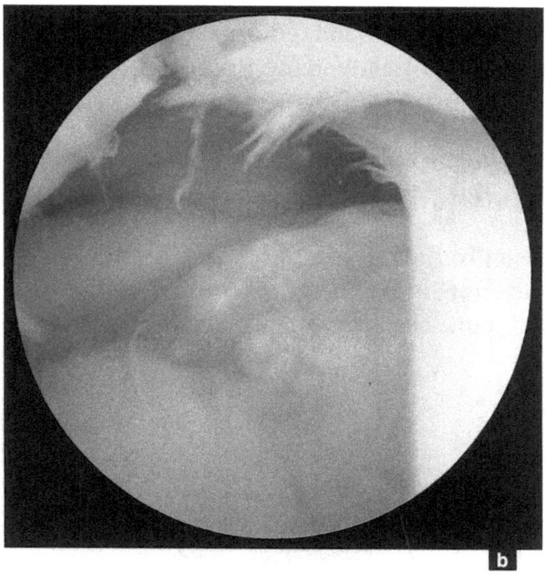
b

Fig. 8-40 a, b. Plica syndrome (medial shelf syndrome).
History: The patient, a 43-year-old male, first experienced medial knee pain 6 years ago. A hypertrophied mediopatellar plica (type III) was found at arthroscopy but was left alone because the femoral cartilage appeared undamaged. Patient has had increasing knee pain for 4 weeks.
Arthroscopic findings: Arthroscopy reveals a type III mediopatellar plica that is duplicated anteriorly and shows fibrillation similar to that in a degenerative meniscus (**a**). The area of the medial femoral condyle in contact with the plica shows grade III chondromalacic change (**b**). Grade II chondromalacia is apparent on the medial patellar facet.
Procedure: Complete arthroscopic resection of the plica

- *Difficulty inspecting the medial recess.* A type III plica can block arthroscope entry into the medial recess. In this situation the knee is maximally extended until a narrow space appears between the medial femoral condyle and the free edge of the plica. If the plica does not move off the cartilage even in maximum extension, the scope is withdrawn to the level of the central depression of the femoral trochlea, swept downward, and advanced straight toward the medial joint space. With the light post at 5:00, the mediopatellar plica can be clearly inspected from below.
- *Iatrogenic perforation of the plica.* Insertion of the sheath can perforate a mediopatellar plica that contacts the medial femoral condyle in the extended knee. This complication restricts the maneuverability of the scope. If the scope is withdrawn and reinserted, a hole will be found in the plica; if the scope is forcibly maneuvered in place, the plica will become lacerated. The examiner should consider the possibility of iatrogenic perforation before declaring that a rare "fenestrated" mediopatellar plica is present.

8.6 Medial Compartment

Position

The knee is slightly flexed. When the extended knee position is used for arthroscopy (see Sect. 4.2.1), the lower leg hangs off the side of the table, and the thigh rests against a lateral post mounted a handswidth proximal to the joint line. This produces a mild valgus strain that opens the medial joint space.

Visualization

Starting from the medial recess, the arthroscope (light post at 2:00) is swept downward with the knee slightly flexed. The medial meniscus (anterior horn, central portion, posterior horn), the medial femoral condyle, and the medial tibial plateau are inspected.

8.6.1 Medial Meniscus

Visualization

Anterior horn. The anterior horn of the medial meniscus is best examined with the knee flexed approximately 40°–60° and the light post positioned at 1:00.

Central portion. With valgus pressure applied, the central portion (middle third) of the medial meniscus is demonstrated by rotating the light post to 2:00 in the slightly flexed knee. The meniscosynovial junction is also inspected (Fig. 8-41).

Posterior horn. Visualization of this segment is particularly important as it is a site of predilection for meniscal tears. The light post is moved to 3:00, and a valgus pressure is applied with the knee *slightly (!) flexed* (approximately 10°) to widely open the medial joint space (Figs. 8-42 and 8-43).

Greater flexion, while relaxing the medial capsule, would lead to posterior displacement of the upper tibia and laxity of the posterior capsule. The posterior portion of the meniscus would recede and disappear from sight.

Technique for visualizing the posterior horn of the medial meniscus:

1. First image the central portion of the meniscus (light post at 2:00).

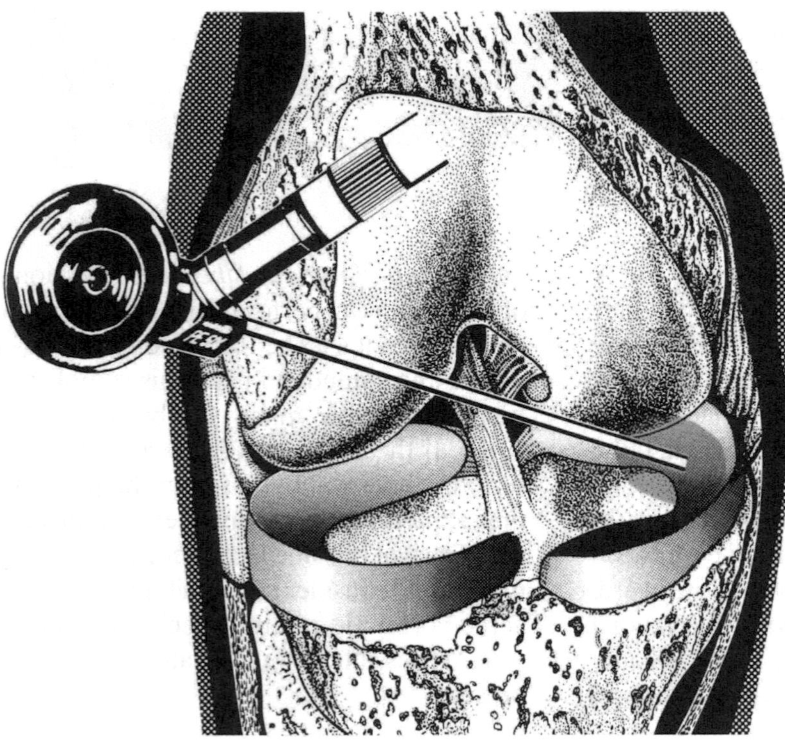

Fig. 8-41. The light post is at 2:00 (10:00 in the left knee) for inspecting the central portion of the medial meniscus

2. Rotate the light post to 3:00.
3. Apply a valgus stress in minimum flexion while externally rotating the tibia.

In tight joints and in osteoarthritic varus knees, it can be extremely difficult to demonstrate the posterior segment of the meniscus. In these cases scrupulous attention must be given to the basic rules for positioning the arthroscope and constructing the instrument portal (see Sect. 6.2.2).

When there is extensive posteromedial and medial capsuloligamentous disruption, the posterior segment of the medial meniscus is easy to visualize (Fig. 8-44). If the posterior horn is easily seen from the medial side, the patient may have a constitutional ligamentous laxity (Fig. 8-45).

Normal Findings
The intact meniscus is yellowish-white, resilient, and exhibits a sharp inner border. Small undulations in the inner border of the meniscus are considered to be a normal finding (Figs. 8-46 and 8-47).

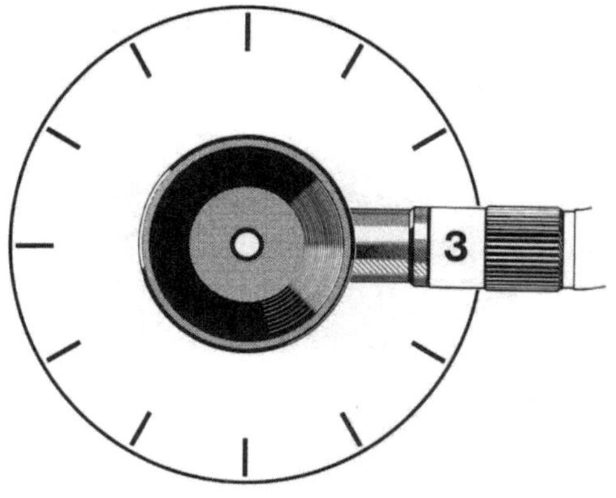

Fig. 8-42. The light post is at 3:00 (9:00 in the left knee) for inspecting the posterior horn of the medial meniscus

The meniscal tissue is inspected to evaluate its color and surface condition and to check for the presence of deposits or tears.

The meniscus consists of 3 circumferential zones:

1. The *inner zone* is avascular and cartilaginous. It encompasses the free inner border of the meniscus.

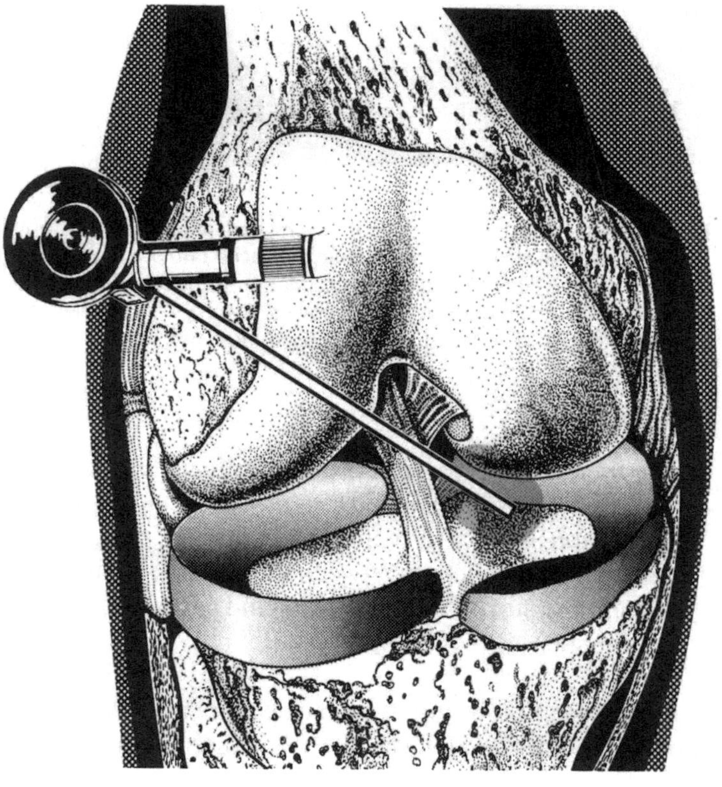

Fig. 8-43. To inspect the posterior horn of the medial meniscus, the light post is placed at 3:00 (9:00 in the left knee) while the tibia is externally rotated and valgus stress is applied

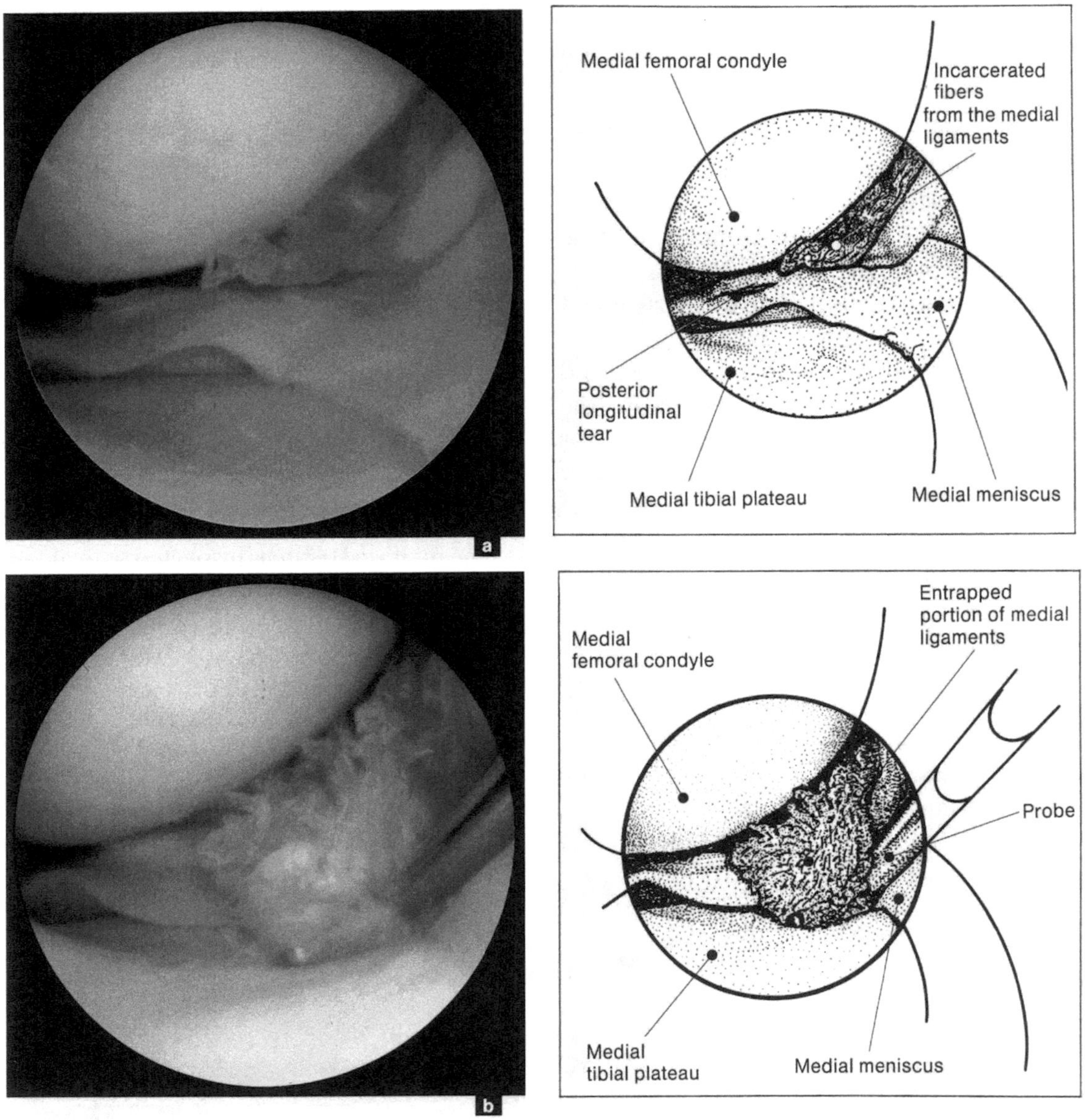

Fig. 8-44 a, b. Marked opening of the medial joint space. A reddish structure has become displaced into the joint space. There is excessive undulation of the inner border of the meniscus, which shows a posterior longitudinal tear. The fact that the meniscus does not elevate off the tibial plateau with valgus strain may signify a rupture of the medial and posteromedial meniscofemoral ligaments (**a**). Some of the torn fibers can be pulled forward with the probe (**b**)

2. The *middle zone* consists of fibrocartilage and is sparsely vascularized.
3. The *peripheral zone* is heavily vascularized and marks the junction between the meniscus and the surrounding synovial and capsular tissue.

This classification is important, since tears in the vascularized periphery of the meniscus can heal following suture repair, and immobilization may be sufficient treatment for minor tears. Repair is a less satisfactory option for tears elsewhere in the meniscus, which are far less likely to heal.

Pathologic Findings

Whereas the meniscus was once considered almost superfluous by knee surgeons, who

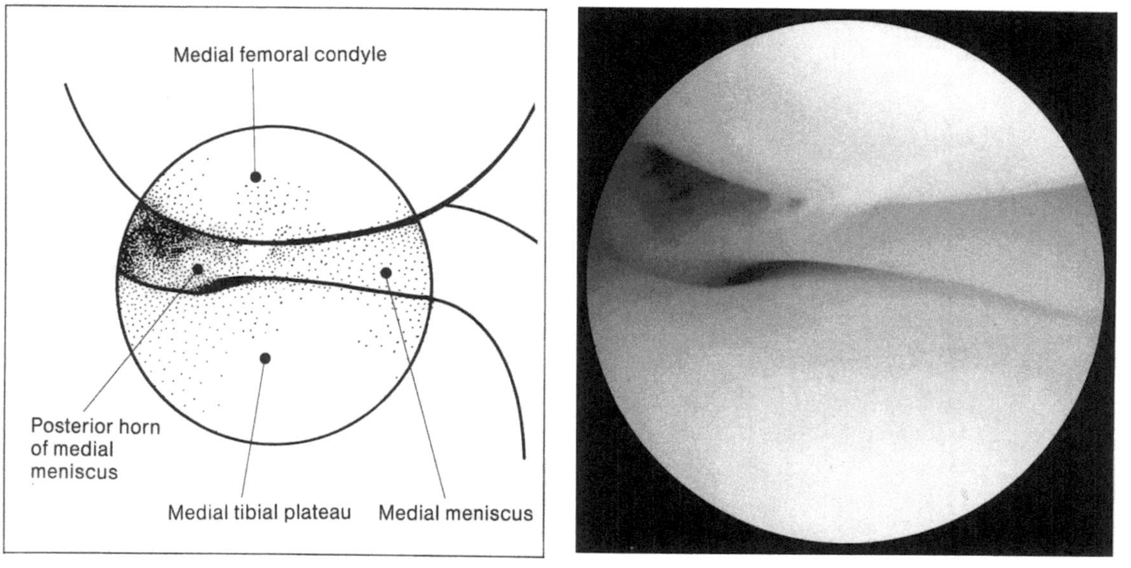

Fig. 8-45. The posterior horn of the medial meniscus is inspected with the knee slightly flexed and under valgus stress, and the tibia externally rotated. The posterior horn of the medial meniscus is completely visualized. Superficial iatrogenic cartilage damage is noted on the medial femoral condyle

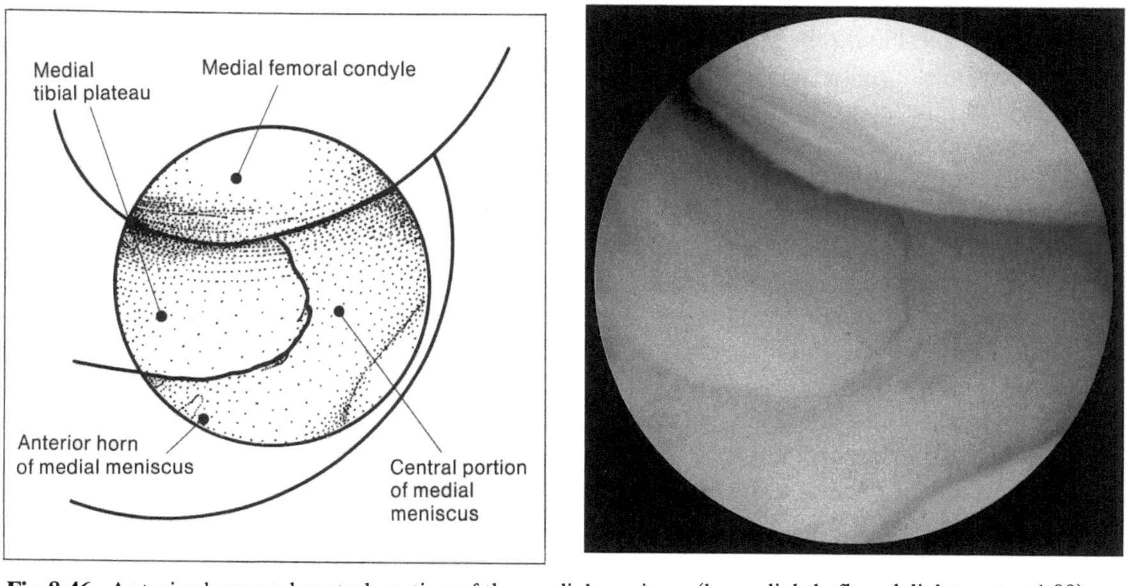

Fig. 8-46. Anterior horn and central portion of the medial meniscus (knee slightly flexed, light post at 1:00)

performed a great many open, total meniscectomies (yielding numerous resected specimens as "hunting trophies"), today the meniscus is credited with performing important stabilizing and proprioceptive functions. As a result, meniscus-conserving therapy has become a worthwhile goal. Increasingly, arthroscopy is becoming the established technique for performing meniscal resections. If a meniscus cannot be salvaged (i.e., cannot be reattached), only the portion of the meniscus that is pathologically altered is removed. The guiding principle in meniscectomies, articulated by Glinz, is to remove *"as little as pos-*

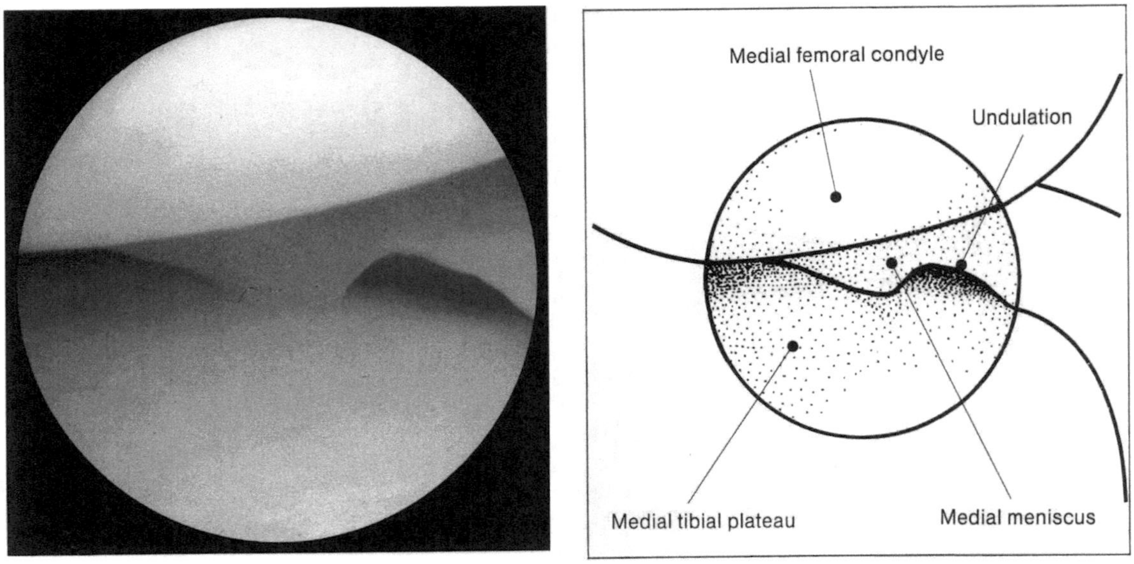

Fig. 8-47. Undulation of the inner border of the meniscus

sible and as much as necessary." A total or subtotal meniscectomy is indicated only if all the meniscal tissue has been destroyed.

The differentiation between normal and pathologic findings is of supreme importance in arthroscopic evaluations of the menisci. Klein (1980) emphasized the marked discrepancies that can exist between the arthroscopic appearance and histologic findings on the one hand, and between clinical findings and subjective complaints on the other. This led Klein to recommend a careful interpretation of arthroscopic findings.

Every meniscal lesion does not need to be widely excised. Especially with nonsymptomatic lesions that are incidentally found, such as transverse tears or fraying of the inner margin, it is best to limit the resection to a simple trimming procedure. With a transverse tear, even the torn portion of the meniscus can still perform a residual stabilizing function.

Old meniscal tears and concealed tears frequently lead to secondary changes ("mirror images") that can direct attention to the tear. Irregularities and/or siderotic changes in the synovium bordering the meniscus, cartilage changes at adjacent sites, and thickenings of the capsule are among the most important of these secondary signs.

If inspection shows no evidence of meniscal pathology or secondary changes, selective palpation with the probing hook is still necessary to confirm meniscal integrity. Difficult to see with an arthroscope, the posterior segment of the meniscus is notorious for harboring lesions that can only be confirmed or excluded by probing (see Fig. 3-32). A blunt obturator does not make a satisfactory probe in this situation (see Sect. 3.6).

The probing hook is useful even if inspection reveals meniscal pathology. Only by selective probing can the examiner establish the true location and extent of the lesion and assess the condition of the meniscal rim. The visible and palpable findings will largely determine the further course of action, e.g., whether the meniscus should be resected or repaired.

If an open meniscectomy is planned, it should still be preceded by arthroscopy. The clinical diagnosis of meniscal lesions has an approximately 15% false-positive rate in terms of identifying the affected side. Preceding the arthrotomy by diagnostic arthroscopy can avoid opening the wrong side of the joint.

The following types of meniscal lesion are encountered:

Longitudinal Tear. Longitudinal tears, which usually involve the posterior portion of the meniscus, are the most common meniscal lesions. In many cases gross inspection reveals no evidence of a tear or shows only slight irregularities in the inner border of the meniscus. Probing is necessary to establish the presence of a tear (Fig. 8-48 and Fig. 3-32).

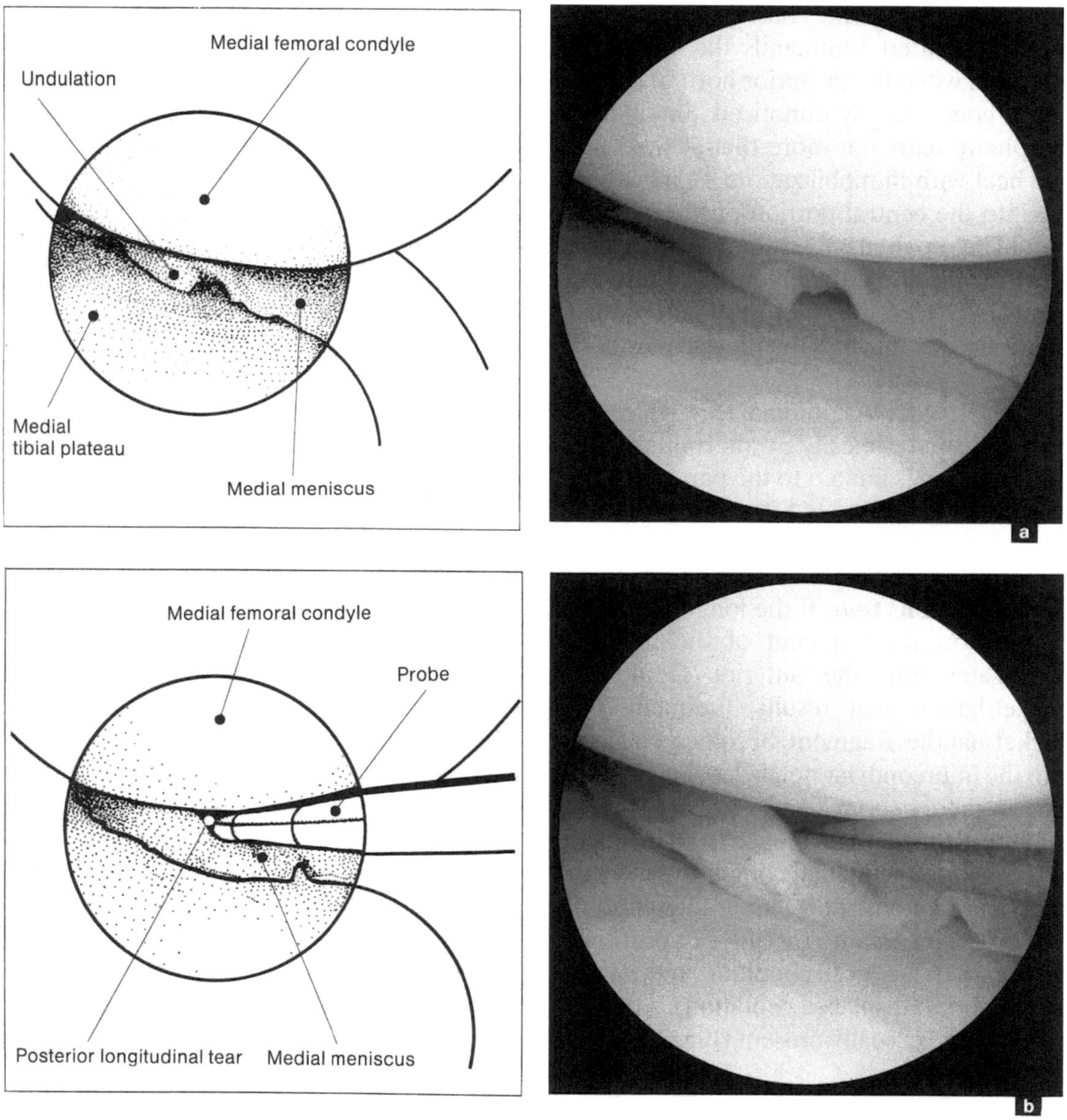

Fig. 8-48 a, b. Posterior longitudinal tear of the medial meniscus.
History: A 17-year-old male sustained a rotational injury 4 weeks ago while playing soccer and afterward felt a snapping sensation in the knee. The patient had sustained a previous knee injury 1 year earlier. He had a positive Lachman test with a soft end point and no intraarticular effusion.
Arthroscopic findings: Superficial inspection shows only an irregularity in the meniscal border (**a**) that resembles a physiologic undulation (see Fig. 8-47). Probing reveals a partially displaced posterior longitudinal tear with degenerative changes (accentuated fiber structure in the meniscal tissue) (**b**). Further inspection revealed an old rupture of the anterior cruciate ligament.
Procedure: Due to the degenerative changes and thinning of the posterior portion of the meniscus, repair is unlikely to be of benefit, so arthroscopic resection is indicated. Anterior cruciate ligament reconstruction would be advised

The meniscus should be probed from its superior *and* inferior surfaces. Often the extent of a lesion can be appreciated more clearly when the meniscus is elevated from the tibial plateau (see Figs. 3-32 d and 8-87 c).

Acute posterior longitudinal tears are frequently combined with a rupture of the anterior cruciate ligament. Thus, the cruciate ligament tear often commands the examiner's attention while the posterior horn of the meniscus goes virtually unnoticed. Small, acute peripheral tears not more than 4 weeks old will heal with immobilization. Tears extending into the central portion of the meniscus should be repaired, and this, too, can be done arthroscopically. If the anterior cruciate ligament is also torn, every effort should be made to preserve as much of the meniscus as possible.

With an older longitudinal tear, which may be manifested clinically by intermittent locking, resection is limited to the part of the meniscus that has separated from the peripheral rim.

Bucket-Handle Tear. If the longitudinal tear of the posterior segment of the meniscus propagates into the anterior segment, a bucket-handle tear results. Frequently the bucket-handle fragment becomes displaced into the intercondylar notch, leaving behind a narrow meniscal rim.

If the arthroscope is moved from the medial recess into the medial compartment of the knee and demonstrates either a longitudinal tear extending far into the anterior portion of the meniscus (reduced condition) or a narrow meniscal rim (displaced condition), a bucket-handle tear is usually present (Fig. 8-49).

If only a narrow meniscus is found, it may represent an expanded, adapted meniscal rim associated with a chronic bucket-handle tear. A displaced bucket-handle fragment will partially obstruct the view of the intercondylar area when the arthroscope is retracted. Also, a fragment that has displaced into the intercondylar notch and undergone fibrous change can be difficult to distinguish from the anterior cruciate ligament. Surgical measures should be undertaken only after the structure has been positively identified by a reduction maneuver.

A bucket-handle fragment may separate from its anterior attachment and become displaced into the posterior part of the joint. Thus, if an abnormally narrow meniscus (thinned peripheral rim) is found, the posterior portions of the meniscus and the posteromedial recess should be selectively explored with the probing hook to check for displaced meniscal fragments.

Transverse Tear. Transverse tears extend from the free inner border of the meniscus toward the periphery. They may involve the superior and/or inferior surface of the meniscus. If the inner border of an apparently intact meniscus rises from the tibial plateau when pressure is applied with a probe, it is likely that an inferior longitudinal tear or transverse tear is present (see Fig. 6-16 b).

Most transverse meniscal tears have a degenerative etiology, and many are incidental findings (Fig. 8-50). These lesions should not be widely excised, for even a torn meniscal rim still performs a stabilizing function. Transverse tears rarely cause locking or other pronounced clinical symptoms.

Fig. 8-49 a–c. Bucket-handle tear of the medial meniscus.
History: Woman 24 years of age sustained an initial knee injury 4 years ago while playing handball, with subsequent locking and intraarticular effusion. Following conservative treatment she experienced recurrent episodes of locking and had to give up sports. She presented with no instability or meniscal signs.
Arthroscopic findings: A peripheral longitudinal tear extending into the anterior third of the meniscus (**a**). On probing, the meniscus (**b**) can be displaced into the intercondylar notch (**c**), confirming the diagnosis of a bucket-handle tear. In its displaced condition, the bucket-handle fragment obscures vision as long as the arthroscope remains in the medial compartment. This is corrected by retraction of the scope (**c**).
Procedure: Arthroscopic resection of the bucket handle

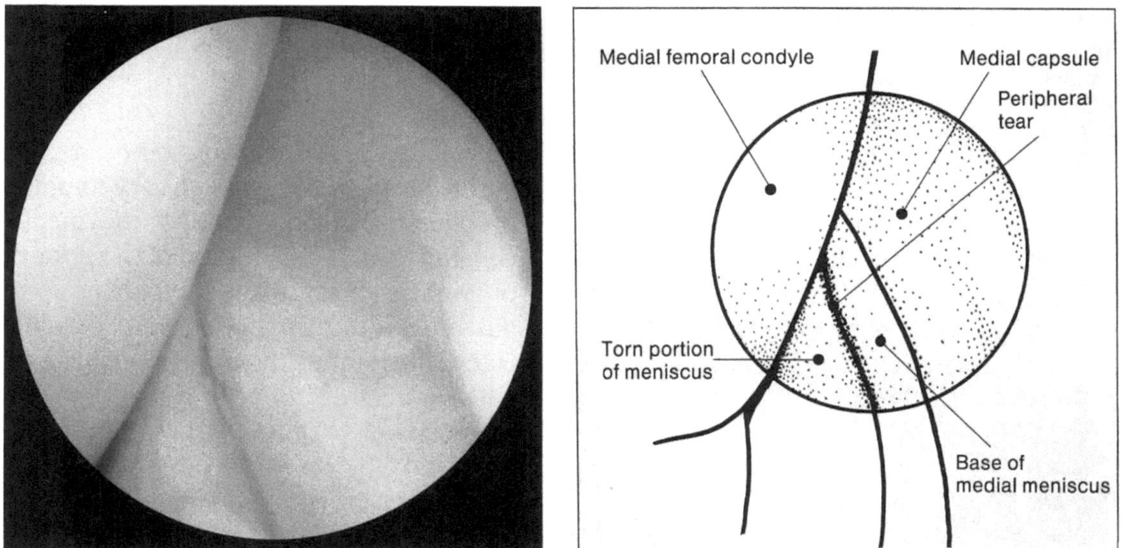
Medial femoral condyle
Medial capsule
Peripheral tear
Torn portion of meniscus
Base of medial meniscus

a

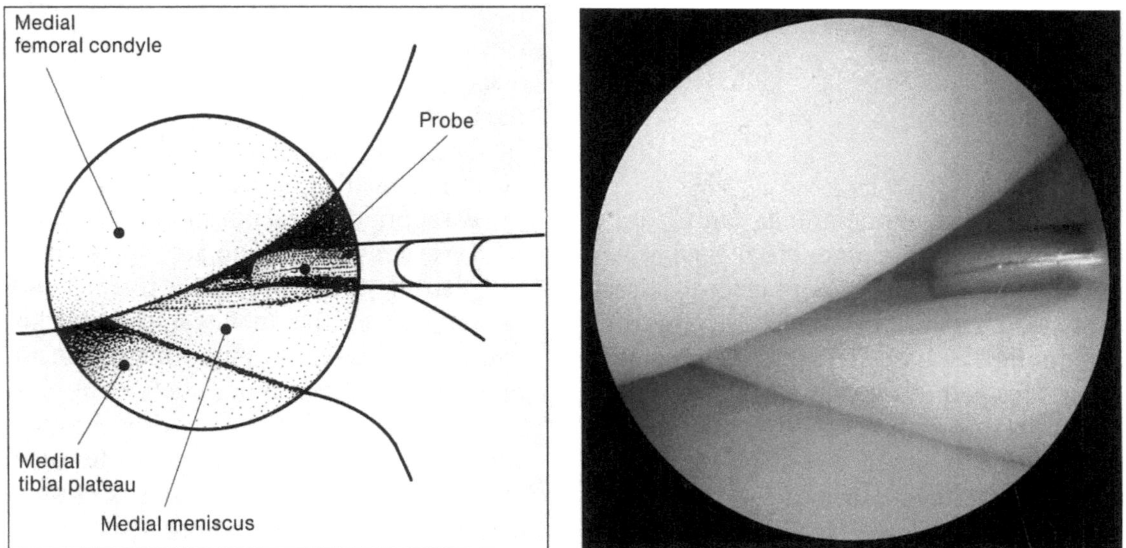
Medial femoral condyle
Probe
Medial tibial plateau
Medial meniscus

b

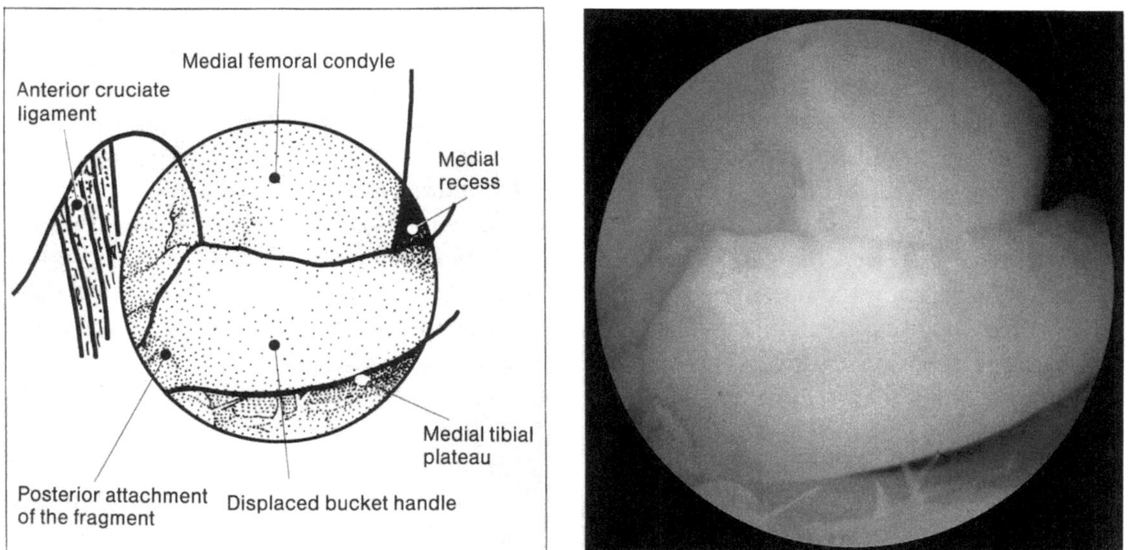
Medial femoral condyle
Anterior cruciate ligament
Medial recess
Medial tibial plateau
Posterior attachment of the fragment
Displaced bucket handle

c

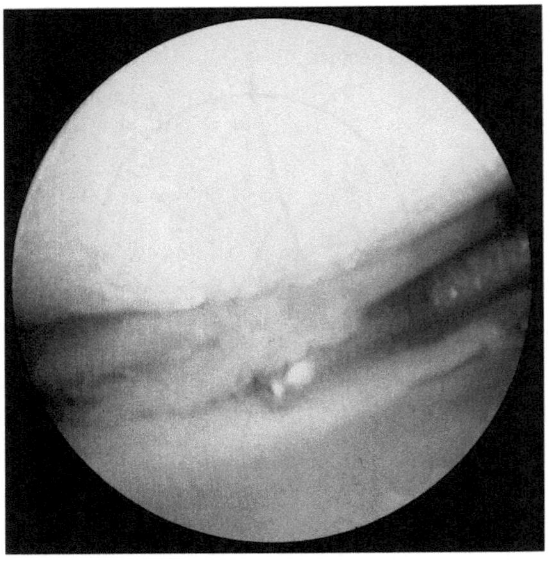

Fig. 8-50. Degenerative transverse tear. The peripheral extent of the tear is determined by probing (monitor image)

Flap Tear. A longitudinal tear can separate from its anterior attachment to form a posteriorly based meniscal flap or tag, or it can separate from its posterior attachment to form an anteriorly based flap. Degenerative changes frequently accompany it (Fig. 8-51). Meniscal flaps with rounded borders are a less common finding.

It can be difficult to locate a posteriorly based meniscal flap that has become displaced into the posteromedial recess. In these cases the posterior segment of the meniscus appears unusually narrow. If the flap cannot be returned to the joint space by manual compression (milking) of the posteromedial recess, the recess should be inspected with the arthroscope (see Sect. 8.7.1).

Degenerative Meniscal Changes. Fibrillation, villous changes, and a coarse fiber structure on or in the meniscal tissue are evidence of degenerative meniscal change. The changes may involve only the inner border of the meniscus or all of the meniscal substance. Several types of lesion may coexist (e.g., fibrillation, transverse tears, longitudinal tears) (Fig. 8-52). Degenerative changes should be distinguished from deposits on the meniscus (Fig. 8-53).

Problems

- *Difficulty visualizing the posterior horn of the medial meniscus.* This is a very common problem in examinations of the medial compartment. Visualization of the posterior horn can be improved by applying a valgus stress to the slightly flexed knee while externally rotating the tibia, applying manual pressure from the posterior side, pulling the posterior horn forward with an instrument, and by lowering the intraarticular fluid pressure (see Sect. 11.8). The light post is positioned exactly at 3:00. Even slight deviations from this optimum position can greatly restrict the visual field.
- *Reducing a displaced bucket handle.* A bucket-handle fragment that has been in the intercondylar notch for some time can be difficult to reduce. If reduction cannot be effected with a probe passed through a medial suprameniscal portal while the joint space is stressed open, an attempt is made to grasp the fragment with a forceps and pull it toward the meniscal rim. If this maneuver fails but the anterior attachment of the bucket handle is positively identified, the fragment is divided anteriorly, grasped with a forceps, and placed under tension. Not infrequently, the fragment is twisted and must be untwisted before it can be reduced to its former position. The posterior attachment also can be severed from a high medial approach while tension is applied to the fragment. Reduction of the displaced bucket handle also serves to distinguish the anterior attachment of the fragment from the anterior cruciate ligament.
- *Meniscal fragment displaced into the posteromedial recess.* Meniscal flaps, posteriorly based bucked handles, or meniscal fragments that have become detached loose bodies may enter the posteromedial recess. If this is suspected, the posteromedial recess is viewed by passing the scope through the intercondylar notch (light post between 8:00 and 10:00, or between 2:00 and 4:00 in the left knee). Through manual

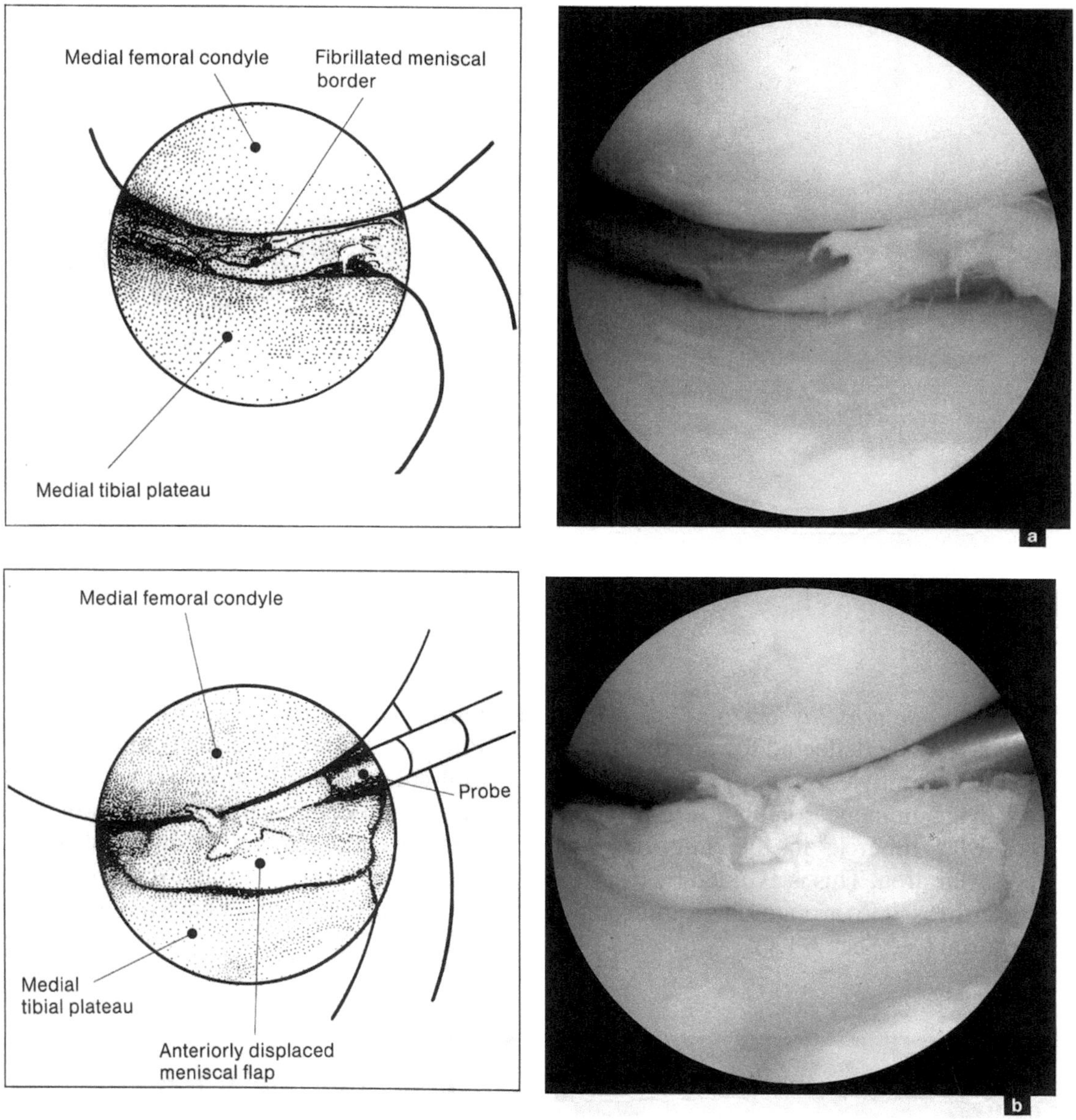

Fig. 8-51 a, b. Posterior flap tear of the medial meniscus.
History: Man 48 years of age had a history of recurring medial joint pain for several months, with pain increasing markedly during the past 6 weeks. He could recall no antecedent trauma to the knee.
Arthroscopic findings: Fibrillation of the inner border of the meniscus (**a**). A large meniscal flap is pulled forward with the probing hook (**b**). The femoral and tibial articular surfaces already manifest chondromalacic change.
Procedure: Arthroscopic resection. The base of the flap is located and partially divided, leaving a small bridge of tissue. The meniscal flap is then extracted with a grasping forceps, rupturing the tissue bridge

milking and suctioning of the posteromedial recess through the arthroscopic sheath with the optic removed, an attempt is made to aspirate smaller meniscal fragments or grasp larger fragments with the suction tip. If this cannot be done from the medial compartment after traversing the intercondylar notch, a posteromedial instrument portal can be added to permit extraction of the meniscal fragments.

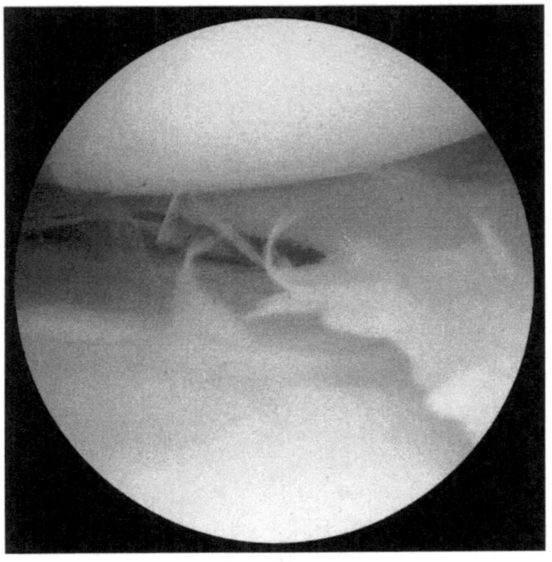

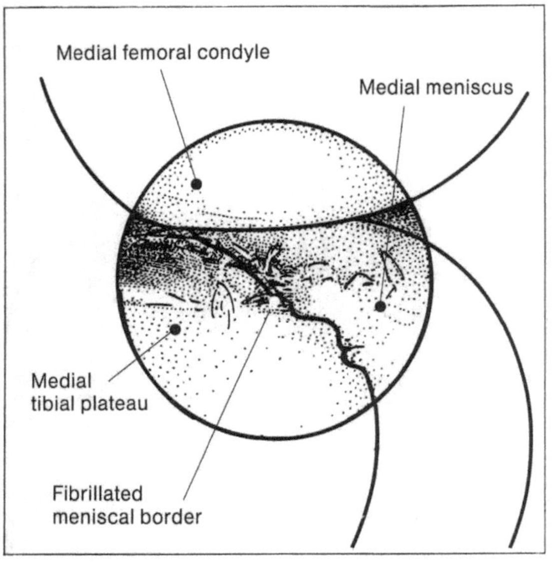

Fig. 8-52. Degenerative fibrillation of the inner border of the medial meniscus

- *Arthroscope portal is too low.* The arthroscope may be deflected toward the medial femoral condyle by a prominent intercondylar eminence or by a tertiary intercondylar tubercle in the anterior intercondylar area. This is avoided by inserting the arthroscope through a high anterolateral portal (see Sect. 6.1.1).
- *Osteophytes on the medial femoral condyle.* Prominent osteophytes on the medial femoral condyle can hamper visualization of the medial compartment. This problem is solved by changing the flexion angle of the knee or by sweeping the arthroscope into the medial compartment at a more anterior location.

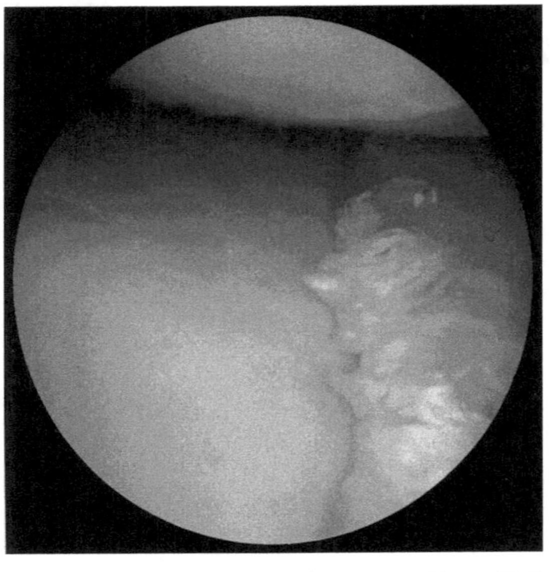

Fig. 8-53. Crystalline deposits (urate crystals) and fibrillation of the inner border of the meniscus 20 years after medial meniscectomy in a patient with hyperuricemia

8.6.2 Medial Femorotibial Joint

Position

The knee is slightly flexed (10°–20°). This position is good for evaluating the cartilage on the anterior portion of the medial femoral condyle (light post at 4:00 and 5:00). Greater flexion (up to 100°) is needed for evaluating the posterior portion (see Fig. 7-14).

Visualization

Medial tibial plateau: Light post at 1:00 and 2:00.
Medial femoral condyle: Light post at 4:00 and 5:00.

Normal Findings

Healthy articular cartilage is smooth, yellow-white, and resilient. The cartilage surfaces beneath the menisci are exposed by elevating the meniscus with the probing hook.

Pathologic Findings

All types of cartilage lesion may be seen on the medial tibial plateau and medial femoral condyle (Fig. 8-54; see Chap. 9 for details). Lesions range from localized areas of softening to extensive chondral defects (Fig. 8-55). Cartilage changes in the medial compartment should always be evaluated in relation to the limb axis. In patients with varus deformity, it is common to find significant cartilage lesions in the medial portion of the joint. Causal treatment consists of corrective osteotomy rather than arthroscopic measures. Loose bodies may be found or, less commonly, multiple chondromas (Fig. 8-56).

Transverse grooves in the articular cartilage of the medial femoral condyle should raise suspicion of anterior cruciate ligament insufficiency. The grooves reflect a disintegration of the rolling-gliding mechanism of the joint and therefore appear on both femoral condyles. They are spaced 2–3 mm apart in the anterior third of the femorotibial joint, below the linea terminalis, and move progressively closer together posteriorly (Menapace 1985).

8.7 Intercondylar Area

Position

Slight flexion.

Visualization

The light post is positioned at 2:00.

To inspect the anterior intercondylar area, the arthroscope is retracted and swept laterally to visualize the anterior cruciate ligament and the infrapatellar plica. The scope can be advanced through the intercondylar notch to view a portion of the posterior cruciate ligament and the posteromedial recess.

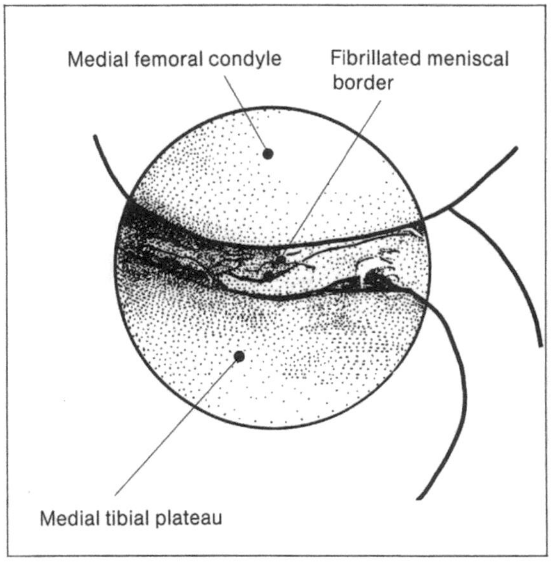

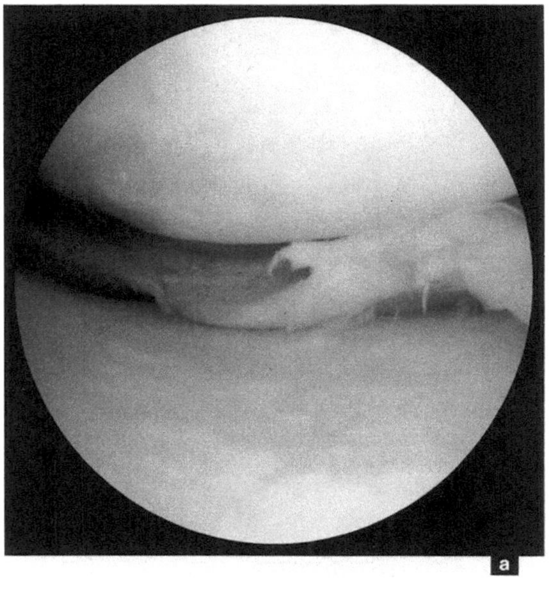

Fig. 8-54. Chondromalacia of the medial femoral condyle.
History: Woman 54 years of age with medial joint pain for several months and bilateral genu varum.
Arthroscopic findings: Grade II chondromalacia on the weight-bearing portion of the medial femoral condyle. Inspection reveals transverse erosive lesions on the condyle with the formation of chondral flaps on the medial side. This is accompanied by a complex degenerative breakdown of the whole posterior segment of the medial meniscus.
Procedure: Partial resection of the posterior horn; corrective osteotomy is recommended

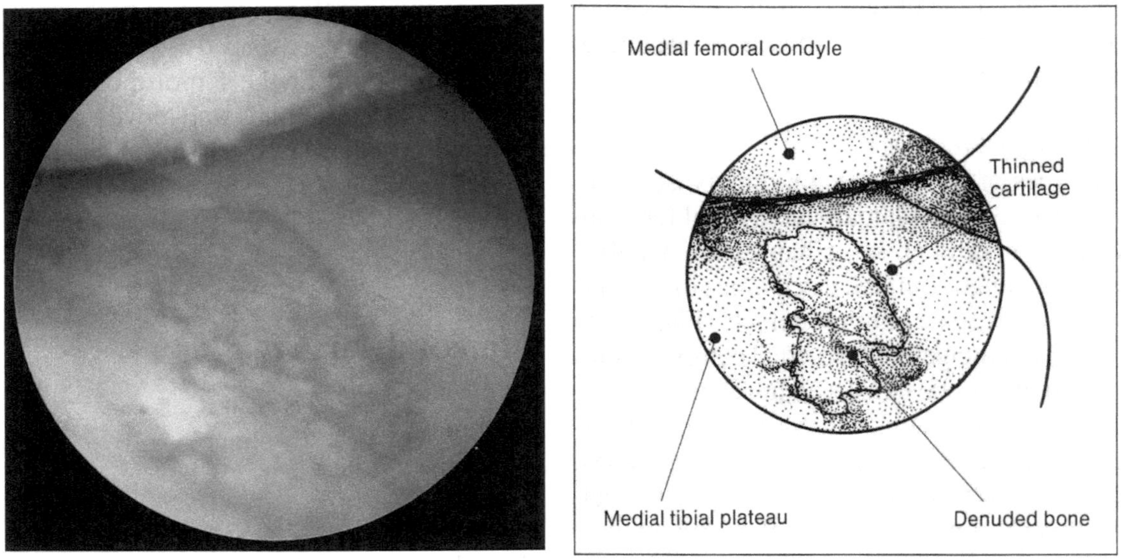

Fig. 8-55. Large, full-thickness cartilage defect on the medial tibial plateau in a patient with varus deformity and degenerative arthritis

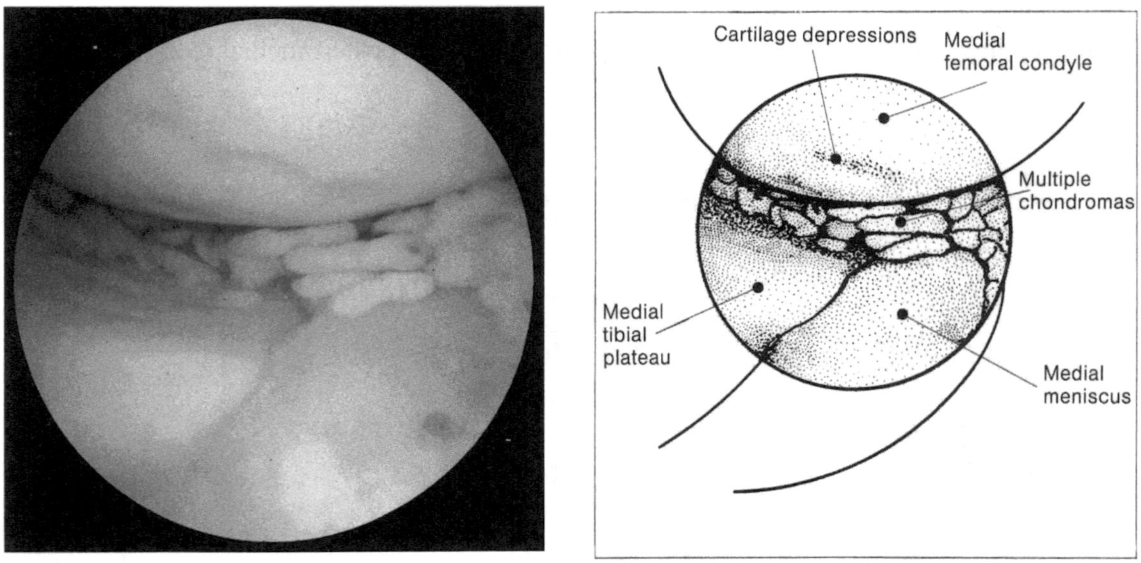

Fig. 8-56. Multiple loose bodies in the medial compartment in synovial chondromatosis. The chondromas have produced numerous depressions in the cartilaginous surfaces of the medial tibial plateau and medial femoral condyle

8.7.1 Posterior Horn of Medial Meniscus, Posteromedial Recess, Posterior Cruciate Ligament

In many cases the posterior segment of the medial meniscus can be viewed directly from the anterior intercondylar area. The intercondylar notch contains a narrow passage bounded medially by the medial femoral condyle and laterally by the anterior and posterior cruciate ligament.

Position

Slight flexion (10°). The narrow passage in the intercondylar notch can be enlarged somewhat by applying a mild valgus stress or by rotating the tibia externally. For inspection of the posteromedial recess, the knee is flexed 90°.

Visualization and Normal Findings

The arthroscope (light post at 10:00) is trained on the space bounded laterally by the medial intercondylar tubercle and posterior cruciate ligament and medially by the medial femoral condyle, medial joint space, and medial border of the tibial plateau (Figs. 8-57 and 8-58). The scope is then carefully advanced posteriorly with a rotating motion.

Degenerative changes may hinder passage of the scope through the intercondylar notch. If the notch must be traversed, the obstructing lesions must be bypassed or removed.

Positioning the light post at 11:00 (1:00 in the left knee) gives a direct view of the posterior horn of the medial meniscus. Even in this situation the examiner should carefully retract the arthroscope to obtain a better general view (Fig. 8-59). In the absence of synovial inflammation, the posterior horn is clearly visualized. Peripheral meniscal tears or meniscosynovial separations are easily verified. For this the knee is flexed 60°–70°, and the scope is again advanced into the posteromedial recess.

For inspection of the posteromedial recess, the knee is flexed to approximately 90°–100°. Inflow through the sheath is left on to distend

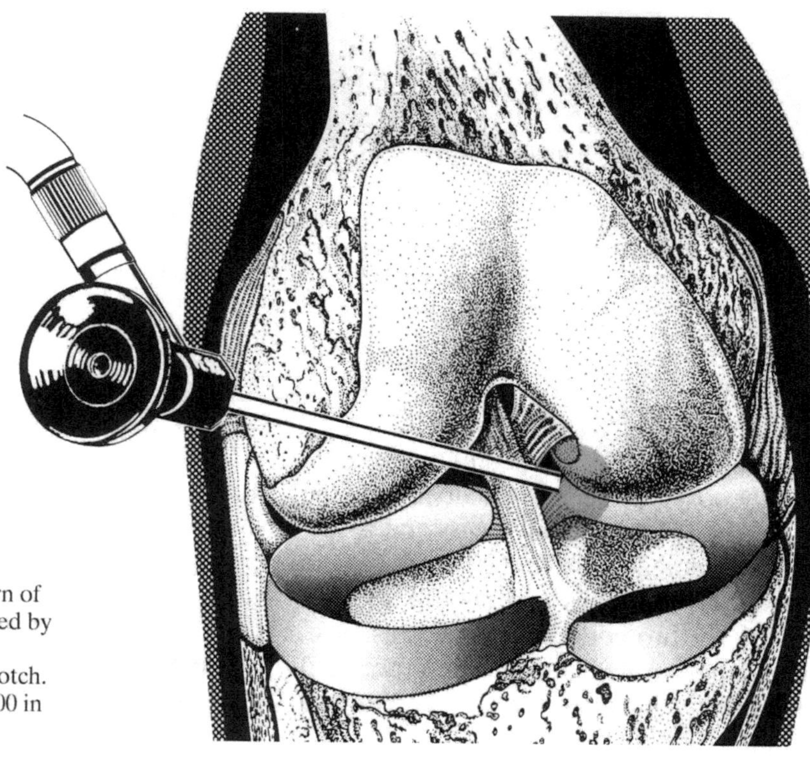

Fig. 8-57. The posterior horn of the medial meniscus is viewed by passing the arthroscope tip through the intercondylar notch. The light post is at 11:00 (1:00 in the left knee)

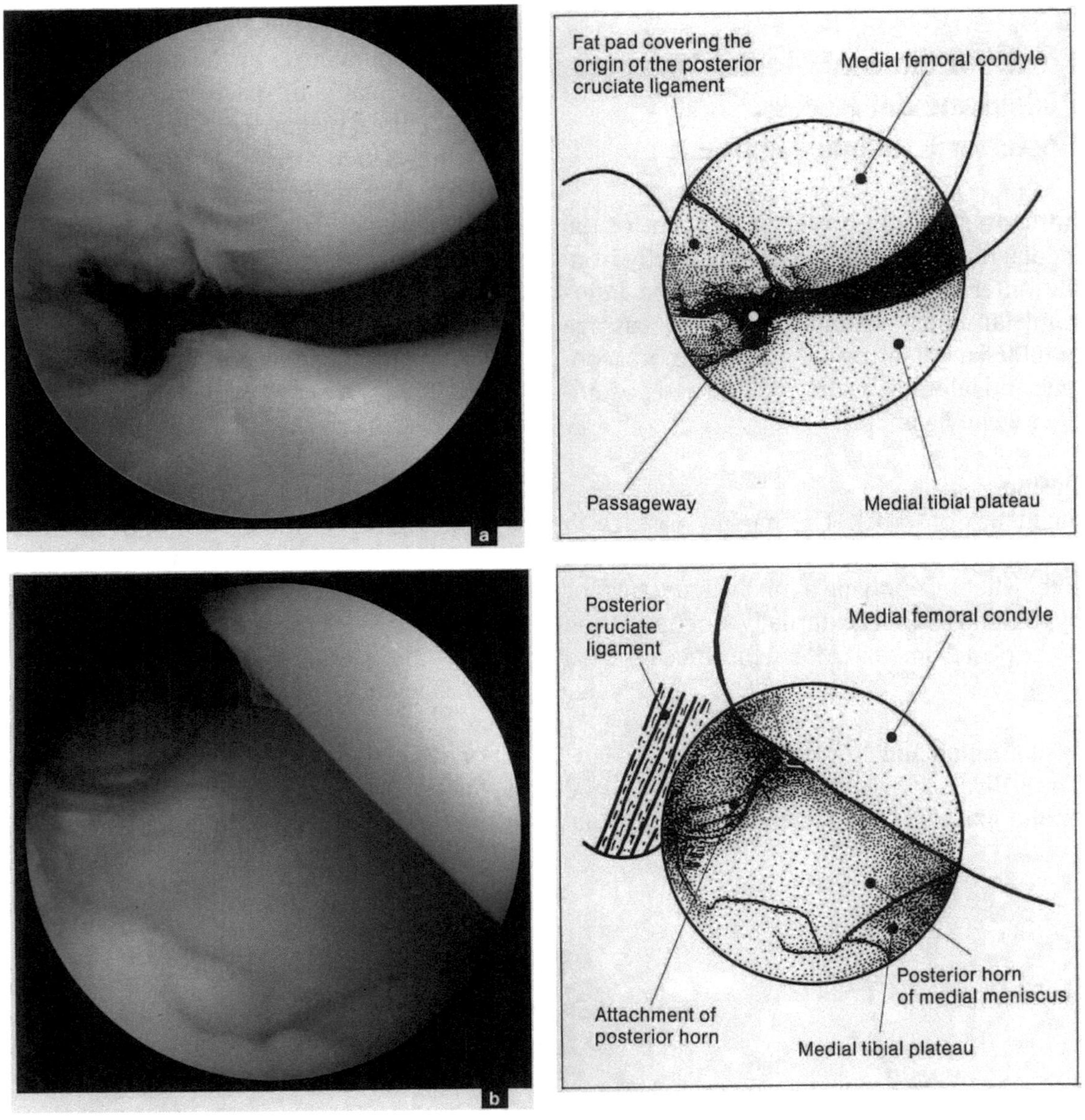

Fig. 8-58 a, b. The passageway to the posterior horn of the medial meniscus is bounded by the medial femoral condyle, the medial joint space, and the medial tibial plateau. The posterior cruciate ligament is in the lateral part of the field (**a**). Direct view of the posterior horn of the medial meniscus (**b**)

the posterior capsule, relaxed by the flexion. The light post is placed at 10:00 to inspect the floor of the posteromedial recess and is successively rotated to 9:00, 8:00, and 7:00 to demonstrate the walls and roof (Fig. 8-60). With the arthroscope and joint thus positioned, a posteromedial instrument portal, if needed, can be created using the cannula technique (see Fig. 6-24).

The integrity of the posterior cruciate ligament can be evaluated to some extent from the posteromedial recess by rotating the telescope to the 2:00, 3:00, and 4:00 positions (Fig. 8-61). The light post is then moved to 1:00 and 2:00 to view the medial fiber bundles of the posterior cruciate ligament and the interval through which the ligament passes to insert on the posterior tibia (Fig. 8-62).

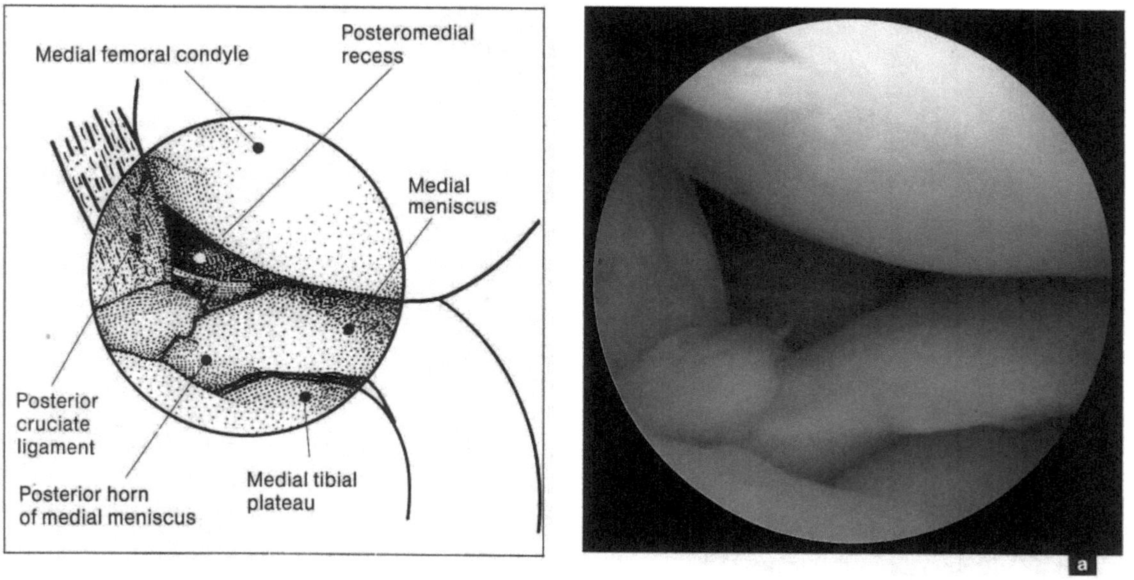

Fig. 8-59. Overview of the posterior segment of the medial meniscus following careful retraction of the arthroscope from the posteromedial recess

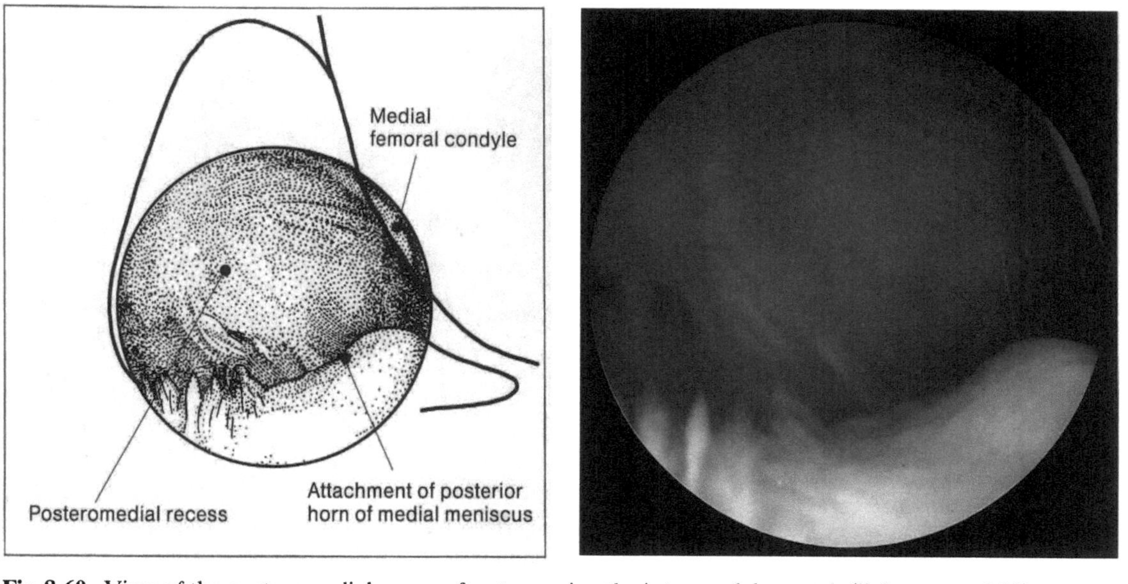

Fig. 8-60. View of the posteromedial recess after traversing the intercondylar notch (light post at 8:00)

Whenever the light post is rotated to a new position, the video camera must remain stationary. Otherwise orientation is easily lost in the hard-to-see confines of the posterior joint region.

Direct inspection of the posterior horn and posteromedial recess is indicated if there is clinical suspicion of a peripheral tear of the posterior horn, but the lesion cannot be verified from the medial compartment. Visuali-

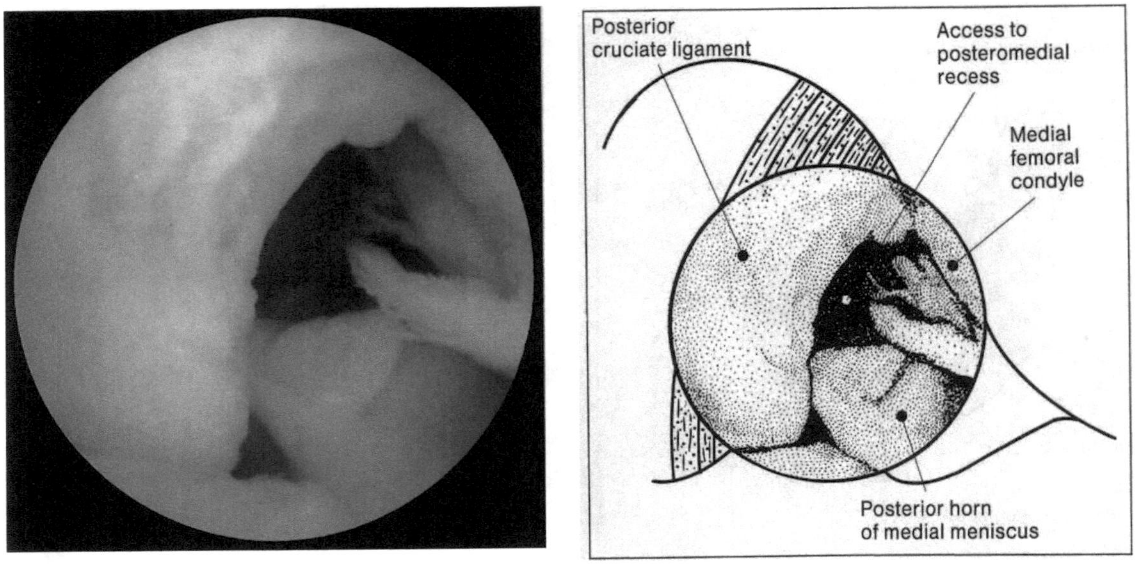

Fig. 8-61. Inspection of the posteromedial portion of the posterior cruciate ligament (light post at 3:00, 9:00 in the left knee)

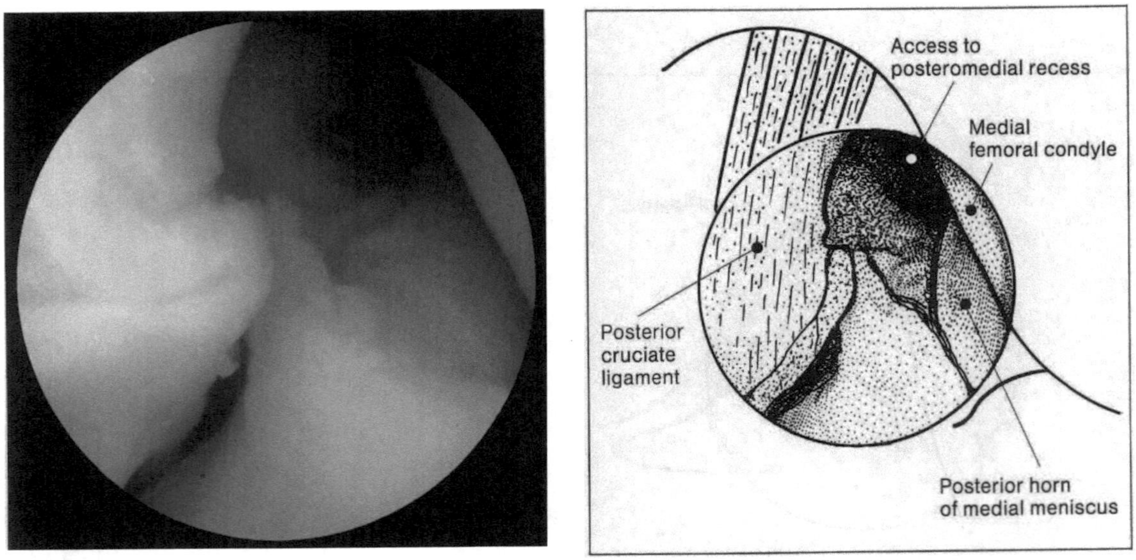

Fig. 8-62. Medial portion of the posterior cruciate ligament. The ligament descends through a slitlike aperture toward its insertion on the posterior tibia (light post at 1:00, 11:00 in the left knee)

zation of the posteromedial recess is also indicated if the recess contains, or is presumed to contain, loose bodies or if a meniscal flap or detached meniscal fragment has entered the recess. The posteromedial recess forms an important site for the gravity-dependent collection of intraarticular loose bodies in the recumbent patient.

Visualization of the posteromedial capsule is part of the procedure for constructing a posteromedial portal using the cannula technique (see Sect. 6.2.5). For direct inspection of the posterior cruciate ligament, the posteromedial capsule can be viewed while a second sheath is inserted under vision into the posteromedial recess. To remove a loose body from the posteromedial recess or for a complete arthroscopic synovectomy, there is no alternative to passing the tip of the scope through the intercondylar notch.

Problems

Several factors can make hamper passage of the arthroscope through the intercondylar notch:

- *Obstructed vision.* As the scope traverses the narrowest part of the notch, it commonly scrapes off cartilage fragments and shreds of synovial tissue. These may totally obstruct vision or at least cause a transient yellow-out, which is self-correcting once the scope enters the posterior compartment.
  The debris may still obstruct the lens even after the scope tip has cleared the intercondylar notch (see Fig. 11-2). There is not enough maneuverability in this position to scrape off the debris on the joint capsule, so the connection between the telescope and sheath is carefully loosened while the saline inflow is still on. This should flush the debris into the posterior portions of the joint. It is usually unnecessary to remove the telescope from the sheath.
- *Osteophytes.* Projecting osteophytes may be sheared off by the arthroscope. It is easier and faster to attempt to negotiate the intercondylar notch in a different joint position, e.g., at full extension or a greater flexion angle. Passage also may be aided by changing the rotational position of the tibia.
- *Synovial hypertrophy.* "Blind passage" of the arthroscope is risky, and it is recommended that hypertrophied synovial villi first be removed with a motorized shaver, taking care to preserve the cruciate ligaments.
- *Unfavorably placed arthroscope portal* (most common problem!).
  - If the arthroscope is introduced through a *far lateral portal,* the scope will enter the anteroposterior passage at too steep an angle. The only way to get through the intercondylar notch is to make a new viewing portal or pass the scope through an existing medial instrument portal directly adjacent to the patellar ligament.
  - If the arthroscope is inserted through an anterolateral *portal that is too low* (at the level of the joint line), the medial intercondylar tubercle will obstruct sagittal entry of the scope, deflecting it toward the medial femoral condyle.

8.7.2 Infrapatellar Plica

Position

The knee is extended, slightly flexed, or flexed to 60°.

Visualization

Light post is at 2:00.

Normal Findings

The infrapatellar plica is a synovial fold of variable prominence located in front of the anterior cruciate ligament. It is a vestige of the ligamentum mucosum, which in embryonic life separates the medial and lateral joint compartments on the sagittal plane. In postnatal life this "septum" regresses to varying degrees and may even be absent, permitting a direct arthroscopic view of the anterior cruciate ligament (Fig. 8-63).

Due to the minor pathologic significance of the infrapatellar plica, there is no point in classifying its numerous forms. It is sufficient to note that three basic types are seen in arthroscopic examinations:

Type I: A bandlike plica that is separate from the anterior cruciate ligament.

Type II: A bandlike plica having some connection with the anterior cruciate ligament. This may hamper arthroscopic evaluation of the ligament.

Type III: A septumlike plica dividing the anterior part of the joint into lateral and medial compartments.

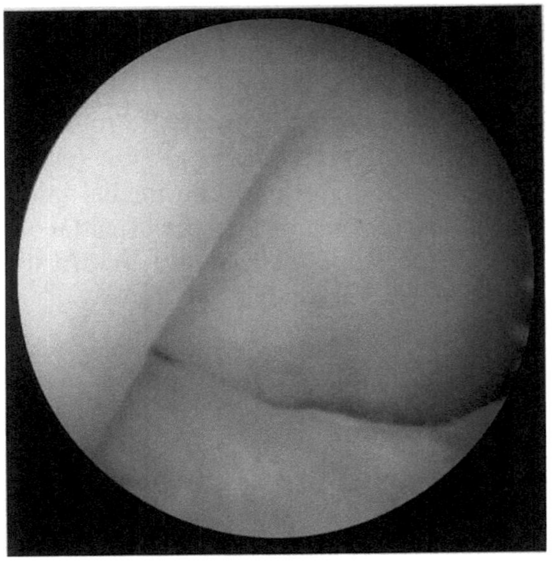

Fig. 8-63. Absence of the infrapatellar plica. The anterior cruciate ligament is directly visualized at the front of the intercondylar notch

In rare cases the infrapatellar plica persists as a complete septumlike structure (Fig. 8-64), making it difficult to demonstrate and identify the anterior cruciate ligament. As a rule, however, the plica forms an isolated fold having no attachment to the cruciate ligament (Figs. 8-65 and 8-66).

The infrapatellar plica shows great morphologic diversity, and bandlike forms can easily be mistaken for the anterior cruciate ligament by an inexperienced examiner (Fig. 8-66).

To visualize the infrapatellar plica and distinguish it from the anterior cruciate ligament, the light post is positioned at 5:00 (7:00 in the left knee) to demonstrate the origin of the presumed anterior cruciate ligament. If the structure arises from the front of the roof of the intercondylar notch, it must be the infrapatellar plica. The anterior cruciate ligament is located by retracting the arthroscope slightly to place the scope tip lateral to the plica. The anterior cruciate ligament lies farther posteriorly and courses at a flatter angle than one would expect. When the knee is flexed 90°, the ligament recedes far into the joint and lies almost parallel to the tibial plateau, whereas the infrapatellar plica forms a column-like structure connecting the anterior roof of the intercondylar notch with the infrapatellar fat pad (Fig. 8-66).

Pathologic Findings

Unlike the medial patellar plica (see Sect. 8.5.1), the infrapatellar plica is not known to undergo pathologic changes lead-

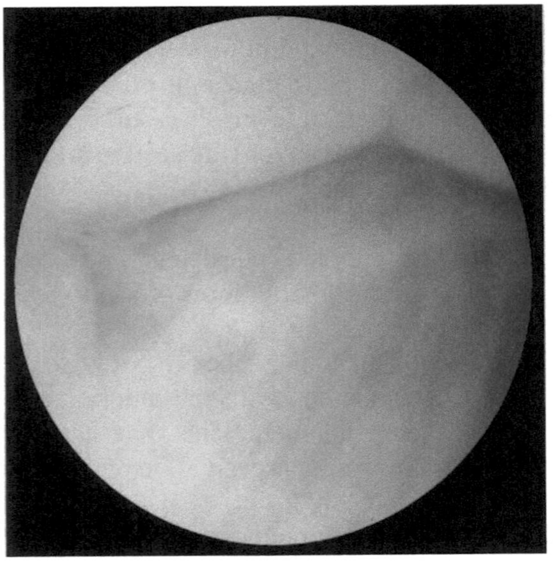

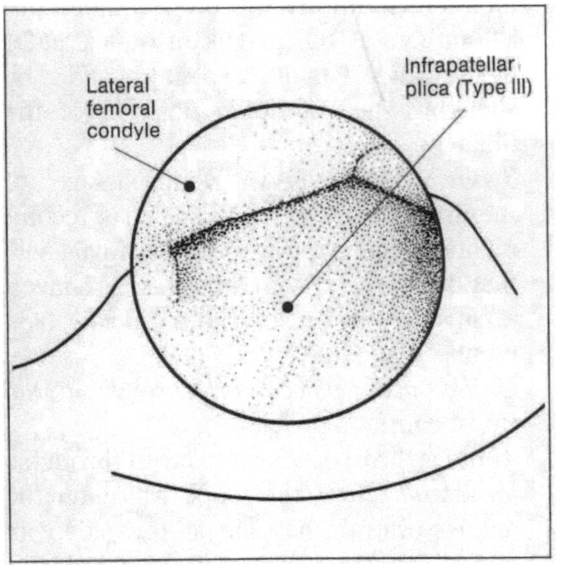

Fig. 8-64. Septum-like (type III) infrapatellar plica. The anterior cruciate ligament is not visible

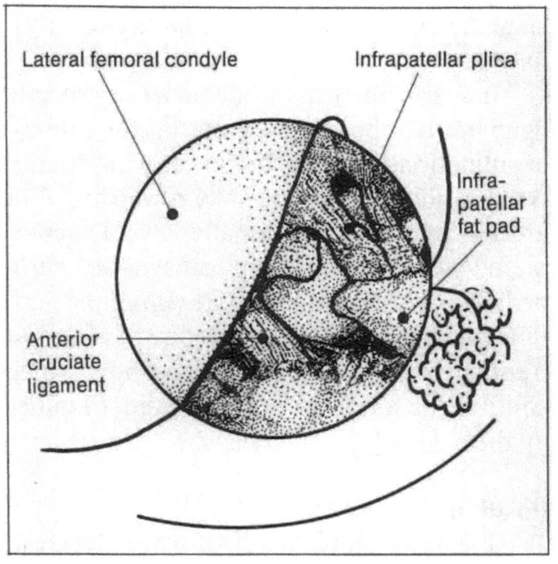

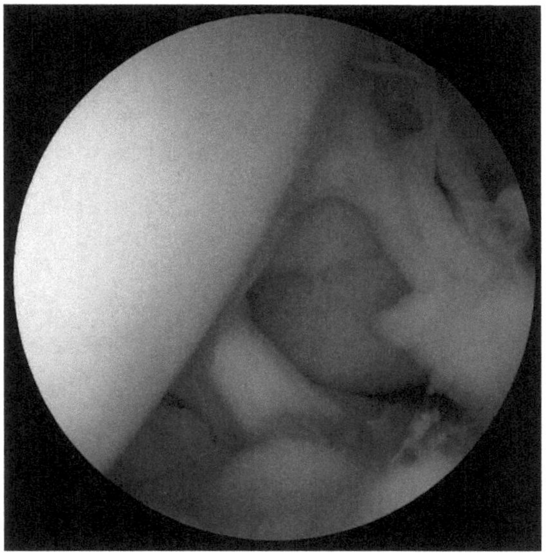

Fig. 8-65. The type I infrapatellar plica is readily distinguished from the anterior cruciate ligament

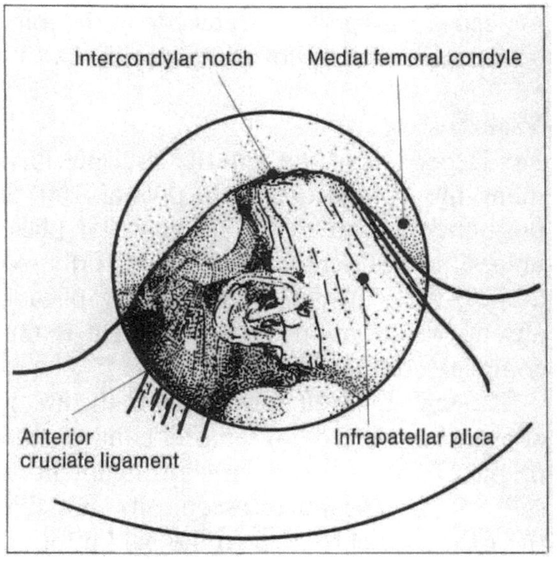

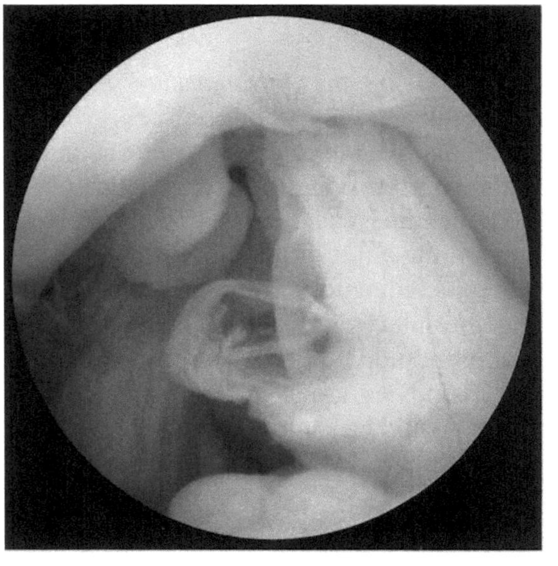

Fig. 8-66. Well-developed bandlike (type I) infrapatellar plica. The anterior cruciate ligament appears in the background

ing to clinical symptoms. However, isolated tears of the infrapatellar plica can occur and may cause hemarthrosis (Fig. 8-67).

Problems

The following measures are helpful in cases where the infrapatellar plica hampers inspection of the anterior cruciate ligament:

- *Creation of a medial instrument portal,* through which the plica can be pulled medially with a probing hook.
- *Sweeping the arthroscope from laterally* to medially toward the anterior cruciate ligament. The slow medial sweep of the scope "loads" the plica onto the sheath and displaces it anteromedially.

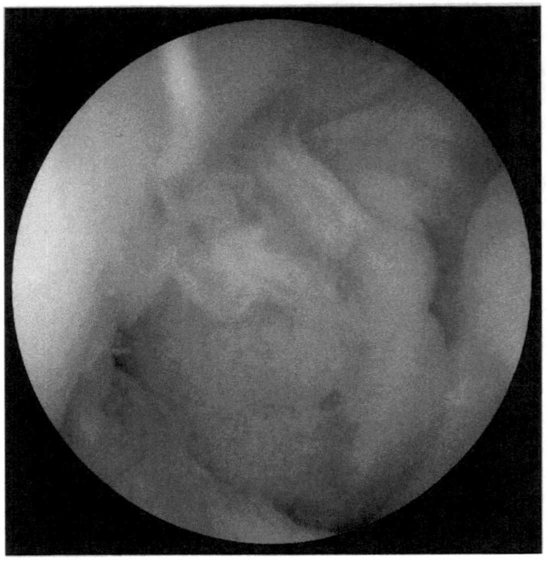

Fig. 8-67. Isolated tear of the infrapatellar plica as a cause of hemarthrosis

- *Removal of the infrapatellar plica.* In doubtful cases, a higher priority is given to evaluation of the anterior cruciate ligament than to preserving the infrapatellar plica. When there is coexisting synovial hypertrophy in the anterior intercondylar area and there is a diagnostic rationale for evaluating the anterior cruciate ligament, synovectomy should be performed in the anterior intercondylar area, and the infrapatellar plica should be removed. If the plica hampers visualization or access for arthroscopic surgery in the lateral compartment, it is partially or completely removed. Removal of the plica is also indicated to improve visualization for arthroscopic cruciate ligament reconstuctions.

8.7.3 Anterior Cruciate Ligament

When we consider the extremely important stabilizing function of the anterior cruciate ligament in the slightly flexed or extended knee, and the frequency of complete and incomplete tears of this ligament, we can appreciate the importance of its differentiated evaluation.

The basic integrity of the anterior cruciate ligament can be assessed during the clinical examination—the Lachman test and end-point resilience are especially rewarding. But arthroscopy can additionally reveal incomplete tears of the ligament, subsynovial hemorrhage, and the approximate age of the tear. Unexplained hemarthrosis is one of the most frequent indications for arthroscopy, which confirms an anterior cruciate ligament injury in more than 60% of cases.

Position

The knee is slightly flexed. The joint is flexed to approximately 60° for inspecting the origin of the anterior cruciate ligament. Usually the knee will be somewhat less flexed when positioned on the table surface than when flexed over the table edge. Greater degrees of flexion cause the ligament to recede in the joint and assume a more horizontal position.

Visualization

For inspection of the anterior cruciate ligament, the arthroscope (light post at 3:00) is positioned lateral to the infrapatellar plica, unless the ligament can be satisfactorily examined from the medial side. If the plica is absent, visualization of the ligament is uncomplicated (Fig. 8-68).

Though sited well posteriorly on the medial aspect of the lateral femoral condyle, the origin of the anterior cruciate ligament is still easy to assess arthroscopically. For this the light post is rotated to the 5:00 position (Fig. 8-68). Flexion of the knee makes the site easier to inspect.

Normal Findings

The anterior cruciate ligament is covered with synovium anteriorly, a consequence of the anterior migration of the ligament during its ontogenic development. Thus the ligament is intraarticular and extrasynovial (retrosynovial). Fine blood vessels can be seen beneath the thin synovium (Fig. 8-69). Sometimes even the fibrous structure of the ligament can be discerned (Fig. 8-70).

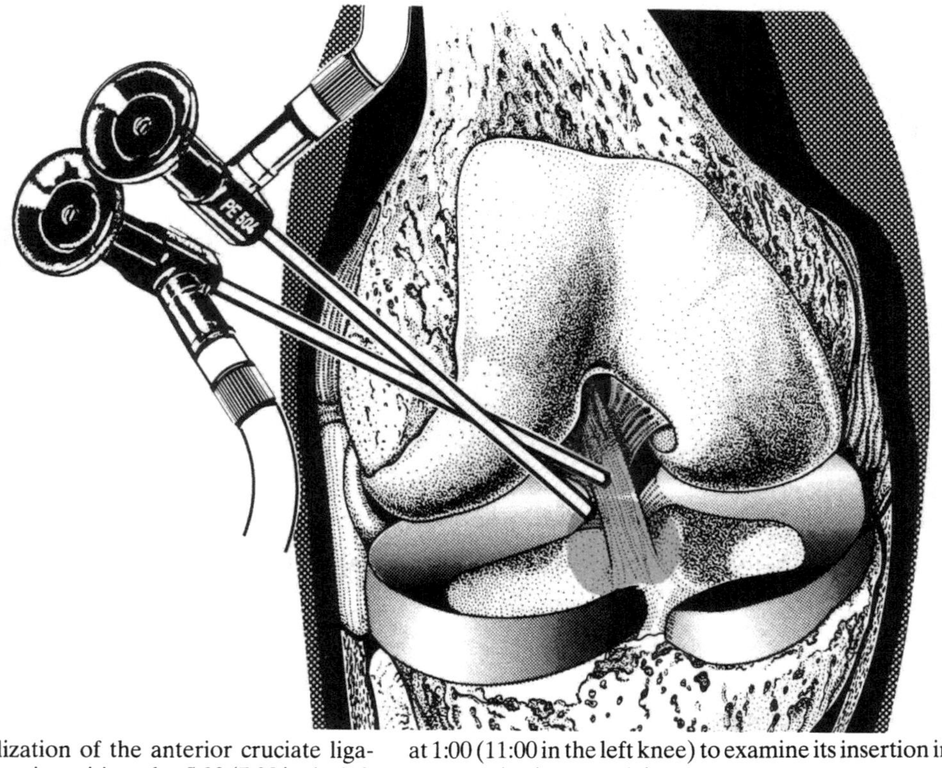

Fig. 8-68. Visualization of the anterior cruciate ligament. The light post is positioned at 5:00 (7:00 in the left knee) to inspect the femoral origin of the ligament and at 1:00 (11:00 in the left knee) to examine its insertion in the anterior intercondylar area

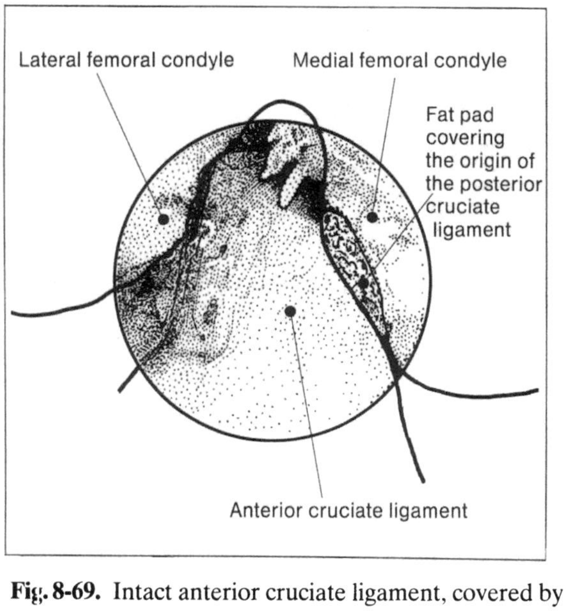

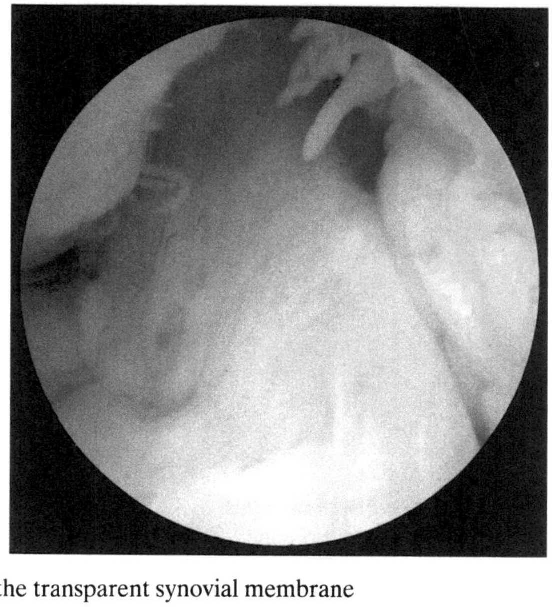

Fig. 8-69. Intact anterior cruciate ligament, covered by the transparent synovial membrane

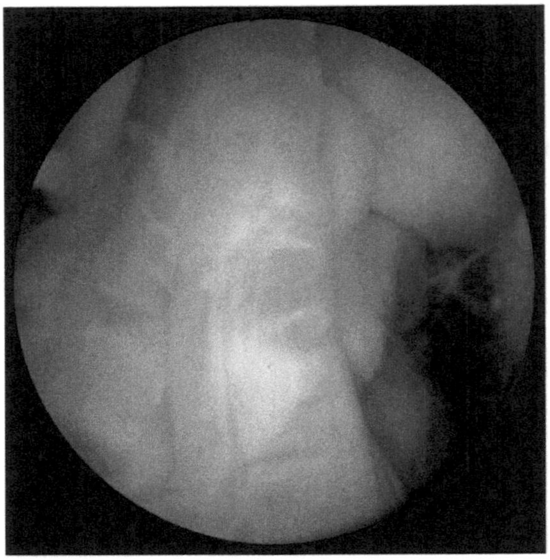

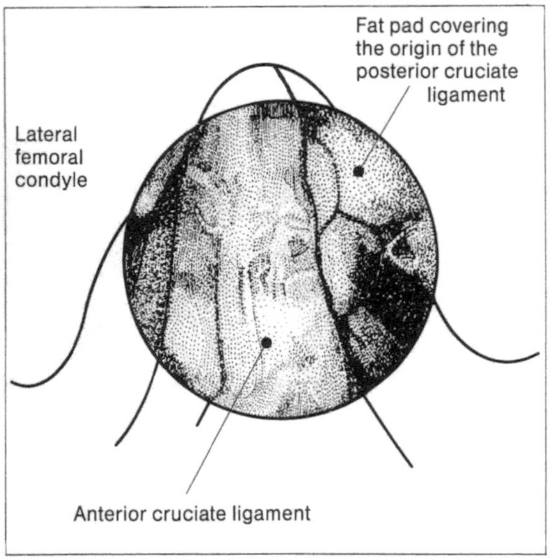

Fig. 8-70. Fibrous structure of the intact anterior cruciate ligament

Pathologic Findings

Abnormalities of the anterior cruciate ligament range from sites of bloody imbibition in the synovial membrane (Fig. 8-71) to diffuse subsynovial hemorrhages (Fig. 8-72) to recent and old complete ruptures and incomplete tears (Fig. 8-73). Particular attention should be given to the course of the cruciate ligament.

In cases where a rupture has been managed conservatively, the anterior cruciate ligament may drape over the posterior cruciate ligament and become attached to it, acquiring a new origin. Inspected arthroscopically, the ligament may appear normal initially, and even its course may appear unremarkable. But selective inspection of its site of origin on

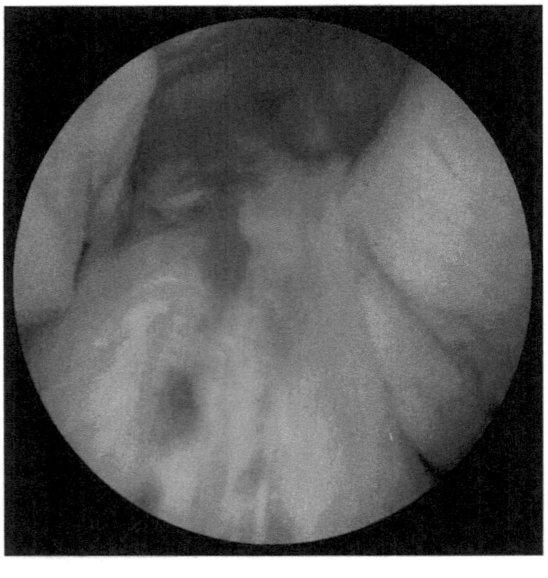

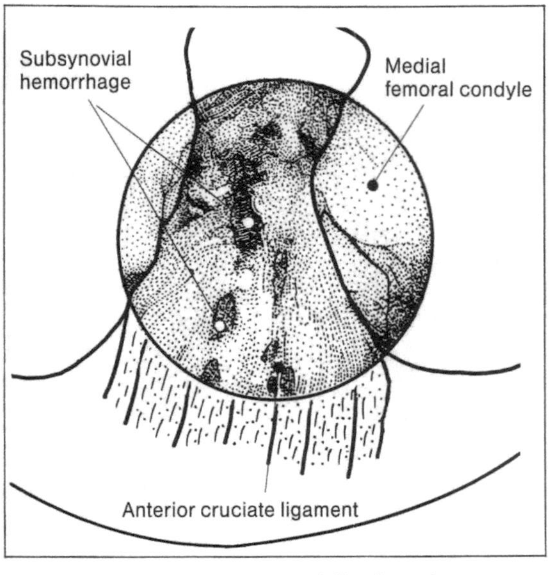

Fig. 8-71. Bloody imbibition of the synovial investment of the anterior cruciate ligament following a hyperextension injury

the medial surface of the lateral femoral condyle will reveal that the ligament has been torn from its proximal attachment. Probing is useful in these cases to demonstrate the draped position of the anterior cruciate ligament over the posterior cruciate and its attachment to it.

Several determinations are important with regard to further treatment planning:

Complete or Incomplete Tear. Incomplete tears usually do not require operative treatment, so it is important to distinguish them from complete ruptures (Fig. 8-73). Small rents in the synovium covering the cruciate ligament may provide subtle evidence of a complete or incomplete tear (Fig. 8-72). Additional information is furnished by palpation with the probing hook. Sometimes the entire stump of the torn ligament will protrude from its synovial sheath through a small slit in the synovium. This form of injury underlies cases where an acutely torn anterior cruciate ligament gives a positive Lachman test but causes no posttraumatic hemarthrosis. Hemarthrosis is frequently seen with acute anterior cruciate ligament ruptures, but it need not be present.

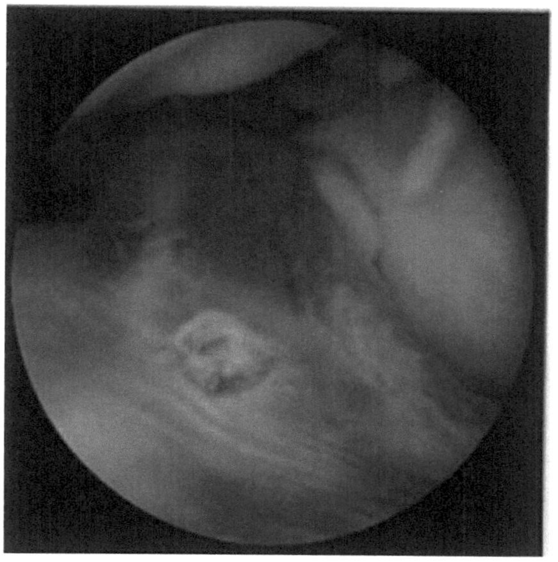

Fig. 8-72. Diffuse subsynovial hemorrhage about the tibial insertion of the anterior cruciate ligament (light post at 1:00) with perforation of the synovium

Location of the Tear. The ligament may be ruptured in its proximal, middle, or distal portion. Osseous involvement is possible distally and proximally (very rare) (Fig. 8-74). While proximal and distal tears are amenable to primary repair, possibly combined with augmen-

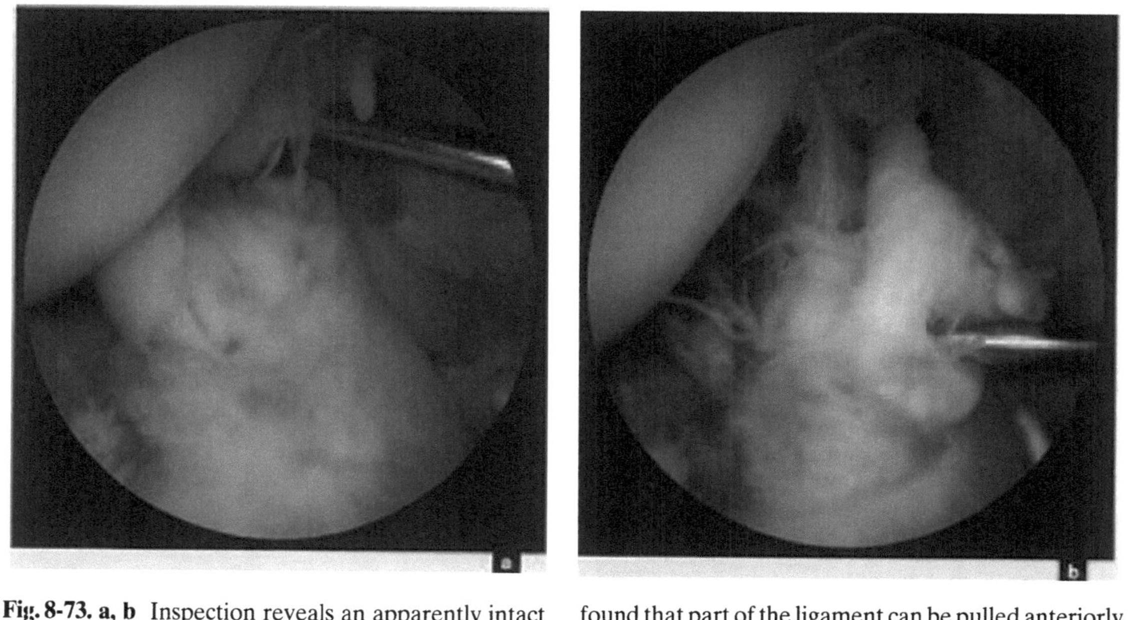

Fig. 8-73. a, b Inspection reveals an apparently intact anterior cruciate ligament (**a**). But on probing it is found that part of the ligament can be pulled anteriorly with the probe, signifying an incomplete tear (**b**)

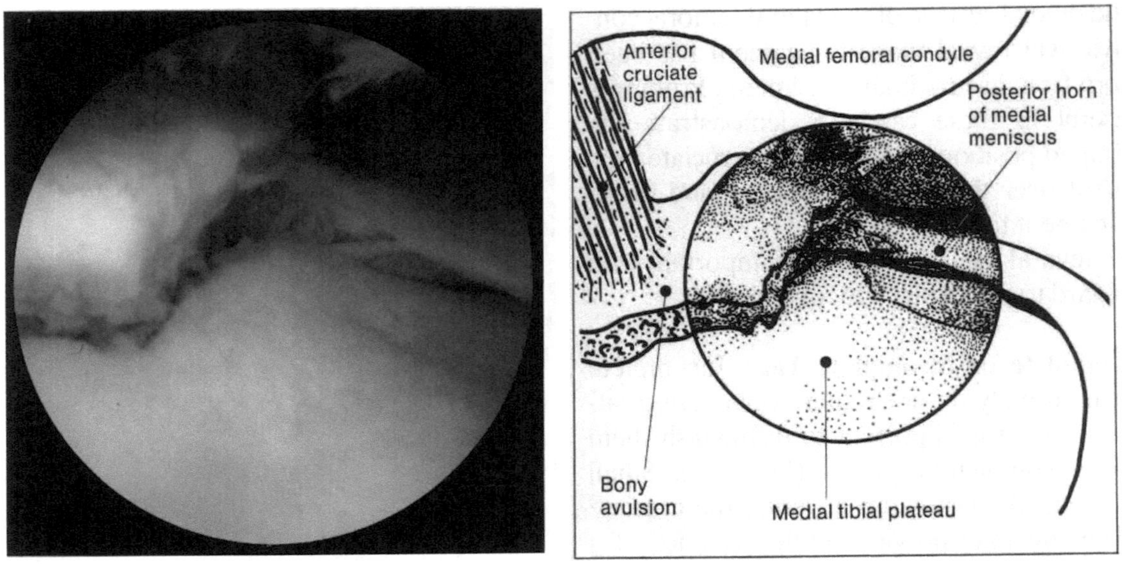

Fig. 8-74. Distal bony avulsion of the anterior cruciate ligament

tation, simple suture repair is not indicated for midsubstance tears due to the relatively poor blood flow to that part of the ligament.

Complex ruptures are also seen, i.e., injuries in which one part of the ligament is torn proximally and the other distally.

In acute injuries, the exact rupture site is determined by probing once the intercondylar area has been cleared of coagulated blood and enlarged synovial villi, and a satisfactory instrument portal has been created.

Age of the Rupture. The acutely ruptured ligament typically presents a horsetail-like fraying of fibers at the torn ends (Fig. 8-75). As the rupture ages, degenerative changes in

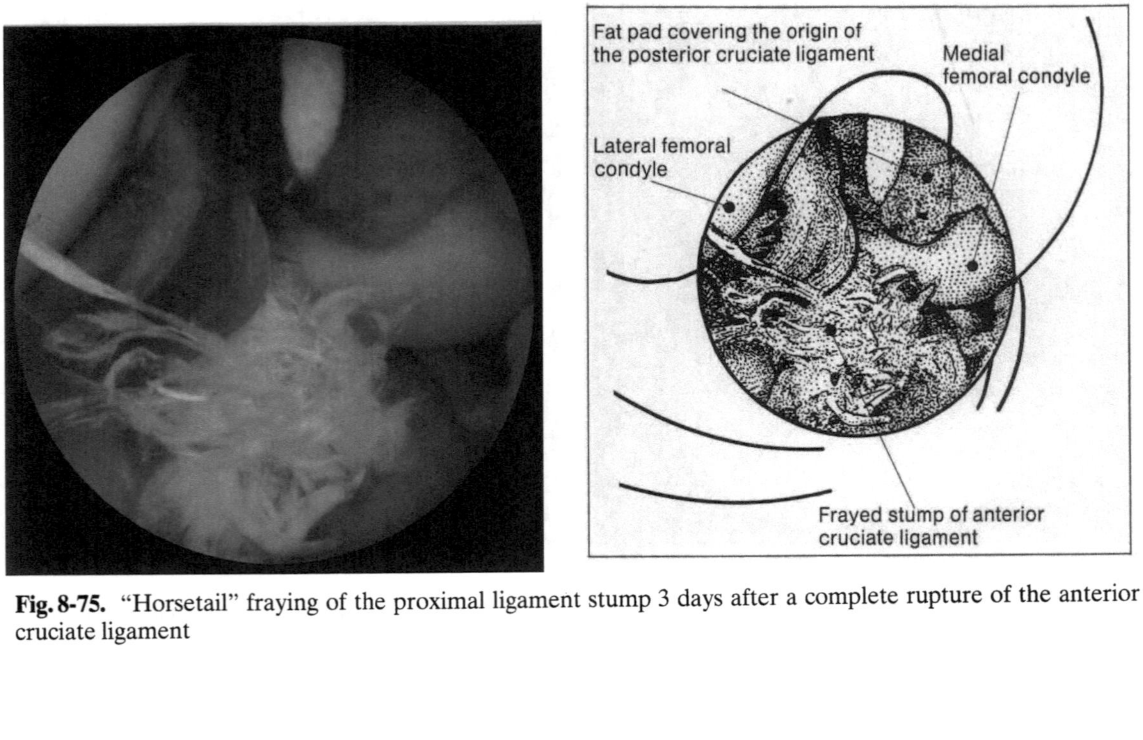

Fig. 8-75. "Horsetail" fraying of the proximal ligament stump 3 days after a complete rupture of the anterior cruciate ligament

the ligament become more pronounced, and the stump becomes rounded. The loss of stability at small flexion angles also causes preosteoarthritic and osteoarthritic changes to develop in other joint regions. After a few months the stumps of the cruciate ligament are thinned and tattered if they have been within the medial or lateral joint compartment. If the stump lies protected within the intercondylar notch, it acquires a stubby, distended appearance (Fig. 8-76).

In other cases arthroscopy performed years after an anterior cruciate rupture may show an empty intercondylar notch with no evidence of the ligament whatsoever (Fig. 8-77). The examiner looks directly at the posterior cruciate ligament.

When an anterior cruciate ligament injury has been diagnosed, a decision must be made with regard to further treatment. Small stumps from an old rupture that do not affect joint mechanics are left alone, since they can guide the surgeon in placing the drill holes for a subsequent open or arthroscopic anterior cruciate ligament reconstruction. Also, most of the proprioceptors in the ligament occur in its proximal and distal portions. Coexisting meniscal injuries often can be treated (by repair or partial meniscectomy) in the same sitting.

During follow-up arthroscopy performed 6–12 months after a cruciate ligament reconstruction, particular attention is given to the synovial investment of the substitute ligament (autologous or alloplastic material), the synovial reaction in surrounding areas (irritative synovitis), and the intercondylar notch (hazardous osteophytes).

Problems

Various factors can make it difficult to visualize the origin of the anterior cruciate ligament:

- *Osteophytic projections* on the roof of the intercondylar notch or on the anteromedial

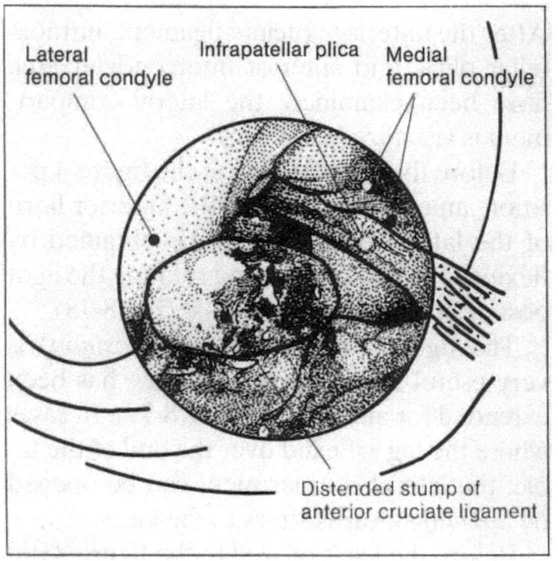

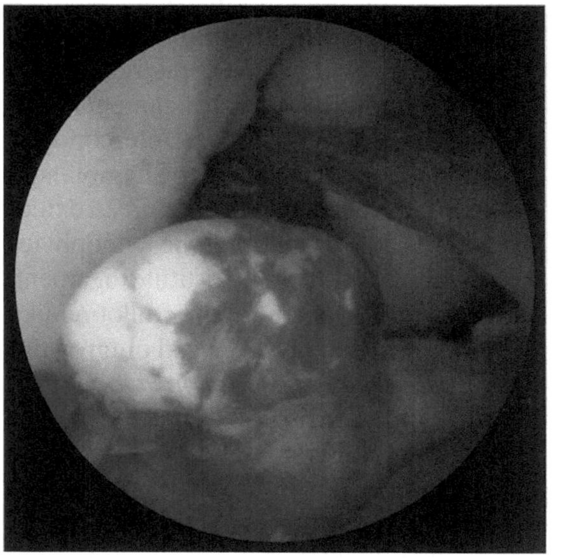

Fig. 8-76. Old rupture of the anterior cruciate ligament.
History: Since sustaining a rotational knee injury 5 weeks ago while playing soccer, the patient, an 18-year-old female, has experienced intermittent locking and pain with mild episodes of giving way.
Arthroscopic findings: Partial rupture of the anterior cruciate ligament (anteromedial fibers). Portions of the posterolateral bundle are still intact. The intercondylar area contains a stubby structure thinly coated with blood. This is not a "tumor" but the distended, clublike anteromedial bundle of the anterior cruciate ligament. The blood results from intermittent catching of the stump between the articular surfaces, which accounts for the patient's symptoms (meniscus-like locking).
Procedure: Arthroscopic removal of the cruciate ligament stump. If a feeling of instability persists, anterior cruciate reconstruction is indicated

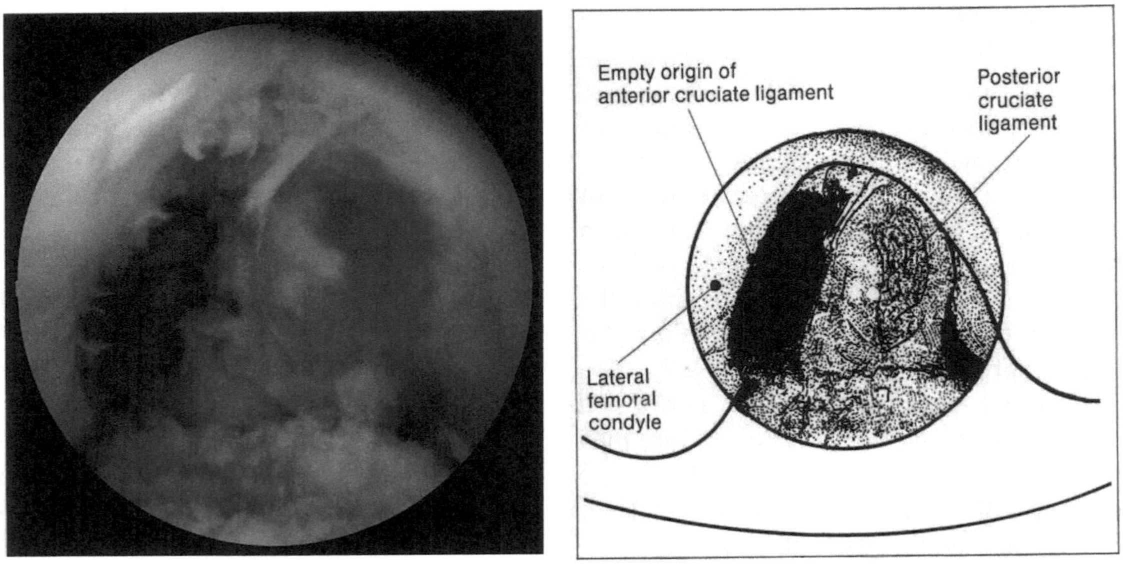

Fig. 8-77. Empty intercondylar notch following an old rupture of the anterior cruciate ligament

border of the lateral femoral condyle. Removal of these osteophytes is indicated when necessary for evaluation of the anterior cruciate ligament. Removal is also indicated to protect the normal anterior cruciate ligament from the (often sharp) bony outgrowths, or if arthroscopic reconstruction of the anterior cruciate ligament is proposed. Osteophytes in the intercondylar notch pose a special threat to an implanted alloplastic cruciate ligament. Forced extension of the knee can bring the osteophytes into contact with the substitute ligament, exposing the ligament to the guillotine-like shredding action of the jagged outgrowths.

- *Arthroscope portal is positioned too far laterally.* The arthroscope, deflected by the lateral femoral condyle, cannot enter the intercondylar notch. It may be possible to insert the scope through a medial parapatellar instrument portal. Whenever there is an inquiry concerning the anterior cruciate ligament, or arthroscopic surgery on the ligament is planned, the arthroscope portal should be placed very close to the patellar ligament.

8.8 Moving the Leg to the Figure-4 Position

After the anterior cruciate ligament, infrapatellar plica, and anterior intercondylar area have been examined, the lateral compartment is visualized.

Before the leg is moved to the figure-4 position, an excellent view of the anterior horn of the lateral meniscus can be obtained by flexing the knee slightly and rotating the light post of the arthroscope to 2:00 (Fig. 8-78).

The figure-4 position (*Glinz position*) is very useful in cases where the leg has been extended for arthroscopy (Fig. 8-79). In cases where the leg is flexed over the end of the table, the lateral compartment can be opened by applying a varus stress to the knee.

Before the leg is moved to the figure-4 position, the examiner trains the arthroscope on the lateral triangle bounded caudally by the lateral tibial plateau, cranially by the lateral femoral condyle, and medially by the anterior cruciate ligament (Fig. 8-80). The light post is at 2:00.

The leg is moved slowly and carefully, always keeping the lateral triangle in view on

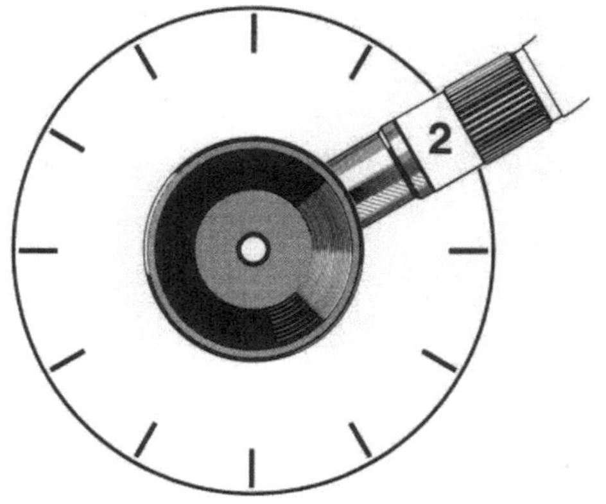

Fig. 8-78. The light post is positioned at 2:00 (10:00 in the left knee) for viewing the anterior horn of the lateral meniscus. It is then rotated to 3:00 (9:00 in the left knee) to visualize the triangle formed by the anterior cruciate ligament, lateral tibial plateau, and lateral femoral condyle before the leg is moved to the figure-4 position

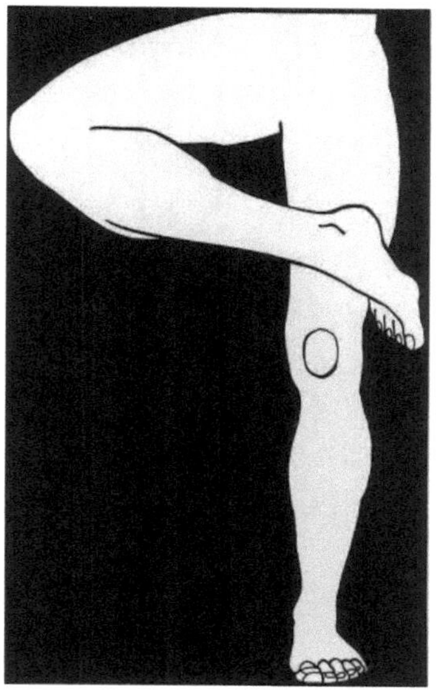

Fig. 8-79. The figure-4 position for arthroscopic examination of the lateral compartment

the monitor. Once the the figure-4 position is reached, the scope will automatically be trained on the posterior horn of the lateral meniscus.

Resting the ankle of the leg to be examined on the contralateral thigh exerts a sufficient varus pressure to open up the lateral joint compartment for examination (Fig. 8-81). The joint space, tilted by the positioning maneuver, is realigned on the monitor by rotating the video camera relative to the telescope.

Problems

- *Loss of visualization of the lateral triangle during repositioning (common!).* The main rule to follow when moving the leg to the figure-4 position is to guide the arthroscope

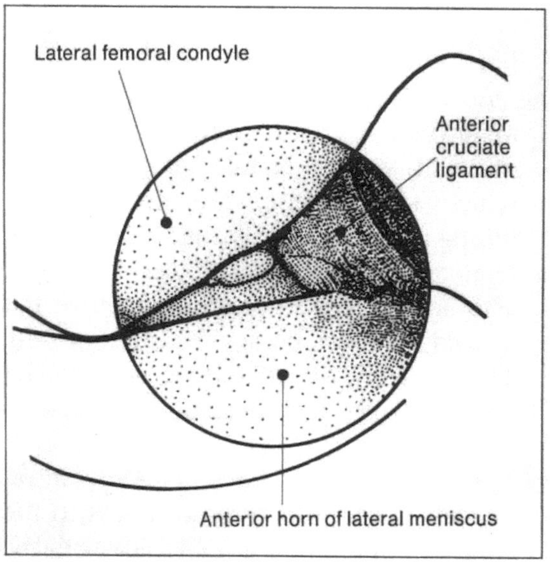

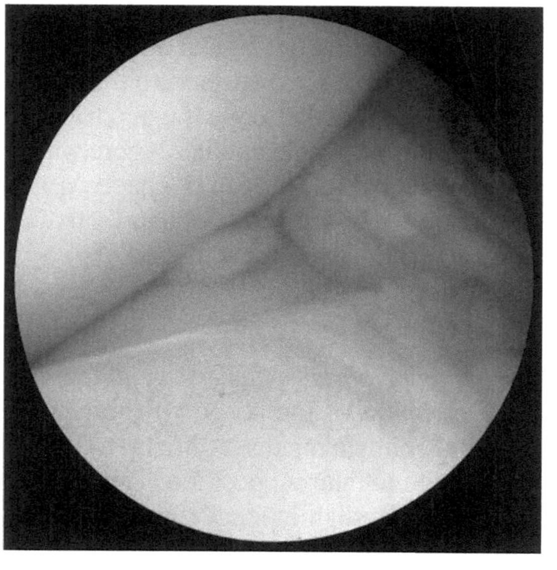

Fig. 8-80. Visualization of the lateral triangle

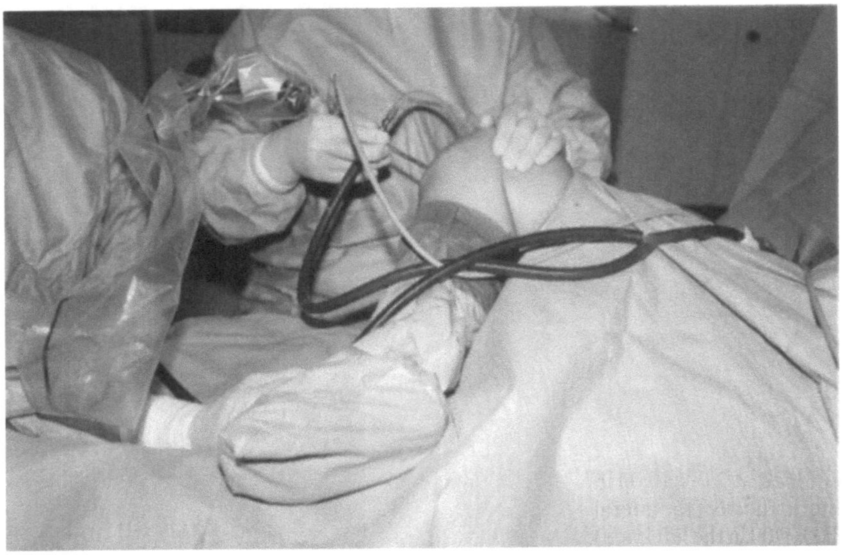

Fig. 8-81. With the leg in the figure-4 position, manual pressure is exerted to open up the lateral compartment

carefully and keep the lateral triangle in view. The long lever arms that become active when the leg is moved to the figure-4 position (often the lower leg is grasped at the level of the ankle joint) can easily lead to severe iatrogenic cartilage damage unless the arthroscope is expertly handled while the knee is moved.

The examiner must follow the movements of the leg with the arthroscope. It is all too easy for the scope to stray laterally or caudally, so that the tip apposes to the anterior horn of the lateral meniscus. From there the lateral compartment cannot be visualized, and a yellow-out is seen on the monitor. The leg must be returned to the original position, and the scope is again trained on the lateral triangle and kept there while the leg is moved. This can be made easier by resting the arthroscope hand on the knee while the leg is repositioned.
The lateral triangle is constantly kept in view as the leg is repositioned.

- *Arthroscope portal is placed too far laterally*. Deflection of the scope by the lateral femoral condyle makes it difficult to move the leg to the figure-4 position. This can be alleviated by slightly lengthening the incision in the fibrous capsule to gain more room for maneuvering.
- *Difficult or obstructed access to the lateral compartment.*

• *Adhesions.* Adhesions in the area of the lateral triangle and anterior intercondylar area are not an uncommon sequel to knee operations or hemarthrosis. Adhesive bands are held aside (probing hook) or, if necessary, divided (punch).
• *Synovial hypertrophy.* Synovitis or hypertrophy of the infrapatellar fat pad makes it difficult to visualize the lateral triangle and reposition the knee. Motorized instruments can be used to perform a partial synovectomy in the anterior part of the joint before the leg is moved to the figure-4 position.
• *Discoid meniscus.* A rare lateral discoid meniscus (incidence approximately 0.5%) or a lateral bucket-handle fragment can obstruct vision into the lateral compartment during repositioning. The lateral tibial plateau cannot be visualized (see Fig. 8-85). The arthroscope is positioned above the discoid meniscus before the leg is moved. The surface of the discoid meniscus can be inspected once the repositioning maneuver is complete.
• *Large infrapatellar plica.* A large infrapatellar plica that obstructs access to the lateral compartment is held aside with the probing hook or, if necessary, divided. In

most cases, however, the infrapatellar plica does not interfere with repositioning.

- *Meniscal flap or cruciate ligament bundle in the anterior intercondylar area.* Rarely a meniscal flap (Fig. 8-82) or torn cruciate ligament bundle (Fig. 8-76) becomes displaced into the lateral triangle. These structures can get in front of the scope tip as the leg is repositioned. The scope can either be maneuvered past the meniscal flap, or the flap can be pushed into the lateral compartment with a probe.
- *Anterior cruciate ligament insufficiency.* This results in excessive lateral joint mobility. As the leg is moved to the figure-4 position, this permits a twisting of the joint members so that the lateral joint space appears significantly narrower. The assistant immobilizes the lower leg to prevent this twisting while simultaneously pulling the upper tibia forward (anterior drawer test).

8.9 Lateral Compartment

The anterior horn of the lateral meniscus is examined in the initial extended leg position, while the central portion and posterior horn of the meniscus are examined in the figure-4 position. The anterior portions of the lateral femoral condyle are evaluated in the initial position (light post at 4:00), in alternating positions of flexion and extension, and also in the figure-4 position.

8.9.1 Lateral Meniscus

Position
Figure-4 position.

Visualization
When the figure-4 position is reached, the arthroscope is trained directly on the posterior horn of the lateral meniscus (light post at 3:00) (Fig. 8-83). A good overview of the lateral meniscus is obtained by carefully retracting and rotating the scope (to 1:00).

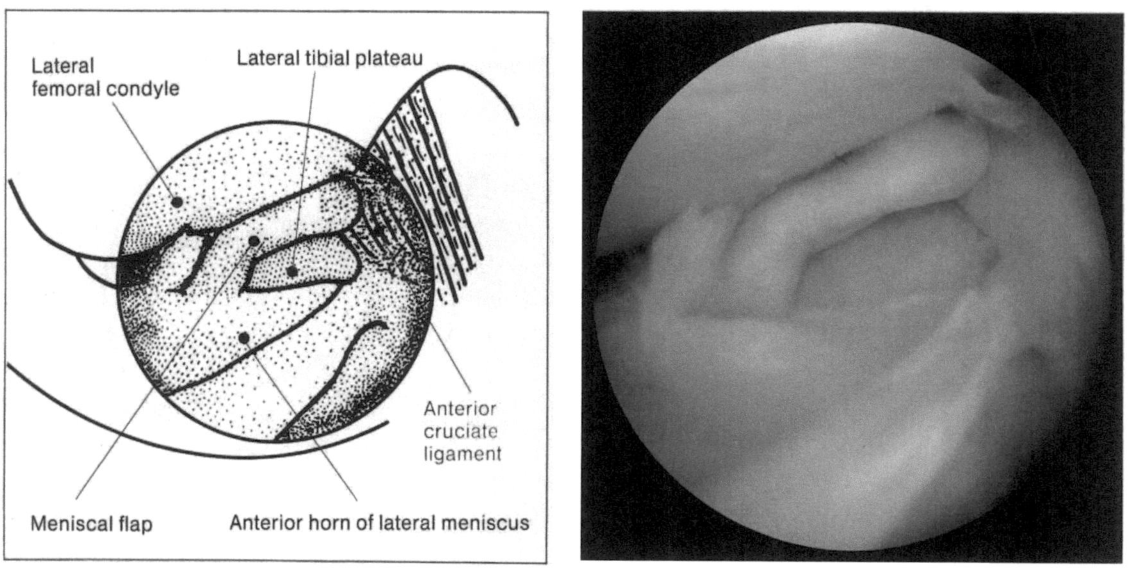

Fig. 8-82. Rounded meniscal flap displaced into the lateral triangle

Normal Findings

The intact meniscus presents a sharp inner border with slight undulations. Minor fraying does not necessitate treatment (Fig. 8-84). The posterior horn of the lateral meniscus may show irregularities, but these have no therapeutic implications. The greater mobility of the lateral meniscus relative to the medial meniscus will be noticed on probing.

In rare cases the lateral tibial plateau is not visualized due to the presence of a complete discoid meniscus (Fig. 8-85). The tibial plateau can be seen only if the discoid meniscus is incomplete or ruptured at its center. It can be difficult to get the scope past the typically distended anteromedial portion of the meniscus to gain entry to the lateral compartment, and the obstructing meniscal segment may have to be removed.

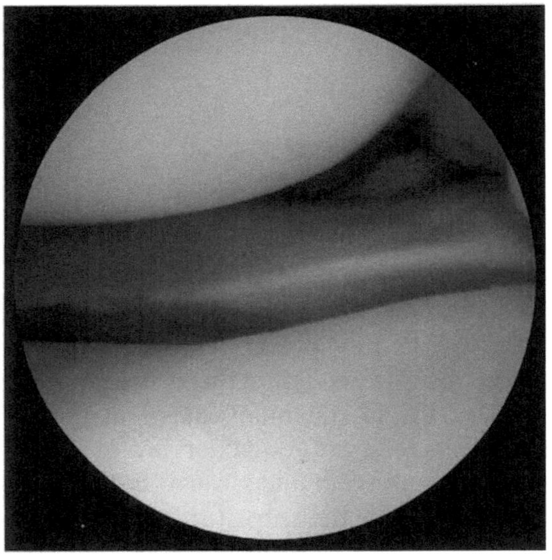

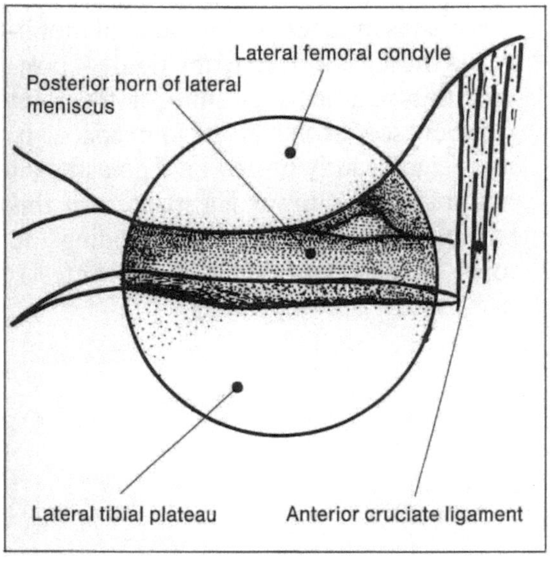

Fig. 8-83. Direct view of the posterior horn of the lateral meniscus with the leg in the figure-4 position

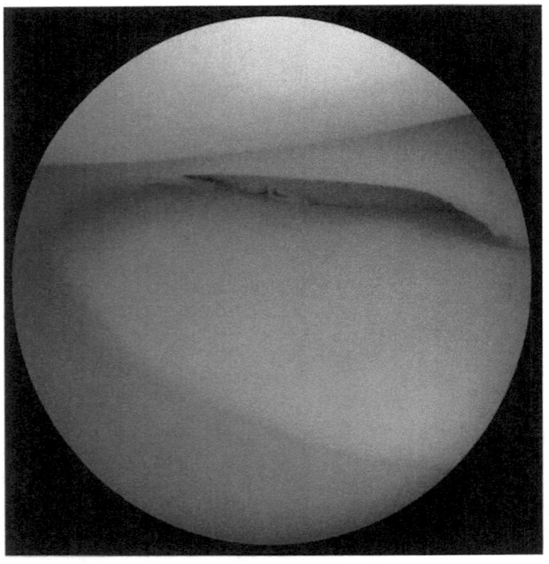

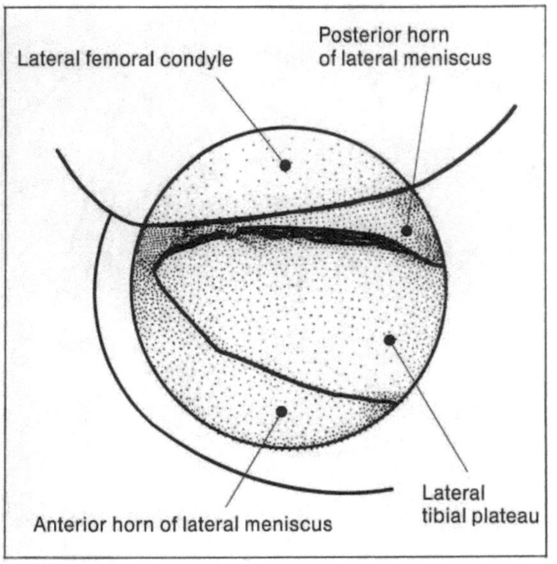

Fig. 8-84. Overview of the lateral meniscus (light post at 1:00, 11:00 in the left knee)

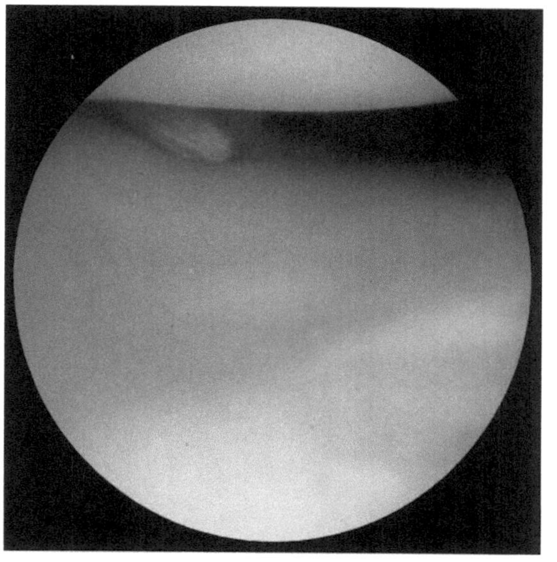

Fig. 8-85. Complete discoid meniscus covering all of the lateral tibial plateau. The popliteus tendon is visible in the background

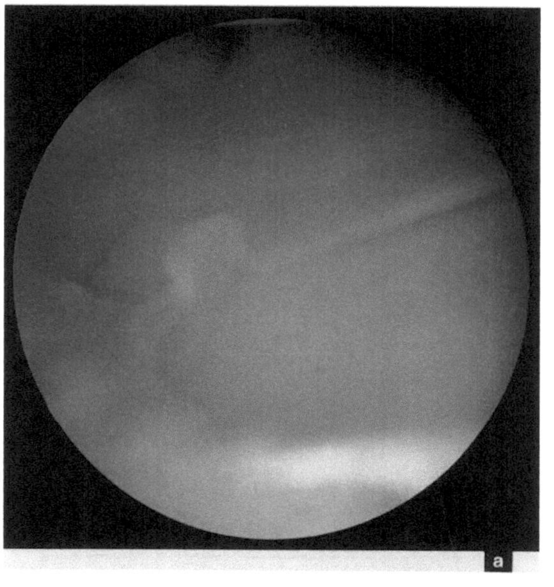

Fig. 8-86 a, b. Radial tear of the lateral meniscus. Inspection reveals increased undulation of the inner border of the meniscus (**a**). Probing uncovers a radial tear in that area (**b**)

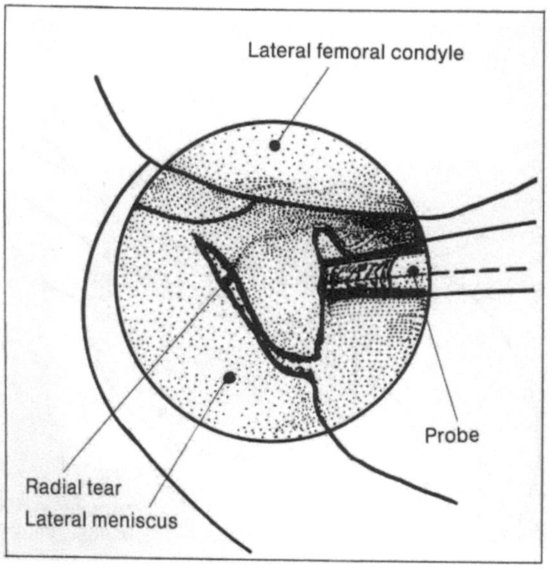

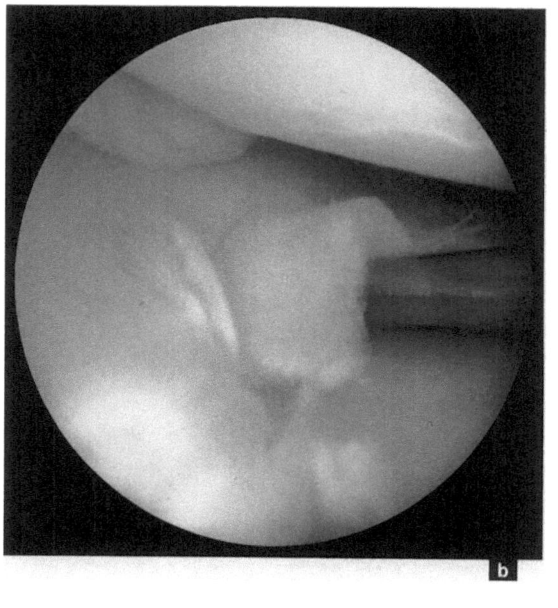

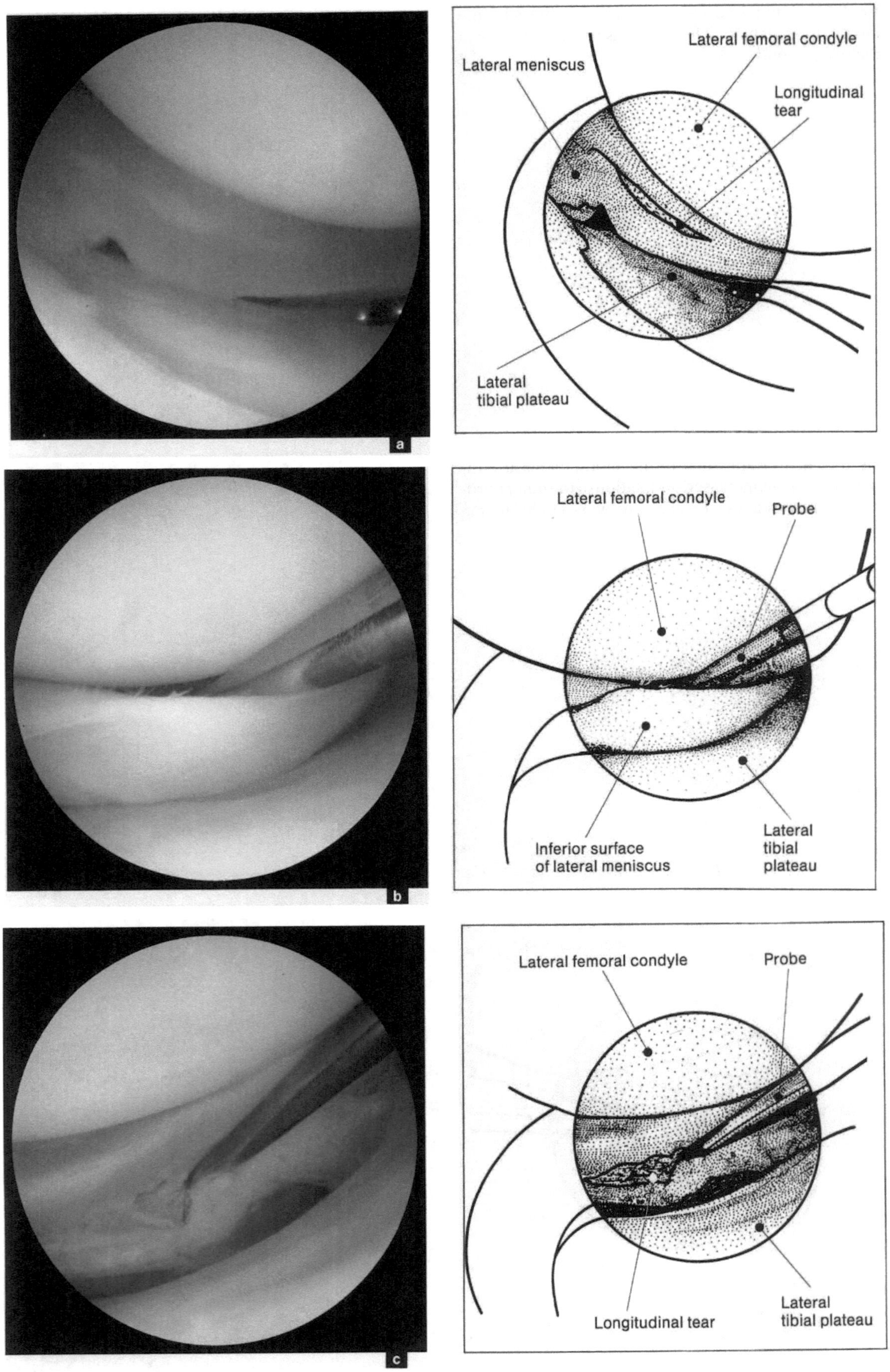
a
Lateral femoral condyle
Lateral meniscus
Longitudinal tear
Lateral tibial plateau
b
Lateral femoral condyle
Probe
Inferior surface of lateral meniscus
Lateral tibial plateau
c
Lateral femoral condyle
Probe
Longitudinal tear
Lateral tibial plateau

◀ **Fig. 8-87 a–c.** Longitudinal tear of the lateral meniscus.
History: A 21-year-old male sustained a knee injury 2 days ago with subsequent hemarthrosis. He has a positive Lachman test with a soft end point.
Arthroscopic findings: Longitudinal tear at the junction of the middle and posterior thirds of the lateral meniscus (**a**). Probing from above (**b**) and especially from below (**c**) is necessary to define the extent of the tear. A coexisting proximal rupture of the anterior cruciate ligament made it difficult to examine the lateral compartment. Probing of the meniscus from above and below is recommended in such cases. Submeniscal probing is essential for defining the extent of the longitudinal tear. The tear does not communicate with the popliteal hiatus.
Procedure: Repair and augmentation of the anterior cruciate ligament. The meniscal tear can be managed conservatively or possibly by arthroscopic repair. Secondary partial resection of the lateral meniscus is indicated if corresponding symptoms appear after the ligament heals and full weight bearing is resumed

Pathologic Findings

Like the medial meniscus, the lateral meniscus is evaluated for pathologic changes (see Sect. 8.6.1).

The typical lesion of the lateral meniscus is the radial tear. It may be hidden by an undulation in the meniscus and is easily overlooked. Probing is frequently necessary to exclude a radial tear (Fig. 8-86).

Longitudinal tears most frequently involve the posterior segment of the meniscus, as on the medial side (Figs. 8-87 and 8-91), but the middle and anterior portions may also be affected. Longitudinal meniscal tears are often combined with ruptures of the anterior cruciate ligament. The posterior horn of the lateral meniscus differs from its medial counterpart in that it is subject to complex tears and contusions. A ligamentum transversum passing into the anterior horn can easily be mistaken for a longitudinal tear.

The lateral meniscus is subject to the same types of degenerative change that affect the medial meniscus (see Sect. 8.6.1) (Fig. 8-88).

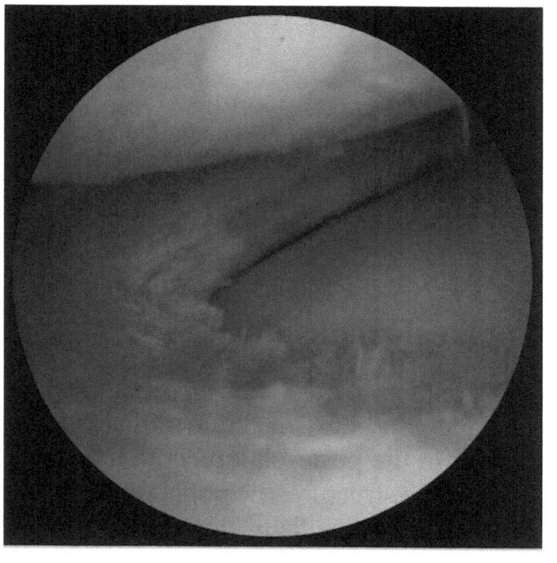

Fig. 8-88. Degenerative fraying of the inner border of the lateral meniscus and a transverse tear

8.9.2 Lateral Femorotibial Joint

All types and grades of cartilage pathology may be found in the lateral portion of the femorotibial joint (see Chap. 9 for details). Aside from proximal tibial fractures, traumatic injuries of the lateral tibial plateau are a rarity. It is more common to find secondary degenerative changes associated with injuries of adjacent structures (Fig. 8-89). Iatrogenic trauma may also be encountered (see Figs. 12-1 to 12-4).

Unlike the lateral tibial plateau, the lateral femoral condyle is a relatively frequent site for traumatic chondral and osteochondral fractures, most often caused by patellar dislocation (see Sect. 9.4.3). Degenerative changes are less common than on the medial side.

If loose bodies are present in the lateral compartment, the leg should be repositioned with particular care to avoid causing additional cartilage lesions. Loose bodies are occasionally lodged beneath the posterior horn of the lateral meniscus (Fig. 7-3). Sometimes they can be displaced into the visual field with the probing hook or by milking the posterolateral corner.

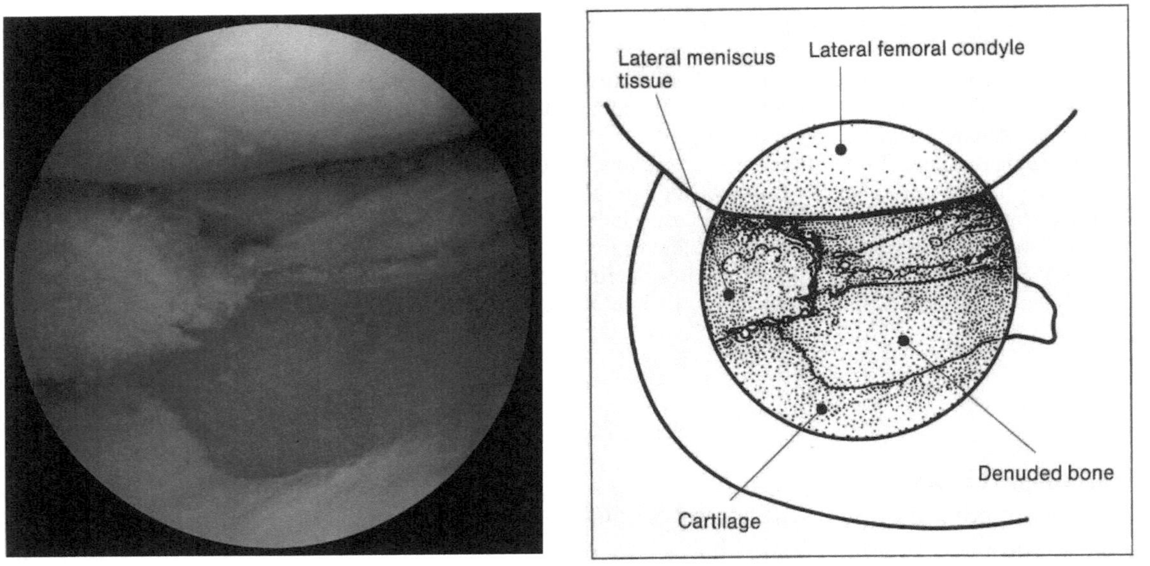

Fig. 8-89. Denuded bone area on the lateral tibial plateau and lateral femoral condyle in a patient with valgus deformity and degenerative arthritis

8.9.3 Popliteal Hiatus

The popliteal hiatus is an approximately 1-cm-wide gap between the meniscal rim and capsule in the posterolateral corner. A whitish cordlike structure, the popliteus tendon, is seen coursing medially downward through the hiatus (Fig. 8-90). When the lateral meniscus is examined, the popliteal hiatus should be explored with the probing hook to define its extent (Figs. 8-90 and 8-91). It may be lengthened as a result of trauma, or it may be involved in a longitudinal meniscal tear. Hemorrhagic areas in the popliteus tendon and meniscosynovial junction are a sign of acute injury.

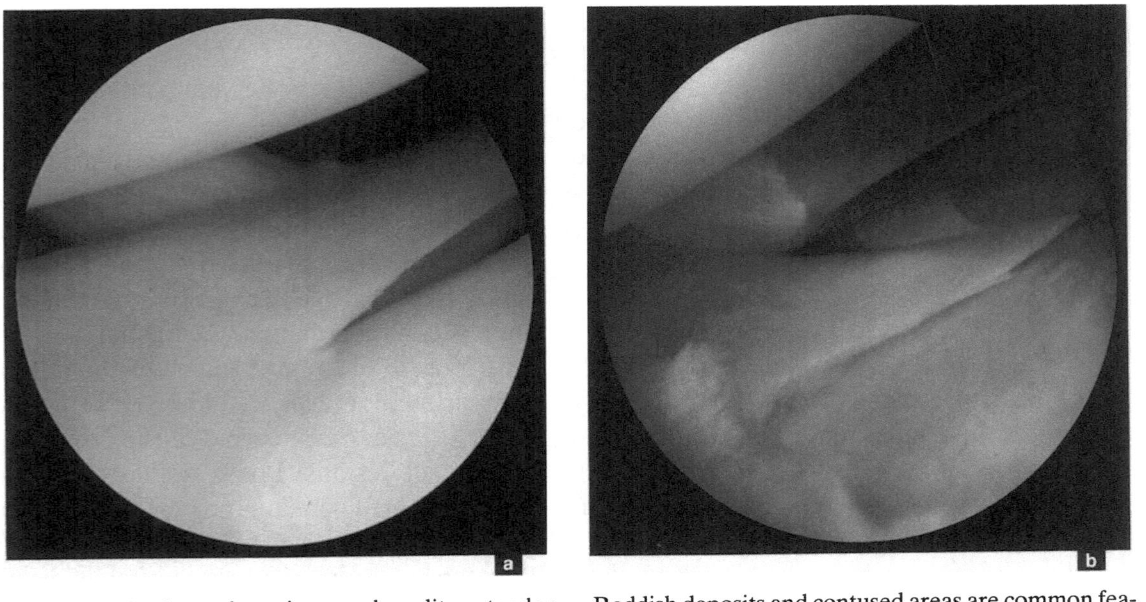

Fig. 8-90 a, b. Lateral meniscus and popliteus tendon (**a**). The popliteal hiatus is explored with the probe. Reddish deposits and contused areas are common features of acute injury (**b**)

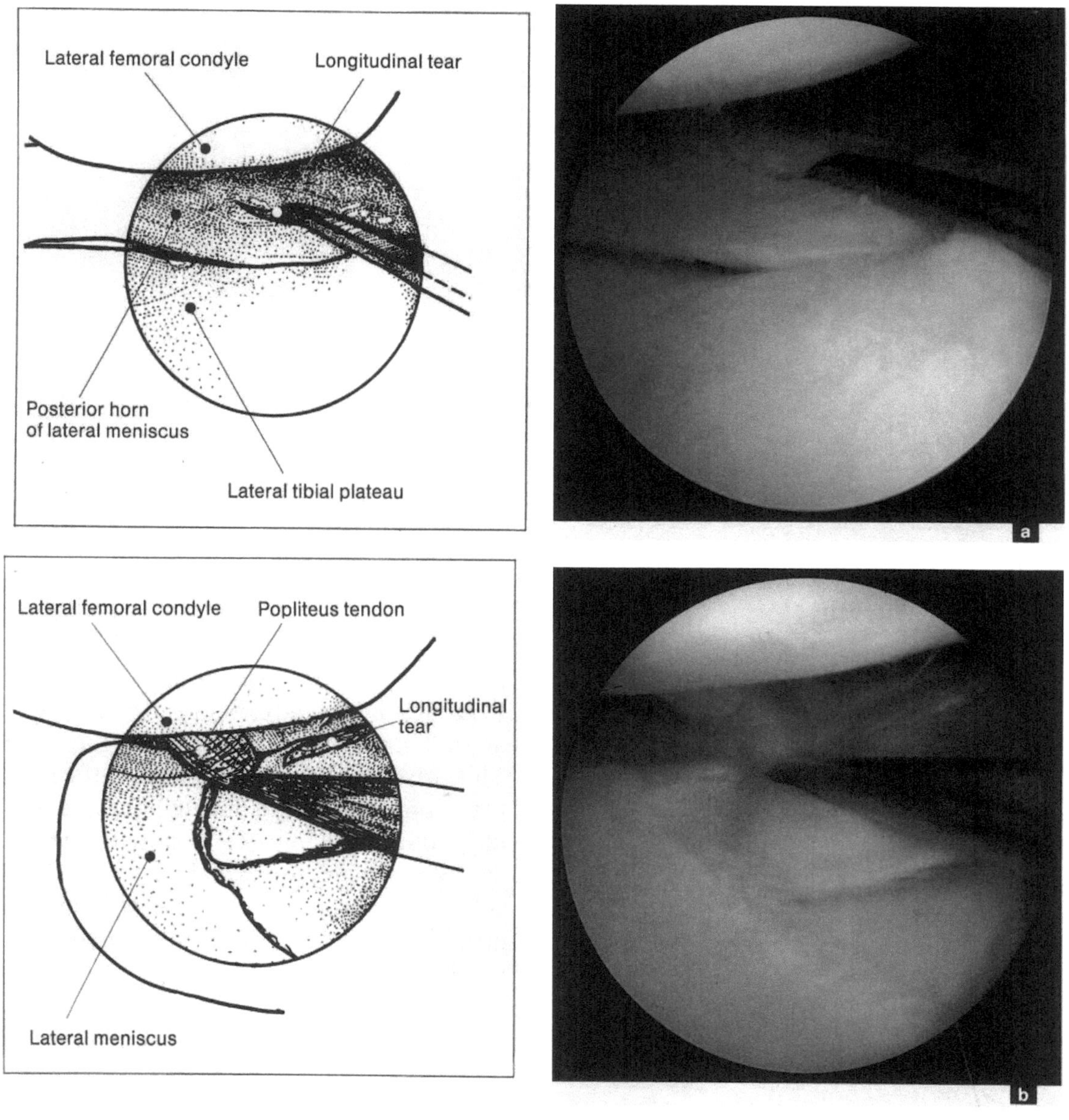

Fig. 8-91 a, b. Probing the posterior horn of the lateral meniscus reveals a longitudinal tear (**a**). The popliteal hiatus is then selectively probed to determine whether the tear communicates with the hiatus (**b**)

8.9.4 Posterolateral Recess

First the posterior horn of the lateral meniscus is visualized, then the arthroscope is advanced posteriorly, past the posterior horn of the lateral meniscus, into the posterolateral recess (Fig. 8-92). The light cable is moved to 5:00 (7:00 in the left knee).

The posterolateral recess may contain loose bodies, which occasionally are large (Fig. 8-93). Small bodies can be aspirated through the arthroscopic sheath with the telescope removed. Larger bodies can either be manually milked from the posterolateral recess or transfixed with a percutaneous needle and removed through an accessory posterolateral portal (avoiding injury to the peroneal nerve).

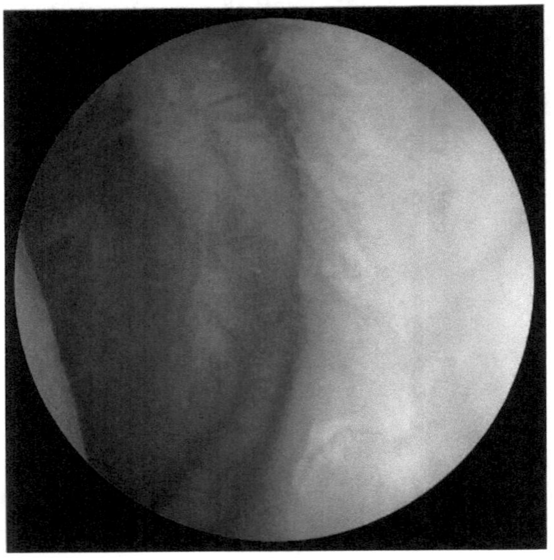

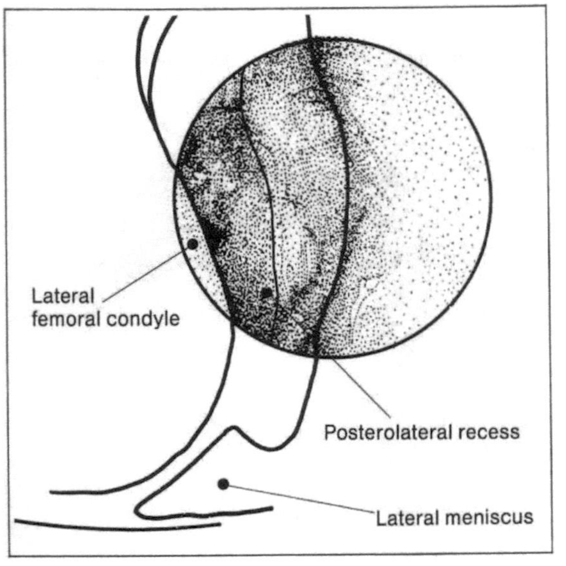

Fig. 8-92. Posterolateral recess

Problems

- *Torn anterior cruciate ligament* (see above).
- *Difficult probing.* The placement of the instrument portal is of key importance. A medial suprameniscal portal may be satisfactory. If there is significant osteophytosis or if the portal has been placed far medially or directly above the meniscal plane, the probe will be deflected toward the lateral femoral condyle and cannot enter the lateral joint space (*ramp effect,* see Fig. 6-21). This is avoided by moving the leg to the figure-4 position before making the instrument portal for the lateral compartment, and then placing the portal on the medial side at the level of the high anterolateral arthroscope portal, directly adjacent to the patellar ligament.

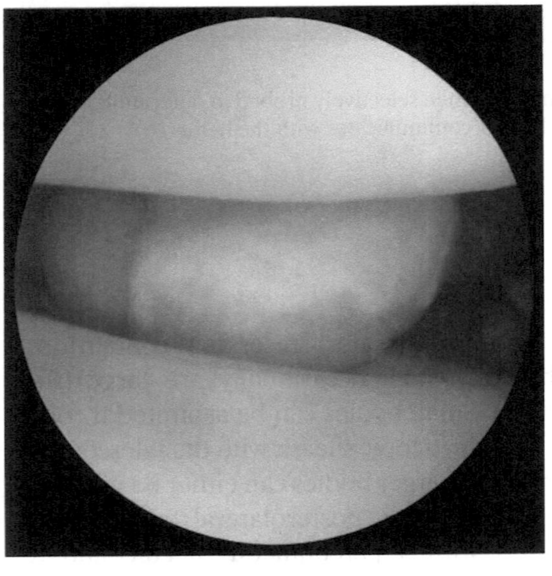

Fig. 8-93. Loose body pushed from the posterolateral recess into the lateral joint space

8.10 Summary

Our standard routine for conducting the arthroscopic examination can be described simply, in a manner that every examiner can reproduce, by referring each step to the rotational position of the light post and the anatomic structures that are visualized (Table 8-3).

Table 8-3. Systematic routine for arthroscopic examination of the *right* (*gray column*) and left knee joints. (Steps marked with an asterisk are reserved for selected cases)

Step	Position of light post		Arthroscope movements, anatomic structures visualized
	Right	Left	
1	6:00	6:00	Orientation. Establish the horizon, displaying the retropatellar cartilage at the top of the monitor (rotate the video camera relative to the telescope).
2	6:00	6:00	Inspect the retropatellar cartilage, patellar ridge, and medial patellar facet.
3	4:00	8:00	Manually medialize the patella to aid inspection of the lateral patellar facet.
4	3:00	9:00	Suprapatellar pouch. Sweep the scope from medially to laterally as far as the entrance to the lateral recess.
5	12:00	12:00	Sweep the scope down into the lateral recess.
6	10:00	2:00	Inspect the synovial attachment of the anterior and central portions of the latera meniscus.
7	9:00	3:00	Inspect the popliteal hiatus and the course of the popliteus tendon.
8	10:00	2:00	Sweep the scope back upward in the lateral recess; inspect the Outerbridge ridge and the lateral part of the femoropatellar joint.
9	5:00	7:00	Advance toward the anteromedial capsule. Alternately flex and extend the knee to evaluate patellar tracking on the femur.
10	5:00	7:00	Inspect the medial portion of the mediopatellar plica.
11	10:00	2:00	Inspect the anterior portion of the medial patellar plica. Flex and extend the knee several times to check for impingement of the plica on the medial femoral condyle.
12	2:00	10:00	Sweep the scope into the medial recess and scan downward until the periphery of the medial meniscus is seen. Inspect the meniscosynovial junction.
13	2:00	10:00	Apply a mild valgus stress to expose the central portion of the medial meniscus.
14	3:00	9:00	Visualize the central portion of the medial meniscus, then apply a maximum valgus stress with the knee flexed about 10° and the tibia externally rotated. Inspect the posterior horn of the medial meniscus. Then retract the scope and inspect the medial compartment.
15	10:00	2:00	Traverse the intercondylar notch toward the posteromedial recess, passing the scope medial to the cruciate ligaments. This gives a direct view of the posterior horn of the medial meniscus and its synovial attachment.
16	8:00	4:00	Flex the knee to approximately 60°, inspect the posteromedial recess.
17	2:00	10:00	Inspect the medial portions of the posterior cruciate ligament. Retract the scope from the posterior joint region.
18	2:00	10:00	Inspect the intercondylar notch. The anterior cruciate ligament can usually be inspected better by positioning the scope lateral to the infrapatellar plica.
19	5:00	7:00	Advance the scope toward the anterior cruciate ligament and examine its femoral attachment.
20	1:00	11:00	Retract the scope and inspect the tibial attachment of the anterior cruciate ligament.
21	2:00	10:00	Inspect the anterior horn of the lateral meniscus.
22	3:00	9:00	Visualize the lateral triangle (medial: anterior cruciate ligament; caudal: lateral tibial plateau, anterior horn of lateral meniscus; proximal: lateral femoral condyle) and move the leg to the figure-4 position.
23	3:00	9:00	In the repositioned leg the scope should point directly toward the posterior horn of the lateral meniscus.
24	2:00	11:00	Inspect the lateral meniscus.
			Construct the instrument portal using the cannula technique, placing it in accordance with intraarticular findings.

8.11 Completing the Examination

After the arthroscopic examination is completed, the therapeutic phase of the procedure is begun. If treatment is unnecessary, the procedure is concluded.

Following arthroscopic operations, and in joints with pronounced synovitis, we conclude the procedure by inserting an intraarticular Redon suction drain (Ch 10). The drainage tube is shortened to 3 holes, sharpened at the tip, and passed into the joint through the arthroscopic sheath following removal of the telescope. While most arthroscopists aspirate all intraarticular fluid from the joint before inserting the drain, others distend the joint maximally with irrigating fluid before or after inserting the drain, and then close. We, too, have had positive results with this technique. The fluid left in the joint has a tamponading effect on blood vessels damaged during the operation, so the tendency toward postoperative bleeding and hemarthrosis is reduced. It takes about 24 hours for all the residual intraarticular irrigating fluid to be absorbed.

We instill 10 ml of a local anesthetic containing epinephrine (e.g., 0.5% carbostesin with epinephrine added) into the joint through the suction drain. Besides the hemostatic action of the epinephrine, the analgesia produced by the local anesthetic provides significant pain relief during the initial hours after surgery.

The portals for the arthroscope and instruments are each closed with a single suture. While the small wounds do not strictly require suturing, it is helpful in that it forces the patient to see his family doctor or the attending physician within 10–14 days to have the sutures removed. This gives the physician an opportunity to assess the therapeutic result. If any complications arise, appropriate countermeasures can be instituted (see Chap. 12).

Finally an elastic compression dressing is applied.

9
The Articular Cartilage – Normal and Pathologic Findings

Lesions of the articular cartilage are the most common pathologic finding in arthroscopy. In the years before arthroscopy was widely used, the diagnosis of cartilage pathology was based on the clinical and radiographic examination. Often this limited the ability of physicians to detect cartilage abnormalities, resulting in a large number of exploratory arthrotomies. No other diagnostic method is as well suited as arthroscopy for evaluating the articular surfaces of the knee. Although MR imaging can determine the thickness of the articular cartilage with high quantitative accuracy, this modality cannot replace arthroscopy (Fig. 9-1). The routine use of MR imaging for the diagnosis of cartilage lesions is not feasible at the present time.

The cartilage changes detected by arthroscopy are described in terms of their:

1. *Location* (e.g., retropatellar, medial femoral condyle).
2. *Type* (e.g., grade II chondromalacia, osteochondritis dissecans, traumatic cartilage lesion).
3. *Extent* (size is stated in cm, using the probing hook for comparison).
4. *Etiology* (e.g., traumatic, posttraumatic, degenerative, or unknown, especially in athletically active patients over 40 years of age. Increasingly this is a source of difficulties in disability assessment).

When an articular cartilage lesion such as an osteochondral fracture is detected by arthroscopy, it should not be reported as an "osteochondral fracture of the patella" but should be described more precisely as, say, an "osteochondral fracture of the medial patellar facet with a 1.5-cm defect." This type of report is especially informative to uninitiated

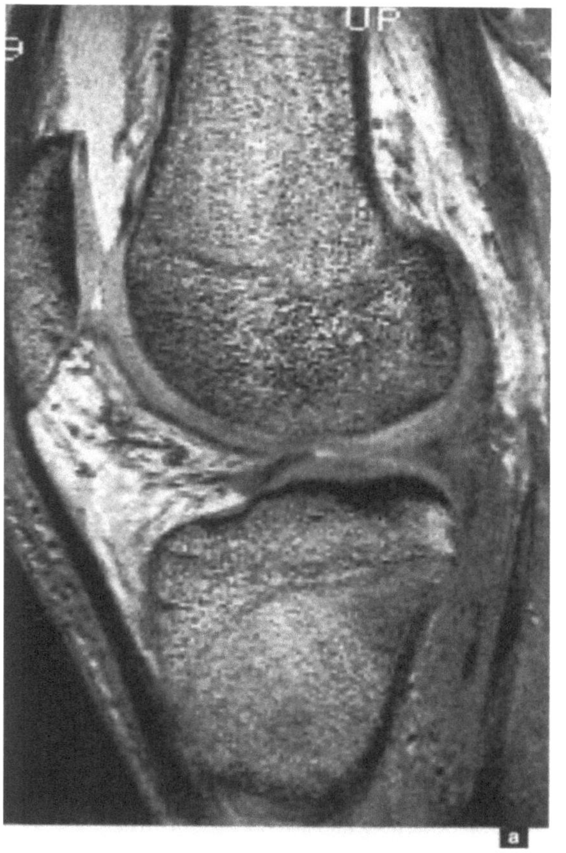
a

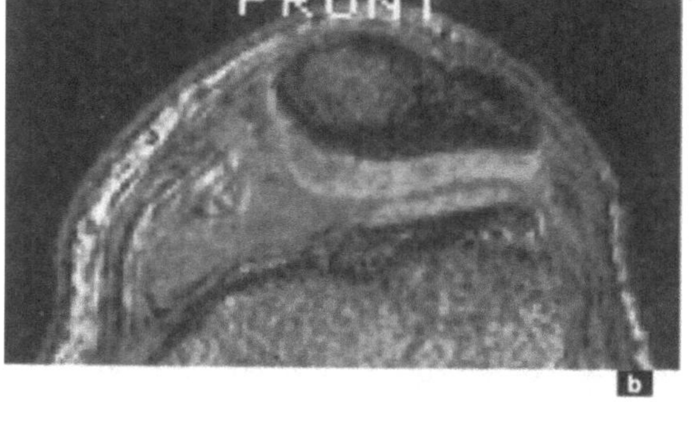

b

Fig. 9-1 a, b. MR images for evaluating the articular cartilage of the knee. The cartilage appears intact on both the sagittal (**a**) and transverse (**b**) planes of section colleagues. Far too often, lesions are diagnosed simply as "chondromalacia" or "chondropathy."

9.1 Normal Findings

On arthroscopy, healthy articular cartilage appears yellowish-white and has a firm, resilient consistency when probed. Chronic cartilage lesions are more common than acute lesions and must be distinguished from them. All types and grades of cartilage pathology may be encountered on the retropatellar surface.

9.2 Chondromalacia

Several different schemes have been used to classify the pure chondral changes associated with chondromalacia (Tables 9-1 and 9-2, Figs. 9-2 to 9-7).

Table 9-1. Outerbridge classification of chondromalacia of the patella (Outerbridge 1961)

Grade 1:	Softening and swelling of the articular cartilage
Grade 2:	Fragmentation and fissuring in an area smaller than 1.25 cm
Grade 3:	Fragmentation and fissuring in an area larger than 1.25 cm
Grade 4:	Erosion of the cartilage down to bone

Table 9-2. Lindberg's modification of the Outerbridge classification, oriented toward arthroscopic findings

Grade 1:	Superficial fissuring and/or softening
Grade 2:	Visible lesion that does not extend to subchondral bone; cartilage fragmentation, deep fissuring
Grade 3:	Cartilage lesion extends to subchondral bone

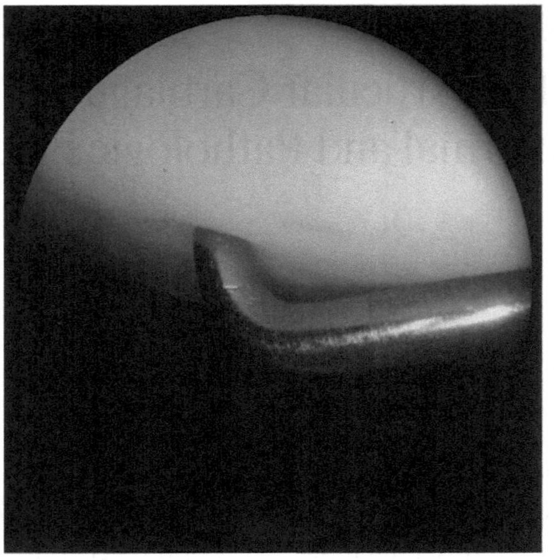

Fig. 9-2. Grade I chondromalacia of the retropatellar cartilage. Probing indicates softening of the cartilage *(most common arthroscopic finding!)*, but the pathologic significance of this finding is questionable. If the cartilage immediately springs back into shape, the finding is normal. But if the indentation persists or if a large area of the cartilage sinks beneath the probe with no resistance ("water bed" effect), it may be inferred that the cartilage is diseased. This is not an indication for operative treatment, however

The spectrum of cartilage lesions following acute injuries range from chondral contusions to large osteochondral fragments.

These classification are not sufficient, however, to describe the multitude of potential cartilage lesions. Degenerative changes are particularly diverse and include fraying, erosion, fissuring, ulceration, and flaking. Combinations of the various types are frequently encountered.

Cartilage changes may be found on the femoral and tibial articular surfaces as well as on the patella. The infracentral portion of the medial femoral condyle and the posterior half of the medial tibial plateau are involved with particular frequency.

Crystalline deposits appearing on the cartilage surface, menisci, and synovium should raise suspicion of hyperuricemia. The crystals can be scraped off with a blunt instrument (e.g., the probing hook) and submitted for

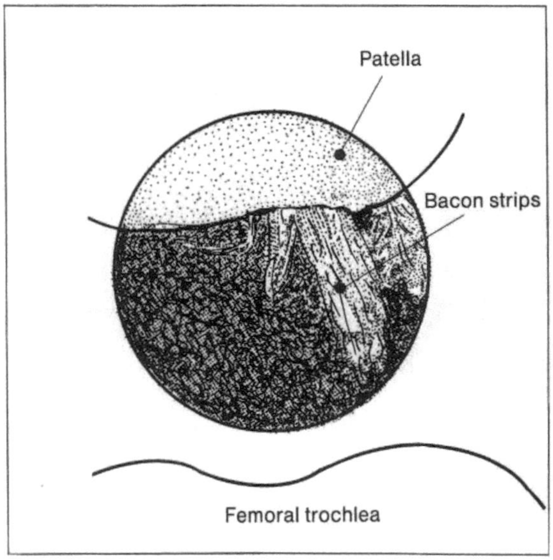

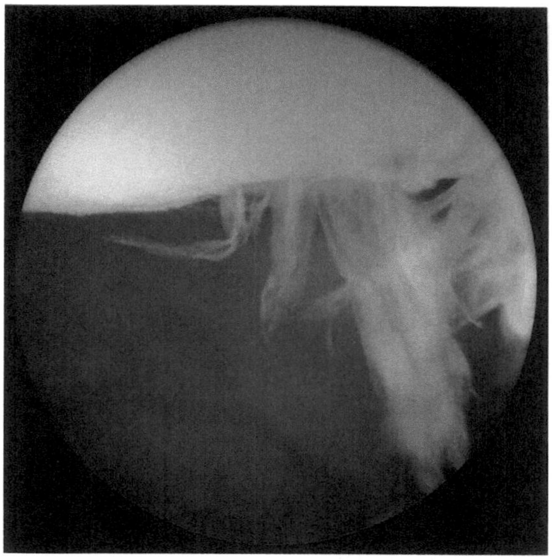

▲

Fig. 9-3. Transparent "bacon strip" exfoliations on the retropatellar cartilage have no pathologic significance. Shreds that obstruct vision may be held aside or removed

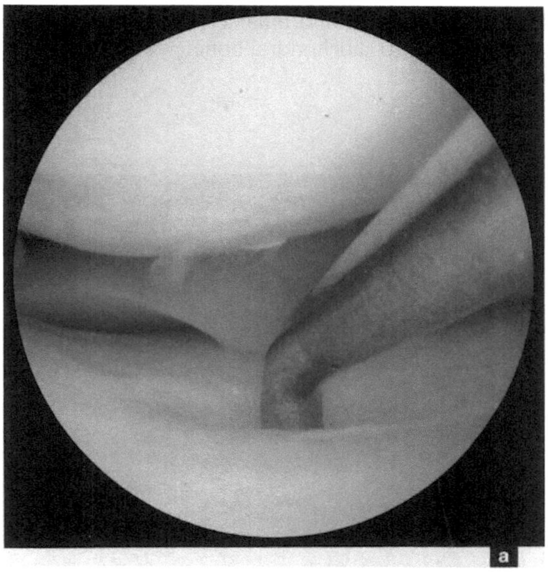

▶

Fig. 9-4 a, b. Grade I chondromalacia of the medial tibial plateau. Pressure from the probe forms an indentation (**a**) that persists after the probe is withdrawn (**b**)

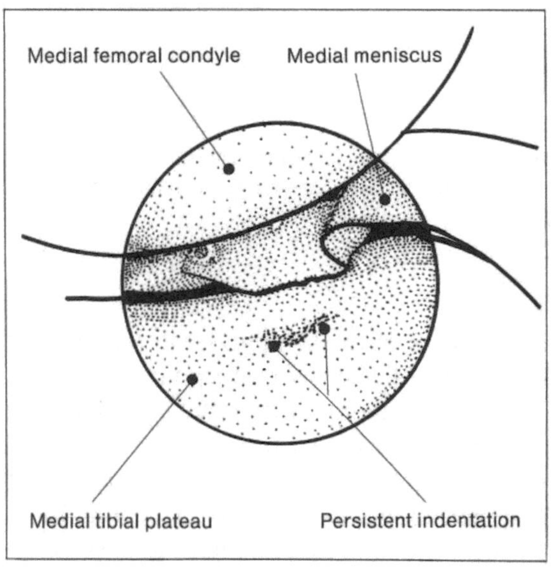

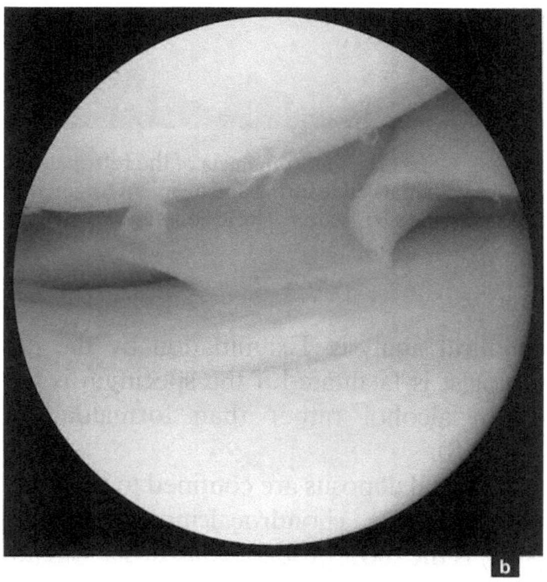

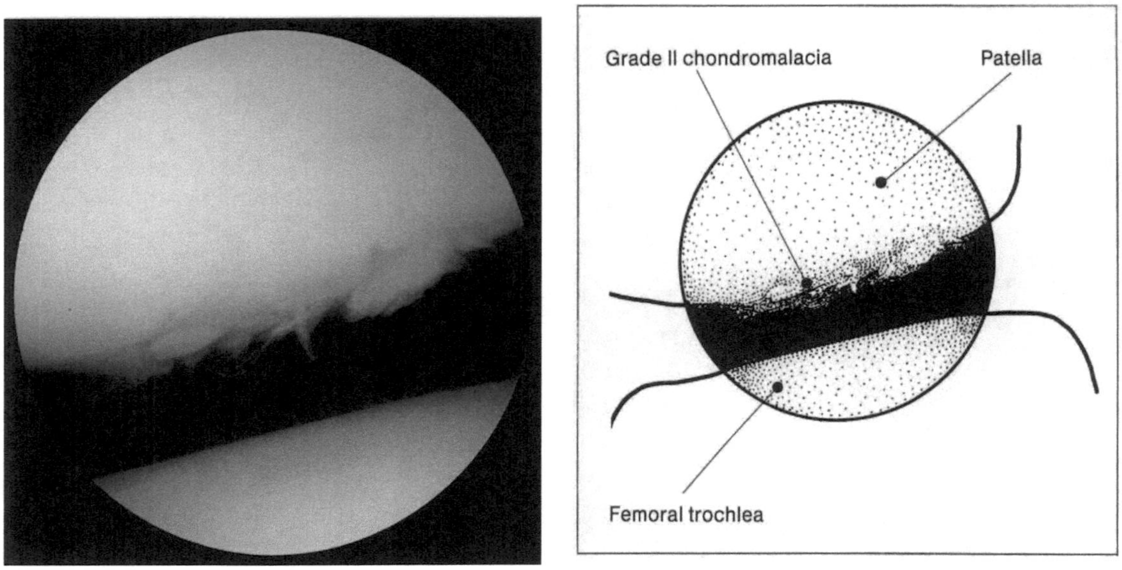

Fig. 9-5. Grade II chondromalacia of the retropatellar surface. Probing is necessary to determine whether the lesion extends to subchondral bone

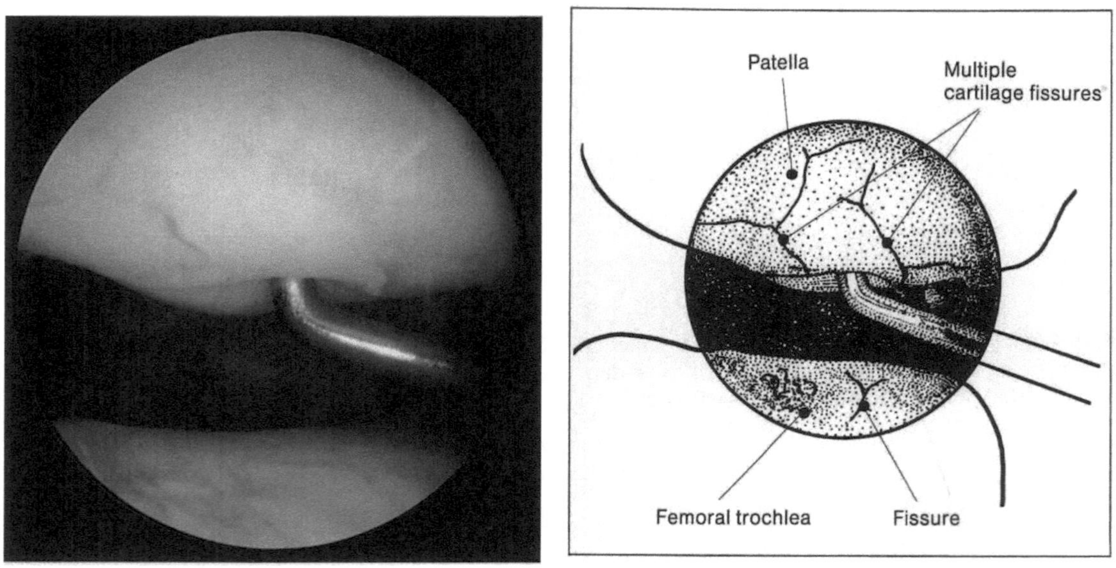

Fig. 9-6. Grade II chondromalacia of the retropatellar surface with marked fissuring and incipient fragmentation involving a large area. The lesions do not yet reach the bone. The opposing articular surface in the femoral trochlea shows partial-thickness cartilage defects

chemical analysis. Examination by the pathologist is facilitated if the specimen is fixed in alcohol rather than formaldehyde (Fig. 9-8).

If crystal deposits are confined to the articular cartilage, chondrocalcinosis (pseudogout) is the most probable diagnosis. Chemical analysis of the scrapings will identify the crystals as calcium pyrophosphate.

If there is overgrowth of the articular cartilage by synovial tissue, a synovial biopsy should be taken at that site and submitted for histopathologic examination (see Fig. 10-7). In these cases there is a high index of suspi-

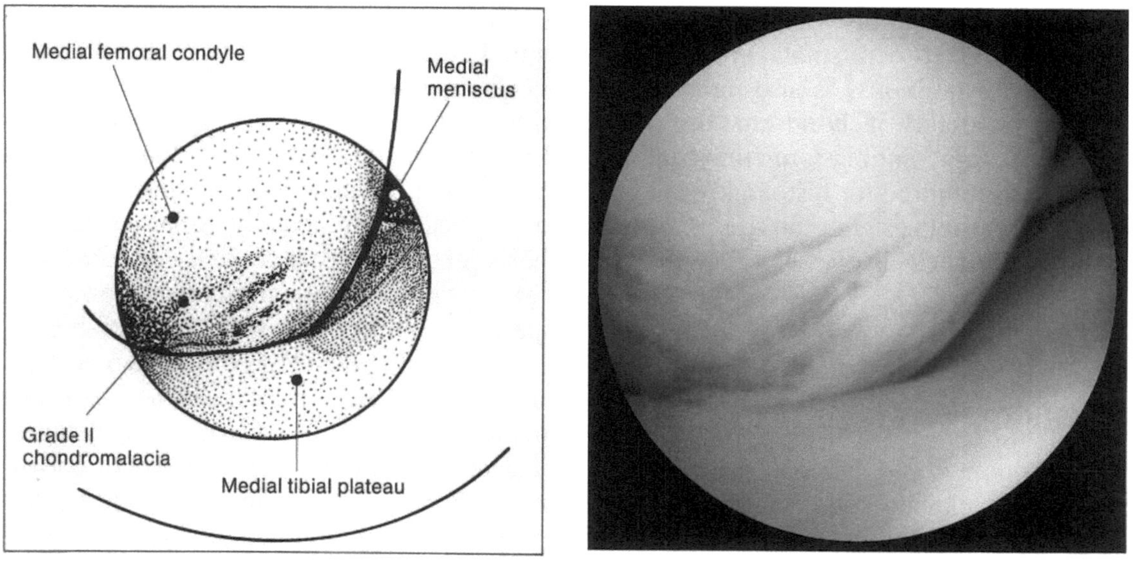

Fig. 9-7. Grade II chondromalacia of the medial femoral condyle. The lesion occurs at a typical site in the principal weight-bearing zone near the intercondylar eminence

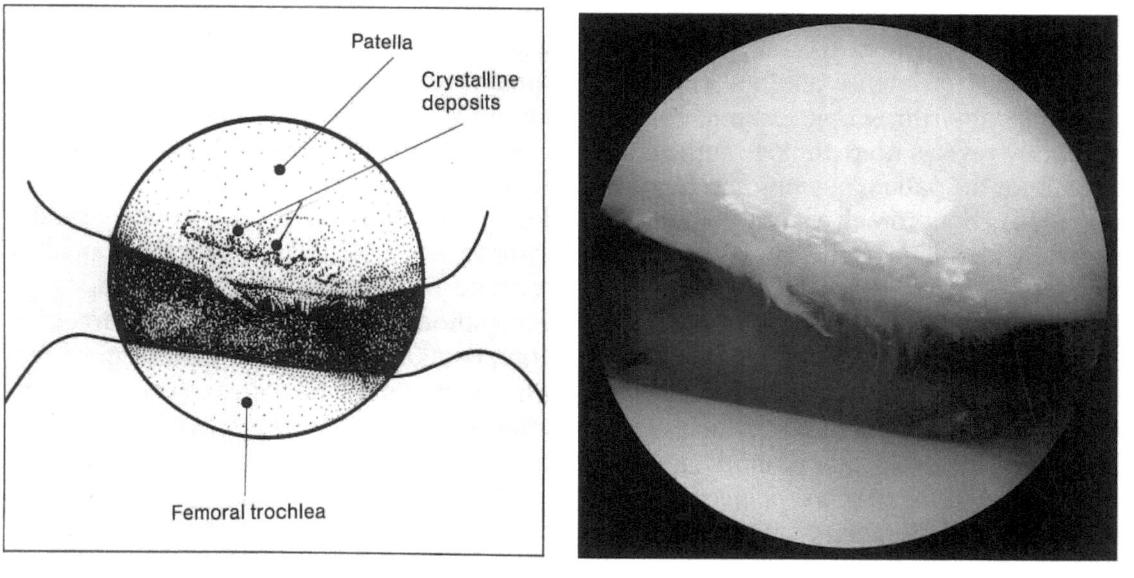

Fig. 9-8. Gouty arthritis.
History: The patient, a 48-year-old male, sustained direct valgus trauma to the knee 2 weeks ago while playing soccer. Since then the joint was repeatedly aspirated by the family physician (yielding a turbid yellowish fluid). Symptoms are consistent with a lateral meniscus injury.
Arthroscopic findings: Crystalline deposits on the retropatellar cartilage with a normal-appearing lateral meniscus.
Procedure: The crystalline deposits were removed (for histologic examination), followed by partial synovectomy and copious lavage. After surgery the patient reported that he had taken gout medications sporadically. His uric acid level was 11.3 mg%

cion for rheumatoid disease. If the articular surface is studded with small cartilage fragments, synovial biopsy is also indicated as there is a possibility of chondromatosis.

If arthroscopic findings are equivocal and material is submitted for histologic examination, the pathologist should be informed about the patient's history.

9.2.1 "Chondropathy"

"Chondropathy" is a catch-all diagnosis applied to unexplained knee complaints, especially those involving the anterior portion of the joint. In this regard it is clinically and therapeutically significant that while pronounced retropatellar cartilage changes are commonly present, clinical symptoms may be very mild or absent. Even large areas of denuded bone may be detected as incidental findings. Conversely, some patients, especially adolescents, will complain of intense anterior knee pain, prompting an arthroscopic examination that frequently reveals no pathology sufficient to account for the patient's symptoms. If grade I or grade II chondromalacia is found, it is immediately identified as the cause of the complaints.

But there is no reason to limit diagnostic and therapeutic attention to the articular cartilage alone, as the term "chondropathy" implies. This painful condition, which mainly afflicts younger patients, is more aptly referred to as *"anterior knee pain"* or *"femoropatellar pain syndrome."* The complaints described by the patient–very severe pain, frequently present at rest and most pronounced after stair climbing or prolonged sitting–and the objective clinical findings such as tenderness to pressure on the patellar facets and a positive Zohlen test can easily direct suspicion toward femoropatellar osteoarthritis. Accordingly, the literature is replete with conservative (physiotherapy, medication, patellar braces, non-weight-bearing) and aggressive surgical treatment options (abrasion, Pridie drill holes, lateral release, transfer of the tibial tuberosity, patellar osteotomies, patellar tethering operations). The operative treatments frequently miss the goal of eliminating the true cause of the pain. Moreover, some extensive operative procedures so traumatize the joint that they not only fail to normalize proprioception and patellar tracking but actually impair them further. These heroic measures leave in their wake patients who manifest significant postoperative abnormalities of patellofemoral tracking accompanied by continued pain. Because the etiology of anterior knee pain remains obscure, and chondromalacic changes detected by arthroscopy often do not correlate with clinical complaints or relate to the complaints in an undefined way, we do not feel that extensive operative treatment is warranted for these patients. Emphasis should be placed, rather, on identifying and treating the possible causes of the increased retropatellar pressure, such as ligamentous or muscular incompetence. This would include anterior cruciate ligament insufficiency, hyperlaxity, quadriceps shortening, and muscular imbalances (Strobel, Stedtfeld 1990).

Arthroscopy is indicated in patients with femoropatellar pain to exclude other pathologic conditions that can produce similar symptoms (e.g., plica syndrome, anterior cruciate ligament rupture, meniscal injury). It is common to see a gradual improvement of complaints following a purely diagnostic arthroscopy. Spontaneous regression of complaints over a period of weeks or months also may occur.

The term "chondromalacia" simply describes a morphologic condition and does not refer to a specific disease entity.

The vague term "chondropathy" should be avoided.

9.3 Degenerative Changes

The osteoarthritic or degenerative joint disorders are characterized by advanced cartilage destruction with associated bone reactions.

Radiographs demonstrate osteophytosis, subchondral sclerosis, cyst formation, and narrowing of the joint space. Arthroscopy reveals a combination of osseous and chondral lesions.

The articular cartilage lesions usually extend to subchondral bone, and some sites may be completely denuded of cartilage, exposing the bone beneath (Figs. 8-31, 8-34, 8-55, and 8-89). Although any part of the joint may be affected, osteoarthritic changes are most prevalent in the femoropatellar joint and medial compartment.

Several therapeutic options may be considered. Arthroscopic irrigation of the joint can itself be beneficial in reducing pain, since the irrigating solution cleanses the joint of enzymes, oxygen radicals, and cellular debris that perpetuate the synovial irritation. If synovitis is advanced, synovectomy may be required. A subchondral abrasion chondroplasty or cartilage drilling (Pridie's operation) may stimulate the formation of fibrocartilage in small defects up to about 1.5 cm in diameter. It is essential, however, that the foregoing procedures be combined with surgery to correct any angular limb deformity that is present.

9.4 Traumatic Cartilage Lesions

The age of a traumatic cartilage lesion can be roughly estimated by watching for several features:

1. *Sharp edges* indicate a fresh lesion that is no more than a few days old.
2. *Rounded edges* indicate that the lesion is at least 6 weeks old.
3. *A round rim* indicates a lesion that is several months old.

If the periphery of the lesion is not loose and adheres firmly to the underlying bone, this is considered a favorable prognostic sign. Undermining of the periphery implies a less favorable prognosis, since further progression of the process is likely.

9.4.1 Cartilage Contusions

Bleeding within the cartilage and sites of reddish discoloration signify a cartilage contusion (Fig. 9-9). The patient should remain under medical supervision, since a symptom-free interval of several weeks or months may pass before the true extent of the damage becomes apparent.

9.4.2 Cartilage Fissures

Fissuring of the articular cartilage may have a traumatic or degenerative etiology. If the fissures run in a sagittal direction, they are probably a result of trauma. Parallel, transverse fissures (see Fig. 8-54) are consistent with degenerative changes secondary to ligamentous injuries, meniscal tears, or other trauma.

9.4.3 Chondral and Osteochondral Fractures

Direct trauma and patellar dislocations are the most common cause of chondral and osteochondral fractures. Clinical manifestations range from a tense hemarthrosis to nonspecific effusion and recurrent locking. Radiographic diagnosis can be difficult, even with a large osteochondral fracture. Often the radiographic changes are subtle and can be correctly interpreted only in retrospect. The history and clinical presentation are helpful initially, but only arthroscopic examination can furnish a definitive diagnosis.

Chondral flake fractures and/or osteochondral fractures involving the margin of the lateral femoral condyle or the medial patellar facet are typical lesions seen after a dislocation of the patella (Fig. 9-10).

Traumatic osteochondral fractures and flake fractures of the cartilage can occur on all cartilaginous surfaces, the defect ranging

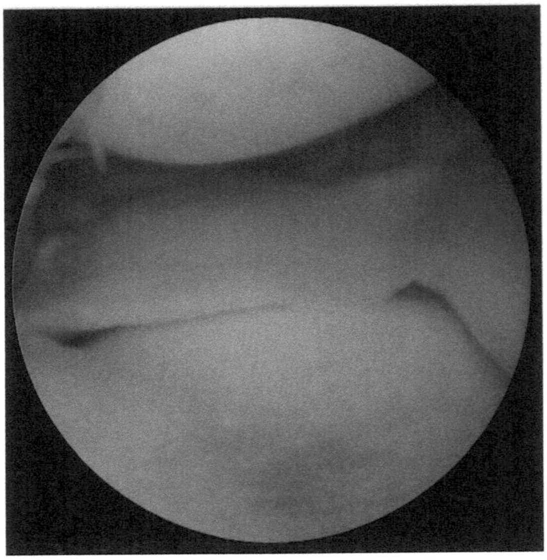

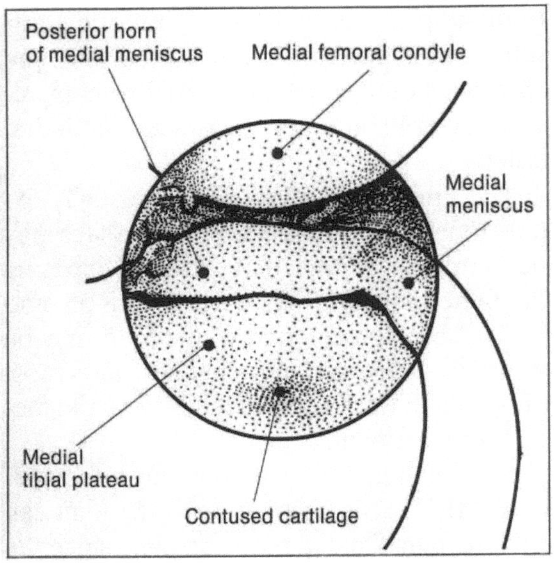

Fig. 9-9. Cartilage contusion in the medial compartment following a complex knee injury. Internal hemorrhage has produced a reddish discoloration of the cartilage. The increased distance between the surface of the medial meniscus and the femoral condyle implies a proximal disruption of the medial capsule and ligaments.
Procedure: Non-weight-bearing is enforced for 8–12 weeks. The final damage cannot be assessed until 6–9 months after the injury

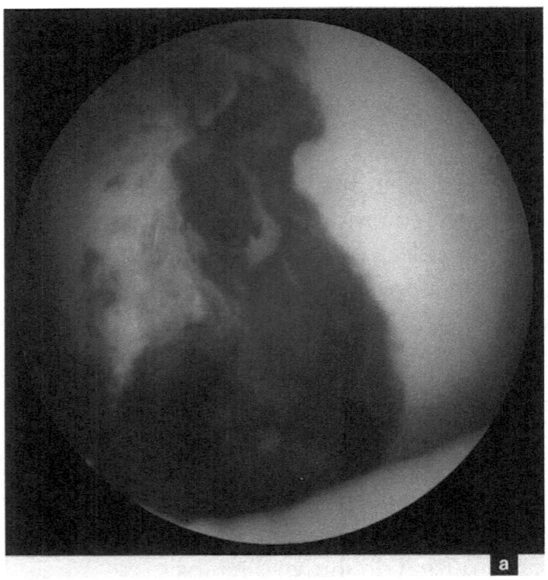

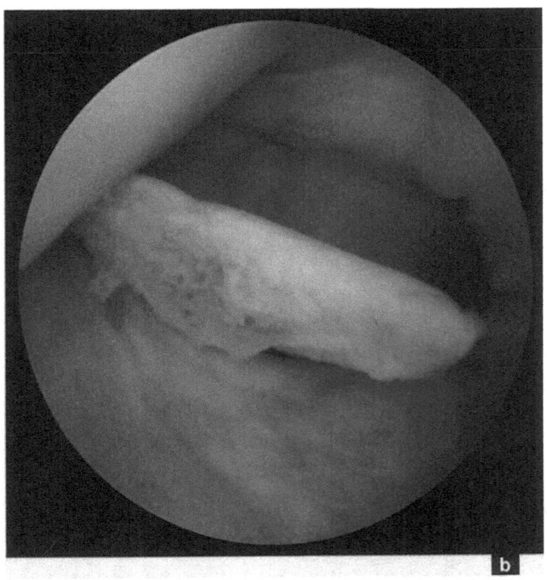

Fig. 9-10 a, b. Osteochondral fracture secondary to patellar dislocation.
History: The patient, a 23-year-old woman, experienced an initial patellar dislocation 3 days ago while dancing. X-rays showed no clear evidence of an osteochondral fragment. Aspiration of effusion yielded blood with fat globules. Clinical examination showed bilateral hyperextension and genu valgum with a positive apprehension test.
Arthroscopic findings: Blood clots adhering to the margin of the lateral femoral condyle (Outerbridge ridge). After irrigation and probing, a small area of exposed bone is found signifying an osteochondral defect (**a**). The flake bed is filled with coagulated fibrin and blood. The detached osteochondral fragment was found in the intercondylar area in front of the anterior cruciate ligament (**b**).
Procedure: Reattachment of the fragment

from a few millimeters to several centimeters in size. In rare cases the cartilage fragment is sheared from the condyle, leaving the subchondral bone intact (Fig. 9-10).

9.5 Osteochondritis Dissecans

The etiology and pathogenesis of this disorder are not yet fully understood. It generally is manifested in adolescents and young adults (Fig. 9-11). The demarcation has been referred to various causal factors including the deficient vascularization of bony convexities, ischemic injury following epiphyseal closure, repetitive microtrauma, unphysiologic loading, fatigue fractures, and enzymatic cartilage destruction. Four stages are recognized in the natural history of osteochondritis dissecans:

Stage I. Radiographs demonstrate a zone of dissection between two sclerosed layers of bone. Arthroscopic examination at this stage may show a slight elevation of the overlying cartilage, which may be softer than its surroundings. Sometimes it shows a greater yellowish discoloration than the surrounding cartilage, or it may show slight roughening. But in many cases the overlying cartilage cannot be identified as belonging to the osteochondritic focus. Contrast between the cartilage and its surroundings can be enhanced by lowering the intensity of the light source or disconnecting the light cable.

Stage II. The joint mouse undergoes demarcation. Already its bed is filling with fibrotic tissue. The fragment is still attached but can be "wiggled" slightly with the probe.

Stage III. The fragment is partially detached and can be swung back and forth like a trapdoor with the probe.

Stage IV. The osteochondritic fragment is completely detached to form a floating loose body. Arthroscopy shows a depression of

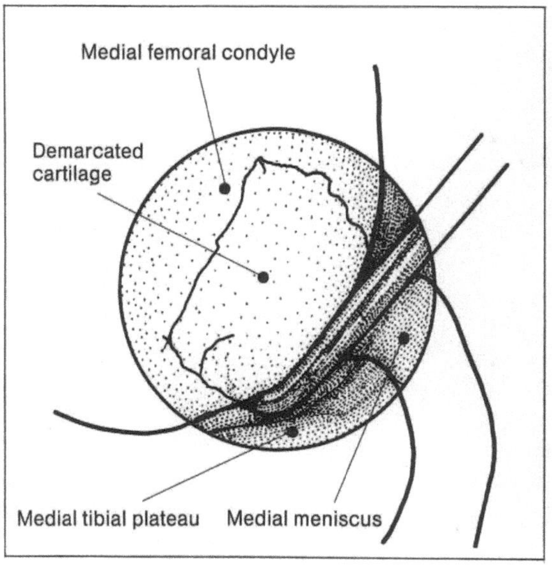

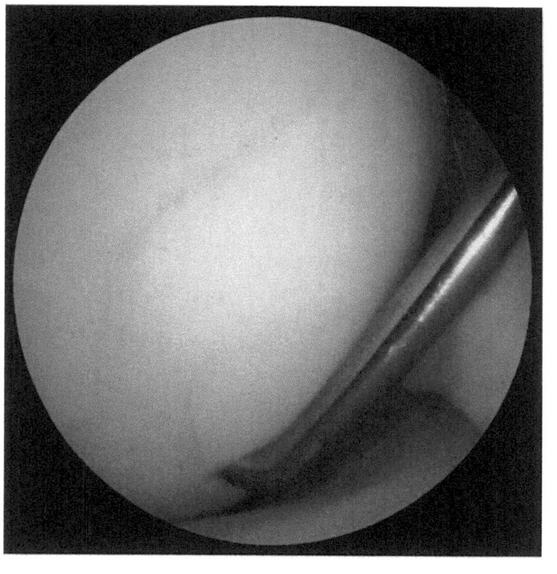

Fig. 9-11. Osteochondritis dissecans.
History: The patient, a 33-year-old competitive skier, had a 4-year history of recurrent medial knee pain. He was referred with a suspected meniscal tear.
Arthroscopic findings: Osteochondritic focus on the medial femoral condyle. Probing clearly indicates demarcation of the cartilage, but the fragment is not yet mobile (stage II lesion).
Procedure: Since radiographs show no sclerotic zones or densities consistent with osteochondritis dissecans, conservative treatment is advised

variable depth that contains varying amounts of fibrous or cartilaginous tissue. In adolescents this filling progresses so far that the defect may fill almost to the level of the surrounding cartilage.

The role of arthroscopy in osteochondritis dissecans lies in the accurate localization and staging of the lesion. These findings provide the basis for treatment planning. Conservative or operative treatment may be necessary for stage I cases. In stage II, the bed should be freshened by subchondral abrasion chondroplasty using a motorized shaver. The fragment can then be secured arthroscopically with a bone screw or pin. In stage III cases the fragment can no longer be reattached, so it is removed. The crater is then freshened as needed by a subchondral abrasion chondroplasty.

10
The Synovium – Normal and Pathologic Findings

Arthroscopy is superior to all other diagnostic modalities in investigations of the synovial membrane.

Because the color of the synovium is an important diagnostic parameter, we always perform arthroscopy under identical conditions (tourniquet control). When a video system is used, careful color adjustment is needed to avoid false interpretations. If a tourniquet or exsanguinating bandage is not used, healthy synovium can easily appear inflamed or hyperemic to the inexperienced examiner. A fluid medium is advantageous for evaluating the synovial villi, as it causes them to float above the general level of the synovial lining. The villi are more difficult to evaluate in gas, because they are flattened against adjacent capsule and bone.

The synovium is evaluated arthroscopically for the following changes (Glinz 1987):

- hyperemia,
- edema,
- hypertrophy,
- fibrosis,
- inclusions,
- crystalline deposits.

The examiner should recognize the limitations of arthroscopy in the differential diagnosis of nonspecific joint inflammations. These disorders are so etiologically and pathogenetically diverse that the arthroscopic and histologic examination alone can contribute little to their elucidation (Klein 1980).

10.1 Normal Findings

The normal synovium appears as a smooth, vascularized membrane lining the articular cavity (Fig. 10-1). The collagenous ligament structures of the medial and lateral capsule and anterior cruciate ligament show through the semitransparent synovial membrane.

In places where the synovium is covered by fatty tissue, as on the floor of the suprapatellar pouch or in the anterior compartment (infrapatellar fat pad), the villi tend to be thicker and more pronounced. In healthy joints the transition between the synovium and the articular cartilage and menisci is smooth and even. When the synovium is affected by a pathologic condition, these junctional areas appear changed.

Histologically, the synovial tissue presents a predominantly folded, fatty, or fibrous appearance depending on the site where the sample is taken (Klein 1980). The synovial cells are modified connective-tissue cells that lack a limiting basement membrane. These cells regenerate from the underlying layers of connective tissue.

Even for an experienced arthroscopist, it is not always easy to describe synovial abnormalities and assign them to a specific pathologic category. Thus we owe a great debt to Klein and Huth, who in their 1980 book *Arthroscopy and Histology of Knee Disorders* presented striking photographic documentation for the known synovial changes that are detectable by arthroscopy and correlated them with histologic findings.

Synovial findings can provide the definitive clue to the nature of the underlying disorder,

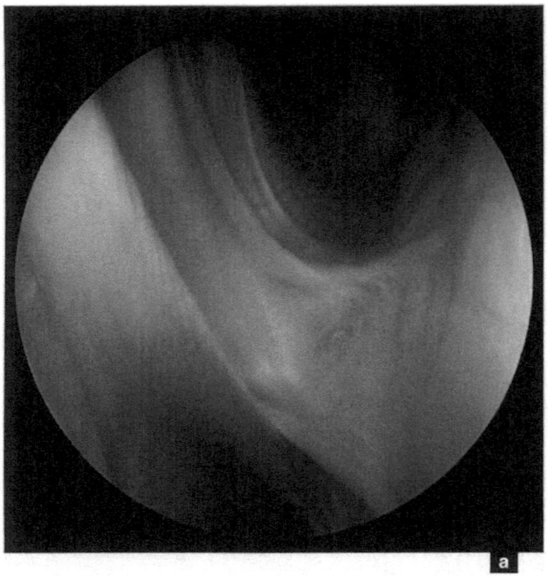

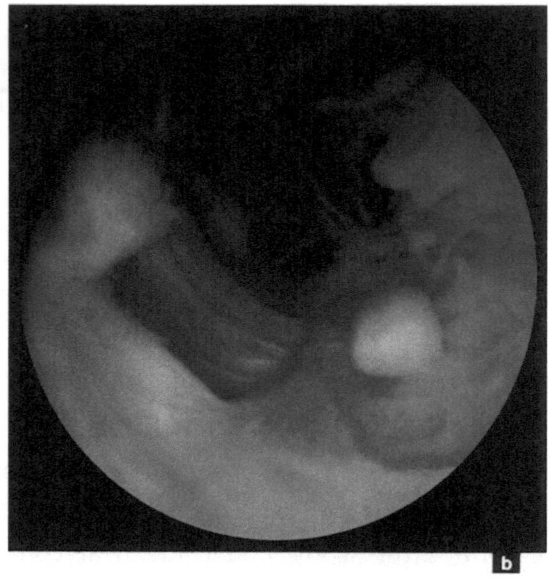

Fig. 10-1 a, b. Normal smooth, transparent synovium in the lateral recess (**a**). Mechanical synovitis and a loose body in the lateral recess associated with grade III chondromalacia and sites of denuded bone (the patient had played soccer for many years) (**b**)

but only if the examiner has sufficient arthroscopic and clinical experience. Synovial findings should always be evaluated in the context of the overall condition of the joint and of clinical findings.

When arthroscopy in performed in fluid, synovial edema may develop a short time after the examination begins. Especially in joints with pronounced degenerative changes or synovitis, this can lead to a rapid, generalized synovial swelling that obscures vision and makes it difficult to continue the procedure. This swelling can be reduced by lowering the fluid pressure, but the best solution is to work swiftly and complete the procedure as quickly as possible.

10.1.1 Synovial Biopsy

Arthroscopic synovial biopsy is a simple procedure, provided the instrument portal is correctly placed (Fig. 10-2) and a small biopsy forceps is used. The most convenient biopsy sites are the floor of the suprapatellar pouch, the capsule bordering the medial and lateral recesses, and the anterior compartment. If the synovial changes are diverse, a representative biopsy site should be selected for each type of change, and the pathologist should be told where the samples originate.

10.2 Posttraumatic Synovial Changes

Arthroscopy in the acutely traumatized knee may reveal lacerations of the synovium as well as areas of direct intrasynovial hemorrhage. These changes are usually confined to the site of the injury, the rest of the synovium appearing normal (Fig. 10-3). Subsynovial hemorrhages due to ligament ruptures are most commonly seen in the area of the anteromedial capsule, medial retinaculum, and anterior cruciate ligament (see Figs. 8-36, 8-71, and 8-72).

Old injuries are usually marked by a generalized synovial response rather than localized changes (Figs. 10-1 b, 10-4, and 10-5).

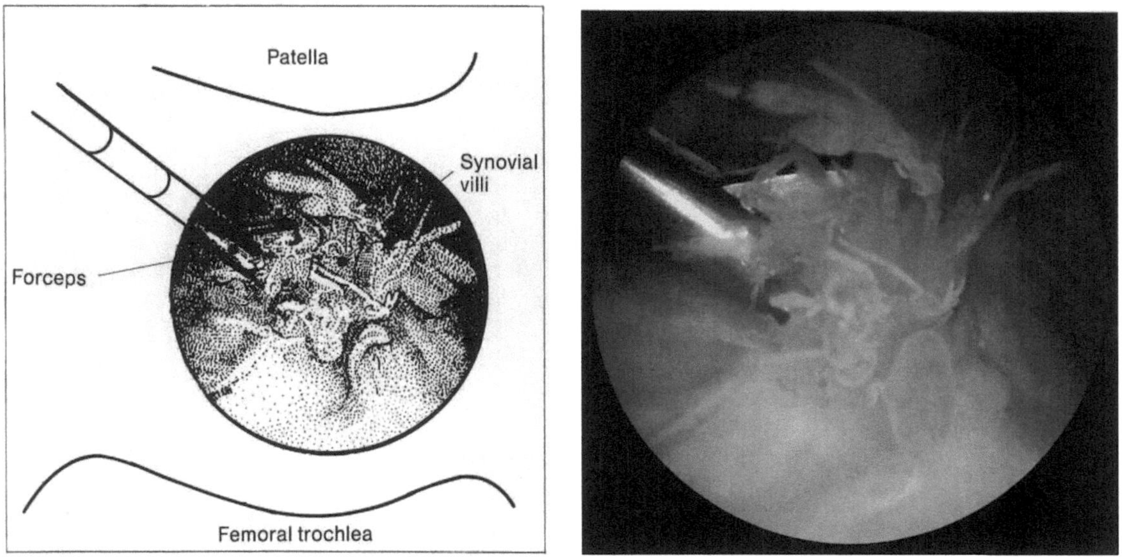

Fig. 10-2. Arthroscopically guided synovial biopsy

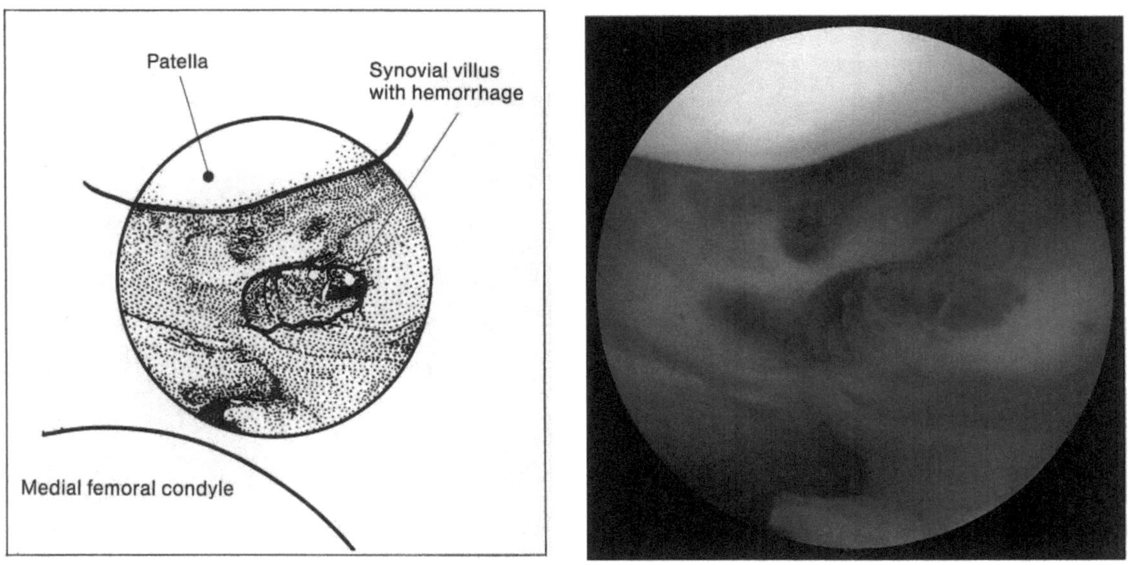

Fig. 10-3. Contusional hemorrhages in fat-pad villi caused by hyperextension trauma

Synovial adhesions are a common sequel to posttraumatic or postoperative hemarthrosis, especially when there has been prolonged immobilization of the knee. Adhesions can partially or completely obliterate the suprapatellar pouch and can seriously hamper the rest of the procedure. If there is a coexisting flexion or extension deficit, creation of the arthroscope portal can itself be extremely difficult due to the constricted femoropatellar joint space.

Nonspecific states of synovial irritation result not just from trauma but also from mechanical irritation like that associated with

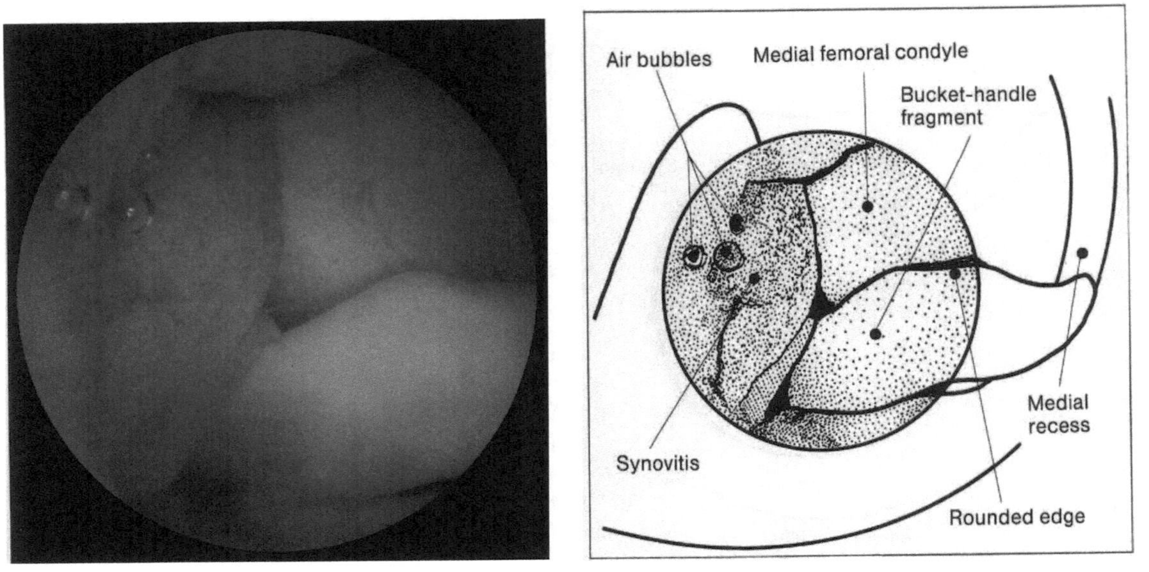

Fig. 10-4. Irritative synovitis associated with a bucket-handle tear of the medial meniscus. The rounded edges of the fragment, displaced into the intercondylar notch, are consistent with an old tear

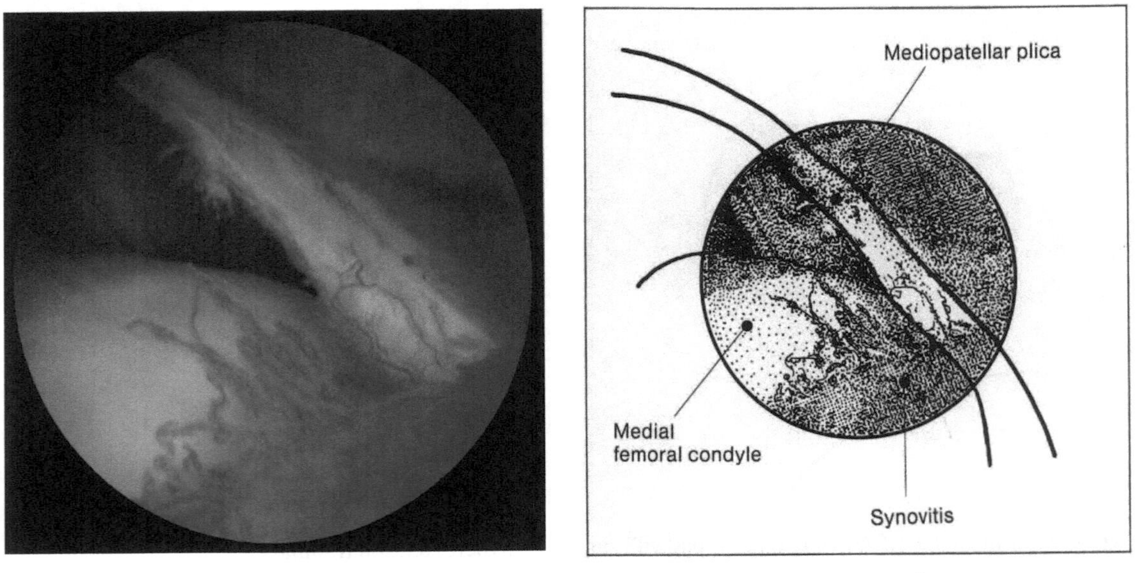

Fig. 10-5. Irritative synovitis associated with a hypertrophied mediopatellar plica (type III)

degenerative arthritis. The synovial villi are thickened, and foci of synovial hyperemia may be found (Fig. 10-6).

In rare cases enlarged synovial fronds may become entrapped and cause locking. Arthroscopy reveals large, partially rounded villi that have become caught between the articular surfaces of the femur and tibia or femur and patella (Figs. 8-29 and 8-30). Treatment consists of arthroscopic removal.

Differential diagnostic assessment of the synovium is difficult in patients who have nor-

Fig. 10-6 a, b. Hypertrophic villous synovitis.
History: Male 41 years of age underwent arthroscopy 5 years earlier for lateral knee pain. A torn lateral discoid meniscus was diagnosed and apparently was partially resected. Afterward the patient was never completely asymptomatic. Knee effusions (serous) had increased in recent months.
Arthroscopic findings: Synovitis with villous hypertrophy is noted in all portions of the joint (**a**). Protruding synovial tissue is even seen above and below the residual lateral meniscus (**b**).
Procedure: Arthroscopic partial synovectomy

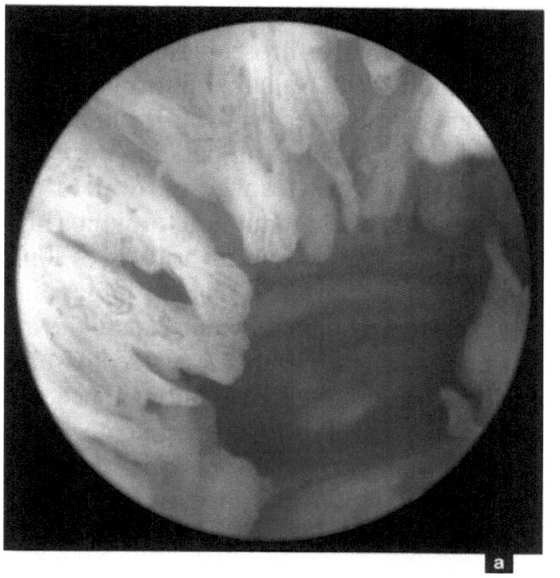
a

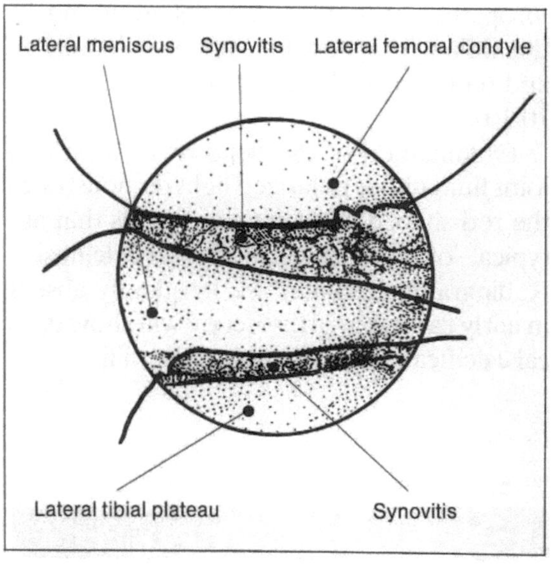

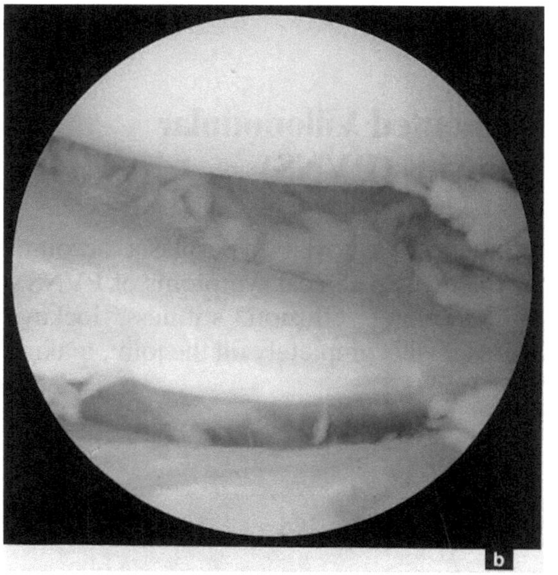
b

mal-appearing articular cartilage and menisci and show no evidence of rheumatoid disease (see Sect. 10.3) or gouty arthritis. These cases additionally require the exclusion of bacterial infections (streptococci, staphylococci, salmonellae, pneumococci, meningococci), viral diseases (hepatitis), vascular inflammations, and collagen diseases (Klein 1980). Close cooperation with an internist, rheumatologist, and immunologist is helpful in pursuing the differential diagnosis.

10.3 Synovial Changes in Rheumatoid Arthritis

The diagnosis of rheumatoid arthritis is based largely on clinical symptoms, the initially subtle radiographic findings, and serologic tests. But only arthroscopy can define the degree of progression of joint damage in terms of synovial changes, pannus formation, and cartilage destruction. Klein and Huth (1980) note that the combined arthroscopic and histologic examination yields valuable information on the aggressiveness of synovial proliferation and is helpful in selecting patients for early synovectomy, which can be performed arthroscopically with minimum trauma (Fig. 10-7). When rheumatoid arthritis is of long standing, the synovial fronds are large, bulbous, and may completely tamponade the intraarticular cavity. If there is a coexisting cloudy effusion, copious irrigation of the joint is indicated. This flushes aggressive enzymes from the joint cavity, restores a normal pH, and very often provides at least a transient improvement of symptoms.

10.4 Pigmented Villonodular Synovitis (PVNS)

Pronounced synovial hyperplasia accounts for the diverse clinical symptoms of PVNS – pain, swelling, effusion, stiffness, locking. Synovial villi completely fill the joint, making it difficult to insert the arthroscope, establish orientation, and complete the procedure. Even so, PVNS is easily diagnosed arthroscopically by its characteristic picture of intensely brown-pigmented synovial fronds and folds that form a "kelplike" mass floating within the joint (Klein 1980) (Fig. 10-8). Nonarthroscopic diagnosis is rarely possible due to the nonspecific nature of clinical signs.

10.5 Gout and Chondrocalcinosis

In gout (urate arthropathy) and in "pseudogout" (chondrocalcinosis, pyrophosphate arthropathy), crystalline deposits are found on the inflamed synovium and occasionally in and on the articular cartilage (Figs. 10-9 and 10-10).

Examination of the deposits or aspirated joint fluid under polarized light demonstrates the rod-shaped, birefringent crystals that are typical of pseudogout (chondrocalcinosis). Radiographic changes are frequently absent in early cases, but arthroscopy will show typical calcifications at the tips of the villi.

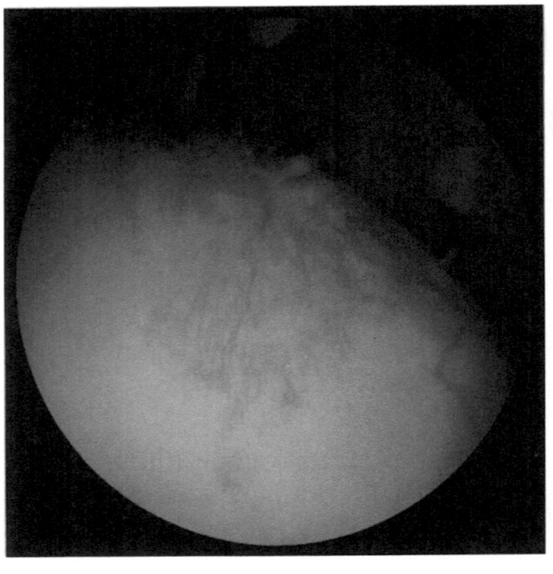

Fig. 10-7. Pannus encroaching on the medial femoral condyle, consistent with rheumatoid disease

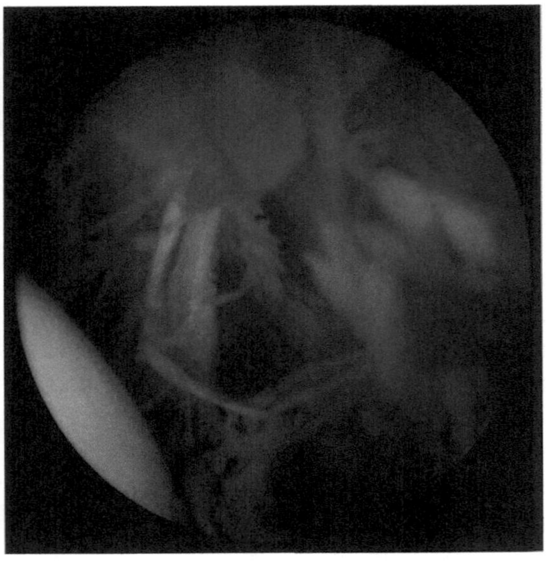

Fig. 10-8. Pigmented villonodular synovitis (photo: W. Klein)

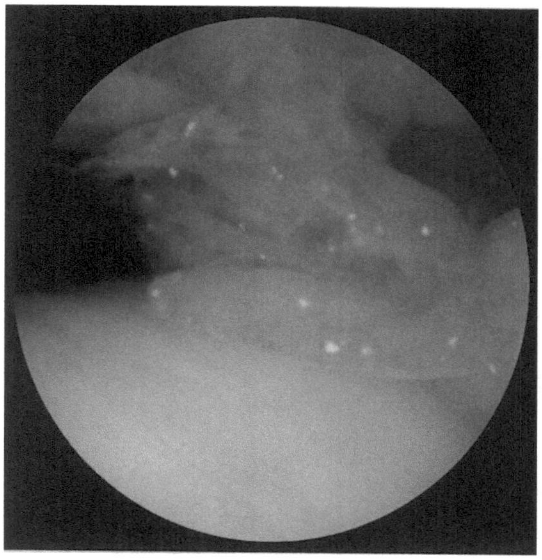

Fig. 10-9. Crystalline deposits (urate crystals) in hyperuricemia (see also Fig. 9-8)

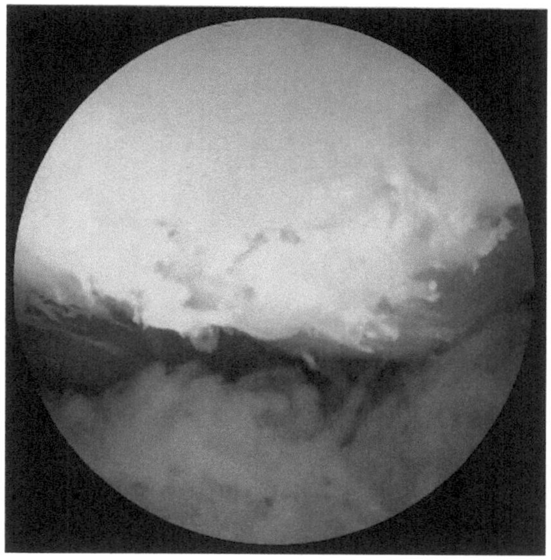

Fig. 10-10. Chondrocalcinosis (pseudogout) with synovitis and massive crystalline deposits and inclusions on the retropatellar cartilage

Klein and Huth (1980) describe the arthroscopic differentiation of gout and pseudogout, noting that the pyrophosphate crystals in pseudogout have a somewhat more patchy distribution than in gout, and that calcified tips of villi are more numerous. The urate crystals of gout typically occur in irregularly distributed, brilliant white aggregates that reflect light more intensely than pseudogout crystals. In both disorders, meniscal involvement is apparent as the process becomes advanced.

10.6 Synovitis Secondary to Psoriasis

Many patients with psoriasis have articular symptoms as their main presenting complaint (Fig. 10-11).

10.7 Postarthrotomy Changes and Reactions to Implants

In patients who have had an arthrotomy several months or even years prior to arthroscopy, it is common to find intraarticular adhesions, isolated adhesive bands traversing the joint, or cordlike elevations in the synovium following the course of the surgical scar (Fig. 10-12).

Adhesive bands have direct pathologic significance only if they limit motion in the femorotibial or femoropatellar joint. Secondary changes in the articular cartilage, especially on the retropatellar surface, are seen following extensive arthrotomies and prolonged immobilization. If a previous arthrotomy (e.g., for repair or reconstruction of the anterior cruciate ligament) has been performed in which the vastus medialis muscle was released, allowing dislocation of the patella (still a common occurrence), the resulting destruction of proprioception will upset the balance of patellofemoral tracking. It is common after such procedures to find exten-

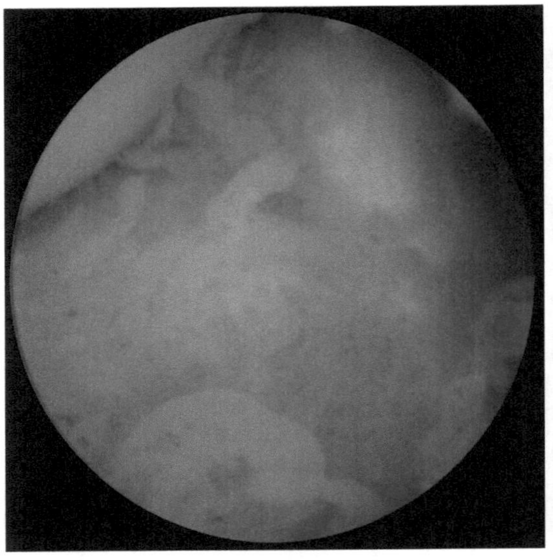

Fig. 10-11. Synovitis in psoriasis vulgaris.
History: Male 37 years of age with no history of trauma experienced symptoms consistent with a posterior horn meniscus tear for 9 months, accompanied by intermittent effusion and a 15° loss of flexion.
Arthroscopic findings: Normal-appearing medial meniscus and articular cartilage. There is conspicuous hypertrophic villous synovitis involving the anterior portion of the joint and spreading to the anterior cruciate ligament.
The Patient reported that he was under treatment by a dermatologist for mild psoriasis of the scalp.
Procedure: Synovial biopsy, synovectomy, medical treatment

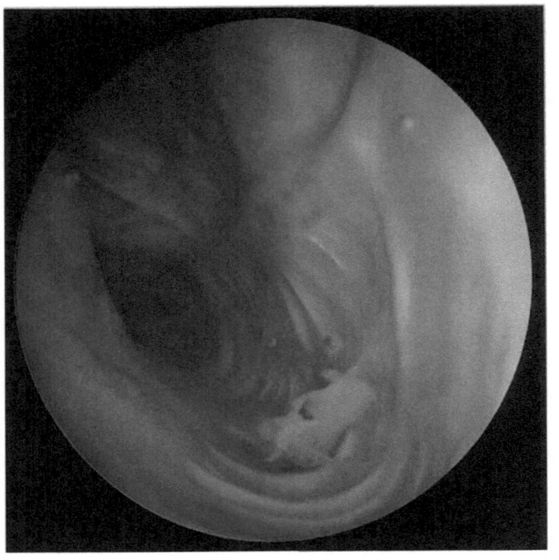

Fig. 10-12. Longitudinal cord in the synovial membrane 4 years following a lateral arthrotomy

sive cartilage lesions on both articular surfaces of the femoropatellar joint.

Implanted plastic materials, such as an alloplastic substitute for the anterior cruciate ligament, can lead to recurrent effusions. Arthroscopy often demonstrates an accompanying reactive synovitis (Fig. 10-13). In

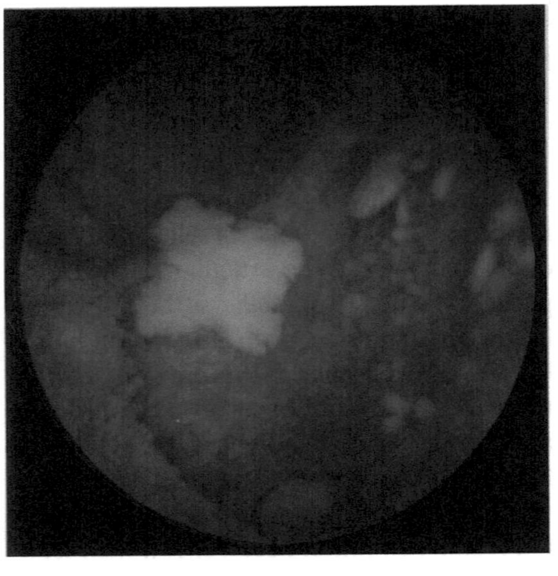

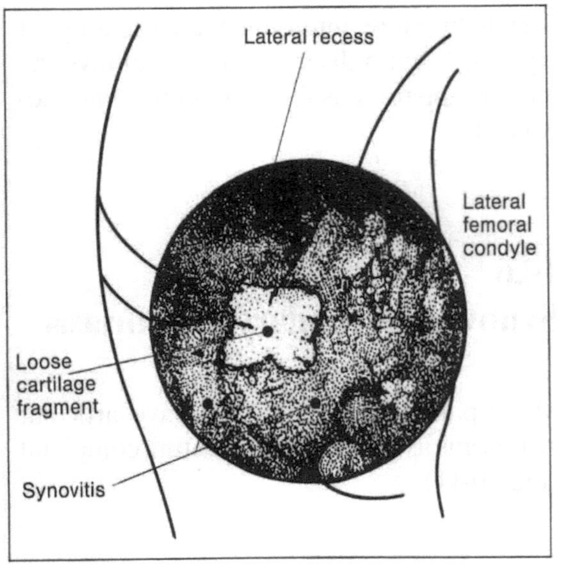

Fig. 10-13. Velvety, rust-colored synovitis with thick villi scattered throughout the joint following alloplastic replacement of the posterior cruciate ligament with a Dacron prosthesis ("Dacron synovitis"). There is a small, detached cartilage fragment at the center of the field

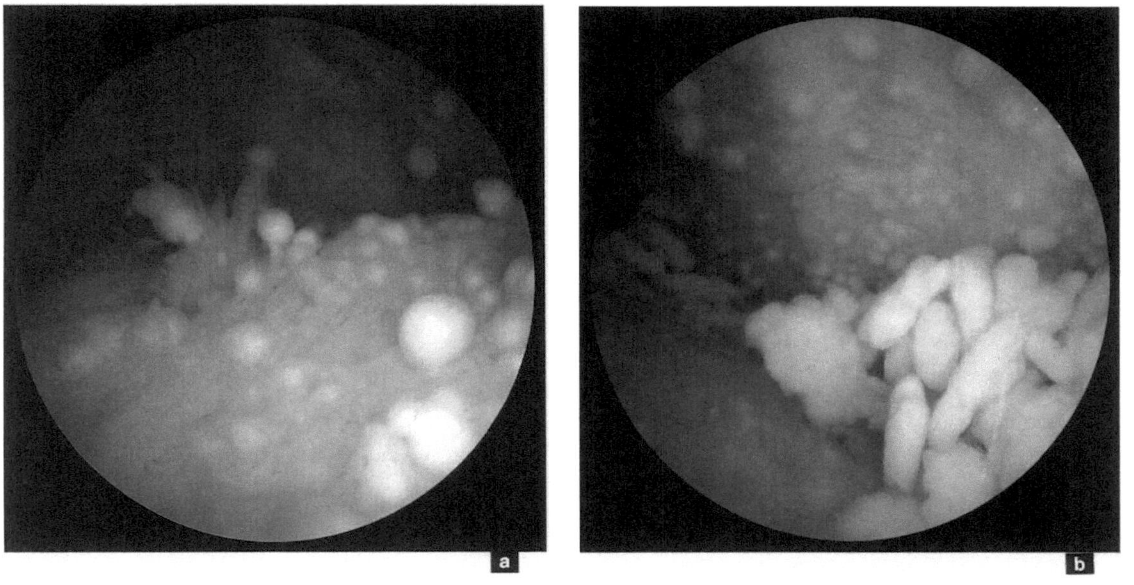

Fig. 10-14 a, b. Synovial chondromatosis. The synovium is studded with chondromatous bodies about to be released into the joint cavity (a). Some of these bodies collect in the suprapatellar pouch (b)

some cases the synovitis results from a partial or complete rupture of the reconstructed ligament.

10.8 Synovial Chondromatosis

Synovial chondromatosis is a rare disorder with conspicuous arthroscopic features. Besides numerous detached loose bodies (up to several hundred), arthroscopy reveals nests of bodies occurring at subsynovial or intrasynovial sites. Many bodies are found still attached to the synovium shortly before they are seeded into the lumen of the joint (Fig. 10-14) (Glinz 1987).

Unlike traumatically detached cartilage and meniscal fragments, synovial chondromas cannot be reabsorbed. The recommended treatment consists in the arthroscopic removal of all loose bodies combined with arthroscopic synovectomy.

11
Problems in Arthroscopy

This chapter deals with the "little problems" that can arise during diagnostic and operative arthroscopy and can be so frustrating to physicians who are just learning the technique. Often the uninitiated arthroscopist works by himself, so he must garner enough practical experience on his own to cope with the frequent and sometimes annoying problems that arise. The seasoned arthroscopist, on the other hand, solves these problems routinely with so little effort that he is scarcely aware of them.

In publications, lectures, and videotape presentations on knee arthroscopy, only the highest-quality images are presented to demonstrate the capabilities of the method. Far more often, however, the images seen in everyday practice are of moderate to poor quality. It is much like the weather: Cloudy days outnumber the clear.

With most problems in arthroscopy, a minor cause produces major effects.

One frequently neglected trouble source is the well-intentioned but overzealous care of electronic equipment (video recorder, monitor, light source) by operating-room and janitorial personnel. Plugs are pulled from sockets and wiped, switches are flipped, and buttons and control knobs are moved, pressed, or turned for a thorough cleaning. The light source, video camera, monitor, and videocassette recorder have to be completely readjusted when handled in this way.

11.1
Poor-Quality Monitor Image

A poor-quality monitor image takes much of the pleasure out of video arthroscopy. It makes findings difficult to interpret and surgical procedures difficult to perform.

11.1.1
Dark Image

Intraarticular structures cannot be clearly identified or differentiated on a dark screen. This can have various causes:

- *Equipment-related causes:* Old, cloudy optics; defective light cable; monitor brightness control set too low; light source set too low; old projection lamp.
- *Anatomic causes:* Since the suprapatellar pouch has nonreflecting walls that "swallow" light, it produces a darker image than more reflective structures like the articular cartilage and menisci.
- *Hemarthrosis:* A murky image due to hemarthrosis can be brightened by thorough irrigation of the joint.

The primary remedial measure for a dark image, besides copious irrigation for hemarthrosis, is to set the light source to maximum intensity. If the image remains dark even when a highly reflective surface (articular cartilage) is viewed, the cause is probably equipment-related. In this case the light cable and/or telescope is replaced during the procedure. A dark image may also result from a dim halogen lamp in a cold-light source or from an improperly positioned lamp socket. This problem is solved by switching to the backup bulb. Finally, a dark image may simply mean that the brightness control on the monitor needs adjusting.

11.1.2 Image too Bright

A very bright monitor image, like that seen when viewing cartilage surfaces or synovial hypertrophy, washes out subtle distinctions of contrast and contour. Also, the bright picture can have a dazzling effect on the viewer.

The brighter the image, the more difficult it is to appreciate structural differences in the cartilage.

Reducing the light intensity (by adjusting the control on the light source) is often sufficient to redefine contours and structural details. If definition does not improve, a white-out or yellow-out situation (with a featureless yellow-white monitor image) may be present (see Sect. 11.3).

11.1.3 Unsharp Image

General unsharpness of the monitor image usually signifies a technical problem. The video camera may be improperly adjusted or defective. Fluid between the eyepiece and camera will cause general blurring or fogging of the image due to evaporation.

This general unsharpness differs from the edge unsharpness caused by the forcible manipulation of a damaged or bent telescope. The image goes out of round and assumes an elliptical shape. A poorly centered or angled connection between the telescope and video camera also causes elliptical image distortion with edge unsharpness localized to one side of the screen.

Small scratches on the distal end of the telescope caused by inadvertent contact with the probe or operating instruments create small, punctate foci of unsharpness on the monitor image. This is usually not serious enough to interrupt the procedure, although the defects may cause a localized refraction that hampers diagnosis.

11.1.4 Foggy Image

In knees with extensive degenerative changes or injury to the infrapatellar fat pad, a foggy image is often seen following fluid distention of the joint. Repeated irrigation is necessary to obtain a clearer view. If a separate inflow cannula is in place or if a large-bore sheath is used with continuous suction, there should be no difficulty in producing a clear field.

If there is intraarticular hemorrhage or if arthroscopy is performed without tourniquet inflation, vision will become obscured unless an adequate fluid flow is maintained. Copious irrigation of the joint is indicated in these cases (Fig. 11-1).

If the video camera is sterilized by soaking in a disinfectant solution, heat generated during operation of the system will vaporize the residual moisture between the eyepiece and camera, and condensation will fog the optical surfaces. This can be avoided by rinsing the sterilized camera and telescope with a sterile solution (physiologic saline, Ringer's lactate) and drying them before use.

When arthroscopy is performed without a video camera, the eyepiece can become fogged by warm breath from the top of the surgeon's mask.

Some CCD video cameras produce a cloudy, grainy, or lined picture if there is inadequate light.

11.1.5 Image Flicker or Flutter

As with an ordinary home television set, flickering or fluttering of the monitor image may signal the "end" of the picture tube. But the most common source of this problem is a defective camera cable. The site where the cable connects to the camera is particularly vulnerable. If that area is damaged, image quality

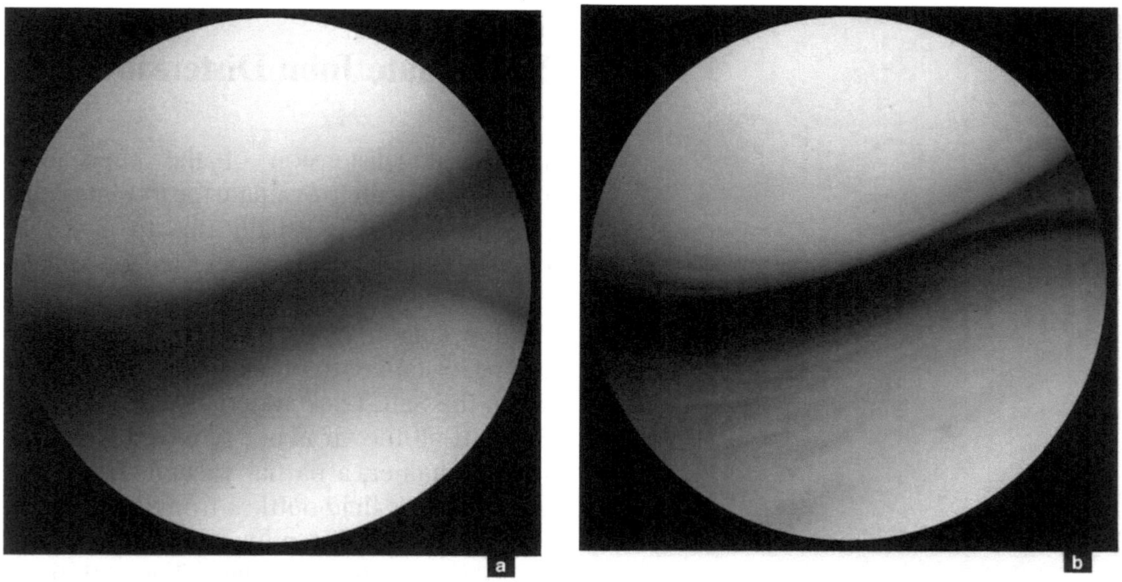

Fig. 11-1 a, b. Cloudy monitor image.
a) Cloudy image due to incipient hemorrhage. The condition of the medial meniscus cannot be assessed.
b) Aspirating the joint and maximally redistending it (by raising the fluid bag to a higher level) restores a clear field. Bloody residue is still visible in the posterior portion of the joint

will be noticeably affected by twisting, pulling, or pressing on the cable connection.

If the monitor image drifts upward or downward with movements of the arthroscope, a loose connection between the telescope and camera is usually to blame.

When electrosurgical instruments are used (electrocautery), the image will become "snowy" if the video camera and monitor are not adequately shielded against interference.

11.1.6 Persistent Image Features

Often a persistent yellowish or whitish structure will appear on the image immediately after the sheath has been inserted and the blunt obturator replaced with the telescope. This occurs when the end of the sheath shears off one or more small pieces of synovium or even articular cartilage, which become caught in the space between the sheath and telescope or sheath and obturator. Forceful insertion of the sheath can even gouge out large cartilage fragments that appear as flakelike structures on the monitor.

First an attempt is made to scrape the offending tissue fragments onto the capsule. If this cannot be done, the joint is maximally distended, the inflow is closed, and the telescope is removed from the sheath. If this does not flush the tissue fragment from the joint, the blunt obturator is reinserted to loosen the trapped fragment. If this, too, is unsuccessful, the sheath should be removed from the joint, manually cleaned, and then reintroduced with the blunt obturator inserted.

If the inflow is interrupted during arthroscopy while suction is inadvertently applied through the sheath, cartilage fragments, blood clots, or synovial villi may become aspirated. Particles too large to pass through the lumen of the sheath are held against the scope tip by suction, where they can obscure much of the optical field. Rotating the telescope (by moving the light post) does not improve the image. Even movements of the entire arthroscope may be unable to scrape off a particle held fast by suction. In these cases the particle

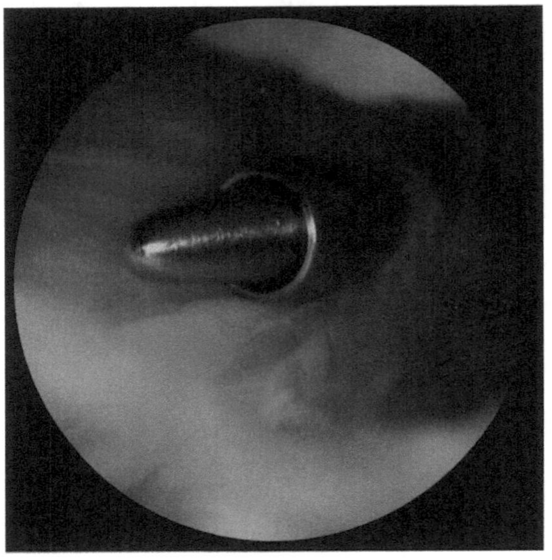

Fig. 11-2. The persistent white features at the top and bottom of the image are pieces of synovium and cartilage picked up by the scope tip as it traversed the intercondylar notch to enter the posteromedial recess. A sheath with blunt obturator has been passed into the recess through a posteromedial portal

can be flushed back into the joint simply by turning the suction off and opening the inflow valve.

When the arthroscope is passed to the posteromedial recess through the intercondylar notch, the tip of the sheath will almost always pick up small flakes of synovium or cartilage (Fig. 11-2). They can be eliminated by following the procedure described above.

A uniformly reddish or whitish image that does not change with movements of the scope probably signifies a red-out or yellow-out (see Sect. 11.3 and 11.4).

11.1.7 Image Off-Center

A crooked connection between the camera and telescope or between the telescope and sheath will cause the monitor image to appear off-center, with its upper or lower edge obscured. A bent telescope can cause the same effect. This problem can usually be corrected by loosening the crooked connections and retightening them in a straight position.

11.2 Inadequate Joint Distension

Inadequate distension of the knee joint makes it difficult to evaluate the intraarticular structures. This is usually due to a simple oversight such as a disconnected or kinked inflow tube, a closed inflow spigot, an open outflow spigot, a closed roller clamp on the tubing, or failure to break off the locking tab when the Safe-Lock system is used (see Fig. 3-24). If all the air is not removed from the fluid container, a partial vacuum is created which retards fluid outflow from the bag.

Thus, if joint distention is inadequate, the examiner should check the inflow path from the reservoir bag to the sheath or from the bag to the inflow cannula. If raising the bag to a higher level does not adequately reinflate the knee, the inflow channel of the sheath may be blocked (remove the telescope from the sheath and flush the channel).

If the joint is filled through a separate inflow cannula (see Sect. 3.5.1), inadequate distention may result from placement of the cannula in the subcutaneous tissue, in dense adhesions, or in the suprapatellar pouch where inflow is blocked by a suprapatellar septum (see Sect. 8.2.1). Inadvertent distension of the subcutaneous tissue can severely complicate the rest of the procedure.

When multiple intraarticular adhesions are present, arthroscope insertion and joint distension can both be difficult to accomplish. The femoropatellar space and suprapatellar pouch in particular may resist expansion due to their frequent involvement by adhesions. The solution is to divide the adhesions while simultaneously raising the fluid pressure (elevating the bag). Arthroscopy of a fibroarthrotic joint with significant loss of motion is by no means a simple procedure and should be reserved for experienced operators.

Motorized instruments of the type used for prolonged arthroscopic operations (e.g., synovectomies or abrasion chondroplasties) require a high fluid flow, so a large-diameter sheath or separate inflow cannula should be used. Fluid consumption can be reduced by turning off the suction during intervals when the shaver system is off (e.g., when the shaver is moved to a new position). When Y-tubing is used for aspiration (see Fig. 3-29), the suction is regulated by an assistant using an adjustable stopcock. If the suction is not adjustable, operation of the shaver system must be stopped intermittently, especially when the joint becomes deflated. If vision is restricted (yellow-out) when deflation occurs, there is the additional danger that intact structures will be inadvertently drawn against the suction tip and damaged.

If very large incisions were made for construction of the portals, a large fluid volume will be needed to compensate for leakage into the subcutaneous tissue and to the outside. The constant fluid loss makes it virtually impossible to establish an intraarticular fluid pressure adequate to distend the joint. Besides flooding the floor of the operating suite, this limits evaluation of the joint interior. Fluid leakage through the instrument portals is prevented by manual compression (assistant), bearing in mind that tentative hand pressure actually increases the subcutaneous extravasation of irrigating fluid. These problems can be avoided by making the instrument portals the correct size. If necessary, a suture can be placed to reduce the size of the opening.

11.3 Yellow-Out

"Yellow-out" denotes a situation in which a featureless, yellowish-white image is seen on the monitor. It is a common problem for beginners (Fig. 11-3).

A yellow-out can have various causes:

- *Incorrect insertion of the sheath.* A sheath inserted tangentially may enter the subcutaneous tissue or dissect between the fibrous capsule and synovium (Fig. 11-4 a). Starting the saline flow causes a balloon-like distention of the subcutaneous tissue, displaces the synovium into the joint cavity, or produces an externally visible swelling. The same situation can occur when the sheath is inserted too horizontally in the direction of the medial joint space (Fig. 11-4 c). The tip of the sheath may pierce and enter the infrapatellar fat pad, distending it with saline and ballooning it into the joint cavity. This hampers or prevents arthroscopic inspection of the anterior compartment.

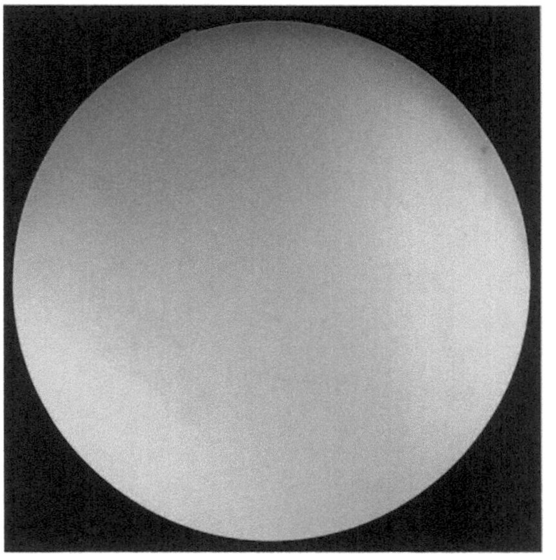

Fig. 11-3. Yellow-out

- *Incorrect positioning of the scope.* A frequent cause of yellow-out is placing the scope tip close to the capsule wall, cartilage, or other soft-tissue structures while the light post is unfavorably positioned (see Figs. 7-10 to 7-12). Thus, the first step in dealing with a yellow-out is to retract the scope carefully (to widen the visual field) and rotate the light post to a different position. Frequently this will bring identifiable structures into view.
  Synovitis or adhesive bands may necessitate debridement of the joint cavity with a motorized instrument (shaver system) before orientation can be achieved.
- *Irrigating fluid not turned on.* Unless the irrigation fluid is flowing, the joint will not distend. The suprapatellar pouch will not expand, and the synovial layers will obscure vision. In most cases the yellow-out will clear at once when the inflow is started.

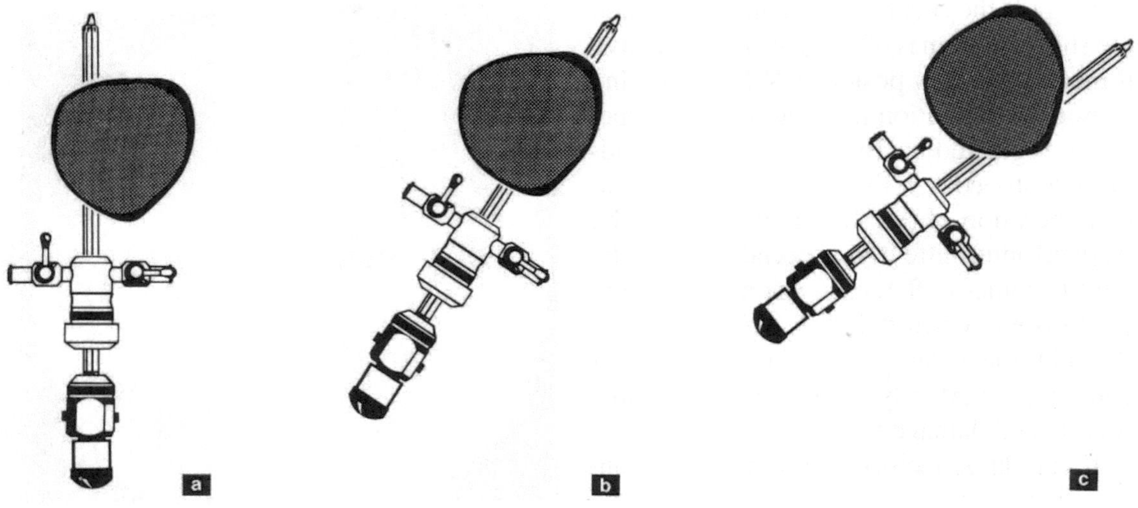

Fig. 11-4 a–c. Direction of insertion of the sheath. **a)** A sheath inserted tangentially, at too high an angle, enters the subcutaneous tissue. **b)** The correctly inserted sheath is directed toward the superomedial pole of the patella. **c)** A sheat inserted at too low an angle enters the infrapatellar fat pad

Extensive arthroscopic surgical procedures involving the use of motorized instruments require a large amount of fluid. If the intraarticular pressure falls in a situation where fluid consumption is high and there is little or no inflow to replace it, the joint will collapse. The remedy is to turn off the suction through the instruments and wait until the joint reexpands before proceeding with the arthroscopy. This problem is avoided by making sure that adequate fluid is provided and that aspiration is matched to the inflow.

- *Tissue fragment held to the scope by suction.* If the suction is inadvertently turned on, it may draw tissue particles against the scope tip and obstruct vision. The problem is solved by turning off the suction and opening the inflow. If the tissue fragment is hung on the tip, removing the telescope from the sheath will help to free it.

Fig. 11-5. Red-out

11.4 Red-Out

Analogous to the yellow-out, "red-out" denotes a condition in which a uniform reddish image appears on the monitor (Fig. 11-5). This situation is encountered with hemarthrosis. The joint should be irrigated until the returning fluid is clear, then the telescope may be inserted. If clots from an organized hemarthrosis are too large to be aspirated through the sheath, the joint should be maximally distended and an instrument portal added for inserting a large-bore aspirating needle, grasping forceps, or motorized instrument (synovial resector, Rosenberg resector). With a motorized instrument, even very large blood clots can be divided and aspirated from the joint.

Diffuse bleeding during arthroscopy can be controlled by increasing the intraarticular fluid pressure (raising the bag), except when there is an extensive capsuloligamentous disruption. If the source of the bleeding is identified, it can be selectively coagulated with electrical knife (electrocautery). If bleeding commences during the examination, the tourniquet should be checked to see that it is correctly positioned on the thigh and inflated to the correct pressure.

11.5 No Picture

If the monitor remains black after insertion of the arthroscope ("black-out"), the power supplies for the monitor, video camera, and light source should be checked. It is confirmed that the monitor and light source are on. and that the light cable is securely plugged into the cable socket on the light source. The brightness control on the monitor should also be checked!

If all the power supplies are connected, the light source is on, and the light cable is securely connected to the source and arthroscope, a dark screen must mean that there is a defect in the video camera, camera cable, or monitor.

Faced with this situation, the arthroscopist used to working from a monitor may find it difficult to switch to the traditional nonvideo technique. In some circumstances an arthrotomy may have to be performed or, alternatively, the procedure may have to be terminated and rescheduled.

But the great majority of camera malfunctions are the result of operator error. The main causes are excessive tension on the camera cable or bending the cable at too sharp an angle, especially at the site where it connects to the camera. Other potential causes of a black-out are improper handling of the shock-sensitive video camera, the entry of water or disinfectant solution into the camera, or the spraying of water into the vent openings on the monitor. Proper conduct on the part of the operator and OR personnel can largely eliminate these trouble sources.

11.6 Extravasation of Irrigating Fluid

The subcutaneous collection of irrigating fluid is a likely outcome when incisions of different lengths have been made in the skin, subcutaneous tissue, and capsule for constructing an instrument portal. The resultant fluid leakage produces a local or diffuse thickening of the soft-tissue envelope. The knee may appear grotesquely misshapen by the end of the procedure. The extravasation can be bothersome during the operation (making it more difficult to insert instruments) but generally does not lead to postoperative complications. Usually the subcutaneous fluid collection is completely absorbed by the second postoperative day at the latest. If the extravasation is exceptionally heavy, the portal sites can be left unsutured so that the dressing can help absorb the subcutaneous fluid.

A subcutaneous fluid collection can seriously hamper an operative procedure, such as an arthrotomy, that is performed in the same sitting. Orientation can be very difficult to establish in the engorged edematous tissue.

When the joint is distended with gas, a large instrument portal leads to an exorbitant loss of intraarticular pressure. This fact alone limits the use of gas in operative arthroscopy. Subcutaneous gas edema or air emphysema can also occur.

11.7 Inadequate Visualization of the Joint Compartments

Inability to visualize the medial and lateral compartments of the knee is most commonly due to errors of operating technique. Use of an improper flexion angle, failure to open the joint space adequately, and especially placing the arthroscope in the wrong rotational position (light post!) consistently lead to inadequate visualization of the articular compartments.

Another error is placing the arthroscope portal too far distally. When the scope enters at the level of the anterior horn of the lateral meniscus, it is difficult to visualize the lateral and medial compartments.

Inspection of the lateral compartment can be hampered by adhesions in the anterior compartment, by a septumlike infrapatellar plica that completely separates the medial and lateral portions of the joint, by a discoid lateral meniscus, a bucket-handle tear of the lateral meniscus, or an enlarged infrapatellar fat pad. Depending on the cause, an attempt is made to bypass the obstruction or eliminate it (remove adhesive bands, resect hypertrophied synovial tissue).

Inspection of the medial compartment can be difficult in the presence of a meniscal bucket-handle tear (see Fig. 8-49 c). A clear view of the compartment can usually be obtained by reducing the fragment or, in some cases, by displacing it out of the way. A hypertrophied mediopatellar plica can obstruct passage of the scope tip from the femoropatellar space to the medial compartment. If the plica impinges on the medial femoral condyle even with the knee extended, the arthroscope is first withdrawn to the level of the patellar ridge and then carefully swept downward to the medial meniscus.

Air bubbles (Fig. 11-6) or cartilage tags (Fig. 11-7) can also restrict the field of vision. Air bubbles most commonly occur in the suprapatellar pouch adjacent to the suprapatellar septum. They can be aspirated, but manual percussion of the joint or slight movements of the arthroscope may suffice to "dispel" them. Small, transparent cartilage tags that obscure vision can be held aside with the probing hook, or they can be removed with a grasping forceps or small hemostat (mosquito forceps).

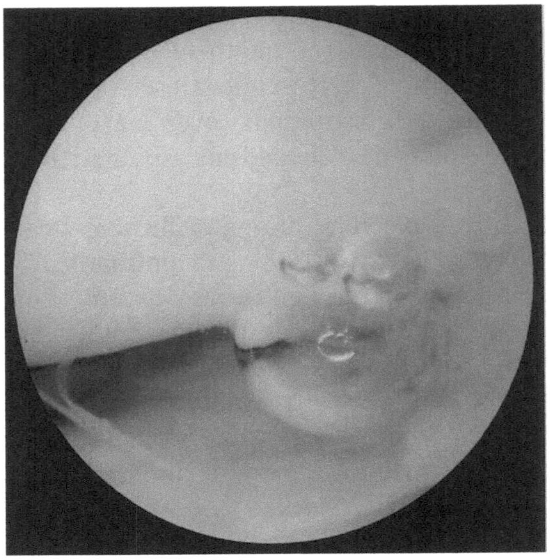

Fig. 11-6. Vision is distorted by the presence of air bubbles

11.8 Visualization of the Posterior Horn of the Medial Meniscus

The posterior horn of the medial meniscus is a difficult structure to view with an arthroscope, especially in very tight joints with little valgus laxity. Because most tears occur in the posterior segment of the meniscus, it is important to obtain optimum definition of that area. Arthroscopic surgery additionally requires satisfactory instrument access. Unfortunately, too many operators proceed with arthroscopic surgery on the posterior horn of the medial meniscus despite inadequate visibility, conducting the procedure "in the dark" without the benefit of clear vision. This can result in significant iatrogenic cartilage damage, resections that are incomplete or exces-

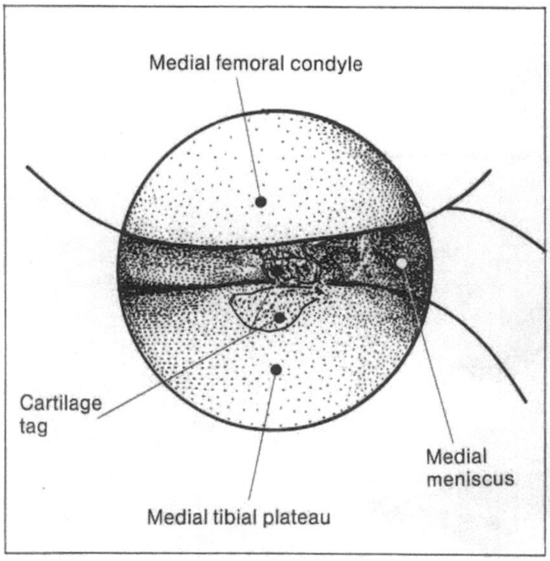

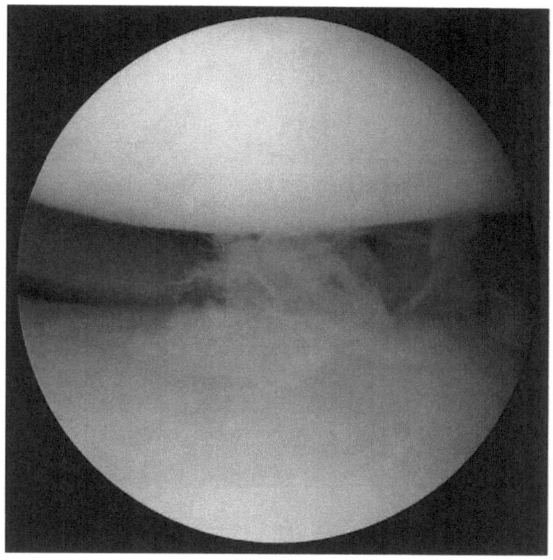

Fig. 11-7. Inspection of the medial meniscus is hampered by a small, transparent cartilage tag on the medial tibial plateau. These filmy tags usually occur spontaneously, but some may result from slight contact between the arthroscope and cartilage

sive, or damage to the posterior capsule with potential injury of the popliteal artery (see Sect. 12.5).

By following the guidelines listed below, the arthroscopist will find it easier to visualize the posterior segment of the medial meniscus and to reach that area with the various instruments used in arthroscopic operations.

11.8.1 Applying Valgus Stress to the Slightly Flexed Knee

A common mistake is to attempt to open up the medial joint space in the strongly flexed knee. The usual rationale is that flexion, by relaxing the medial capsule and ligaments, increases valgus mobility (Fig. 11-8). However, as the knee is flexed the posterior horn of the medial meniscus undergoes a disproportionate posterior recession in the initial degrees of flexion. This is due to the combined rolling-gliding mechanism of the knee, in which gliding predominates near extension while rolling predominates at higher flexion angles. As a result, when the knee reaches about 30° of flexion, the posterior segment of the medial meniscus is very difficult to visualize. Moreover, the increasing laxness of the posterior capsule with flexion reinforces the posterior movement of the medial meniscus. This is because a high intraarticular fluid pressure distends the posterior capsule, causing a posterior pull to be exerted on the meniscus.

As the knee extends from the flexed position, the posterior portion of the medial meniscus reemerges. Simultaneous external rotation of the tibia places tension on the medial capsule and ligaments–especially the posteromedial capsule, which provides the posterior attachment for the medial meniscus. In this situation the intraarticular fluid pressure can no longer push the taut capsule and attached medial meniscus posteriorly.

Strong flexion also has the effect of causing an undesired rotation of the femur upon the tibia, regardless of whether the leg is immobilized in a leg holder (see Fig. 4-2) or stabilized against a lateral post (see Fig. 4-1). A valgus stress can easily produce internal rotation of the femur, while a varus stress can produce external rotation. A minimally flexed knee position is the key to preventing undesired rotation of the leg.

Accordingly, a valgus stress applied to the slightly flexed knee (no more than 10°) com-

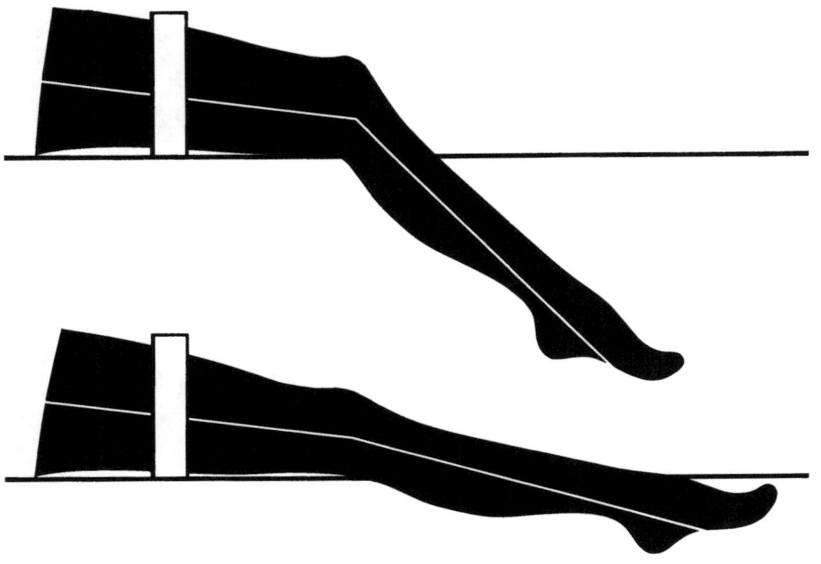

Fig. 11-8. Opening the medial joint space to visualize the posterior horn of the medial meniscus is difficult in the strongly flexed knee (top). This is more easily done when the knee is almost extended (bottom)

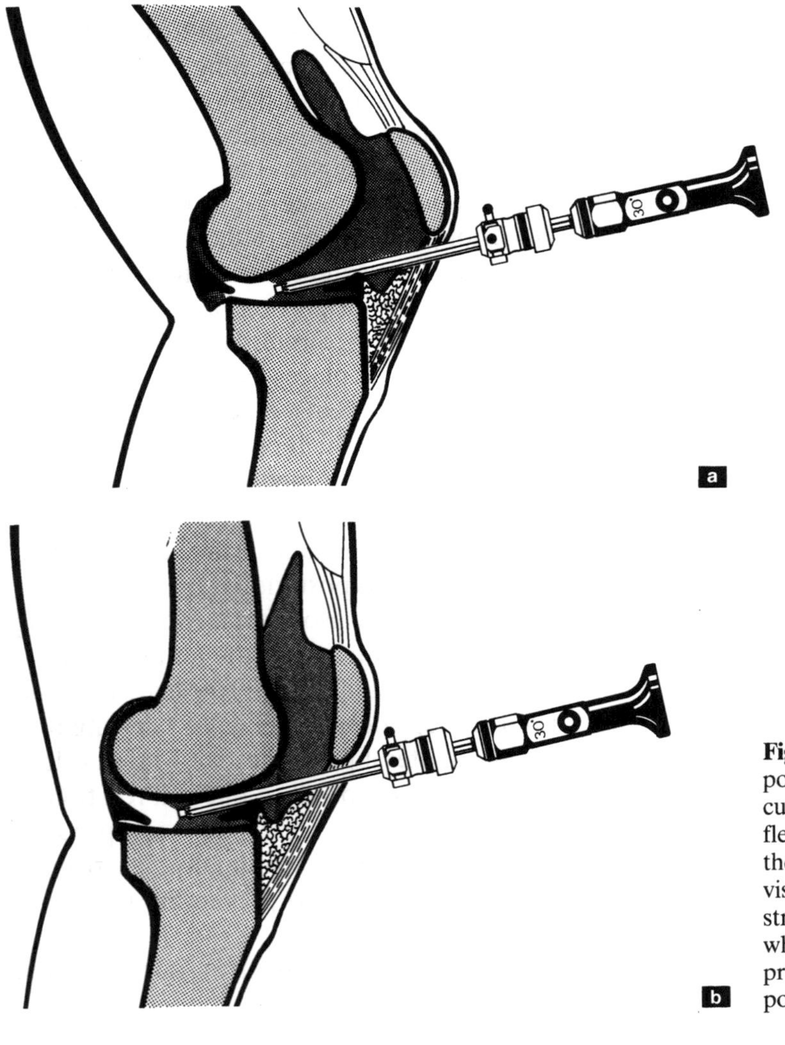

Fig. 11-9 a, b. Visualization of the posterior horn of the medial meniscus. **a)** Medial opening in 30° of flexion. The posterior segment of the medial meniscus is poorly visualized. **b)** Applying a valgus stress in the slightly flexed knee while externally rotating the tibia provides a much clearer view of the posterior horn bined with external rotation of the tibia is the optimum technique for visualizing the posterior horn of the medial meniscus. First the central portion of the meniscus is inspected with the knee extended. Then the tibia is externally rotated and the knee slightly flexed. Usually this will provide a satisfactory view of the posterior horn of the medial meniscus (Fig. 11-9).

Accurate positioning of the light post is essential for examination of this difficult area. The light post should be precisely at 3:00 (see Fig. 7-11), or at 9:00 in the left knee. Any deviation from this optimum position will significantly reduce visualization of the posterior horn.

11.8.2 Applying Manual Pressure from the Back of the Joint

When a valgus stress is applied to the slightly flexed knee while the tibia is externally rotated (see Sect. 11.8.1), direct manual pressure can be applied at the level of the posterior joint line to push the meniscus anteriorly (Fig. 11-10).

11.8.3 Optimum Placement of the Instrument Portal

To gain access to the posterior third of the medial meniscus for probing and other instrumentation in a very tight joint, the instrument portal should be placed just anterior to the medial collateral ligament at a level immediately above the superior surface of the meniscus.

The more resistant the joint is to medial opening, the more important it is to place the instrument portal precisely anterior to the medial collateral ligament.

With a more anterior portal site, the medial femoral condyle would obstruct access to the posterior meniscal segment, and it would be extremely difficult to probe the meniscus effectively (see Fig. 6-20 a). If the portal were too high, the instrument would impinge against the medial aspect of the medial femoral condyle (see Fig. 6-18).

If moderate valgus laxity is present, the posterior segment of the meniscus can also be reached through an anteromedial suprameniscal portal. The farther the medial joint space can be stressed open, the more anteriorly the instrument portal may be placed (see Fig. 6-20 c).

The posterior horn is directly accessible through a high medial portal placed directly adjacent to the patellar ligament, just distal to the patellar apex (see Fig. 6-22).

In tight joints, two instrument portals are often necessary for adequate treatment of the meniscus. In this case a portal placed just anterior to the medial collateral ligament on the immediate suprameniscal plane is supplemented by a high medial paraligamentous portal (posterior horn of medial meniscus).

11.8.4 Instrument Manipulations

With an optimally placed instrument portal, an attempt can be made to pull or push the posterior meniscal segment anteriorly with the probing hook. Johnson (1986) manipulates the meniscus by inserting a percutaneous needle into the posterior horn.

11.8.5 Manipulating the Meniscus with Suction

When the joint is maximally distended, the intraarticular fluid pressure tends to pull the posterior capsule and medial meniscus posteriorly. Thus it can be helpful in some cases, after obtaining the best possible view of the meniscus, to aspirate irrigating fluid through the arthroscopic sheath. This draws the meniscus into the visual field of the scope, making it easier to detect meniscal flaps or peripheral degenerative lesions.

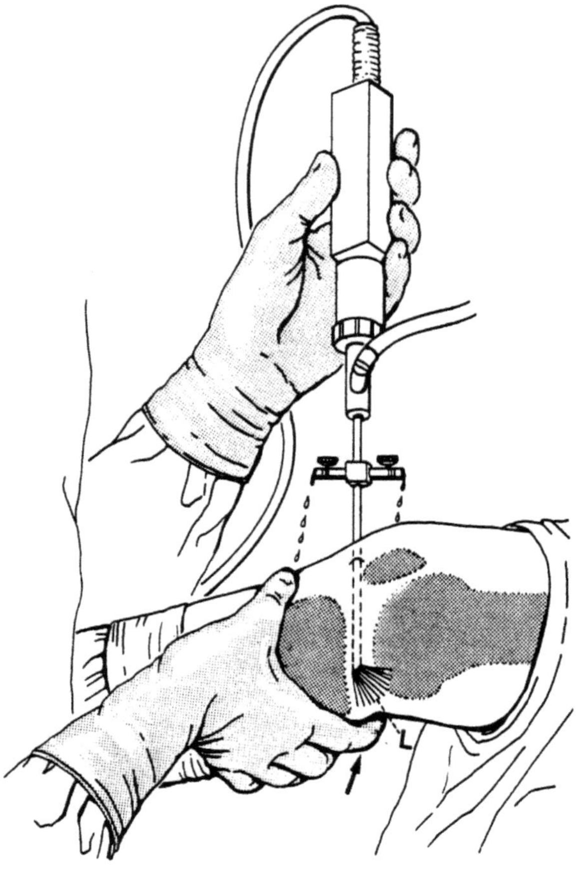

Fig. 11-10. Manual pressure on the posteromedial and posterior joint line pushes the posterior segment of the medial meniscus forward (L = arthroscope beam). The light post is positioned at 3:00 (9:00 in the left knee) (from Chassaing 1988)

If the posterior horn of the medial meniscus cannot be optimally visualized, laxity of the posterior capsule may be a contributing factor. In these cases the medial meniscus can usually be drawn into the visual field by closing the inflow and turning on the suction. This maneuver may have to be repeated several times.

11.8.6 Instrument Selection

Surgical procedures on the posterior segment of the medial meniscus call for the use of small instruments. Due to the concavity of the tibial plateau on the sagittal plane, the posterior horn of the meniscus lies on the ascending portion of the plateau. Thus, straight instruments can be used on the posterior horn only if the joint has good valgus laxity. Angled instruments whose jaws are directed upward can be used in this situation with less risk of cartilage injury. Flexible instruments, such as the electrocautery, can be advantageous in difficult situations.

In operations on the posterior horn, the "suction technique" (see Sect. 11.8.5) can be used to draw the meniscus into the working range of the instruments. Although motorized shaver systems are relatively bulky, once the tip has been positioned in front of the posterior segment of the meniscus, the meniscal tissue can be simultaneously shaved and aspirated.

12 Complications

Though their rate of complications is low, diagnostic and operative arthroscopy are not complication-free. Given the increasing therapeutic applications of arthroscopic techniques, this fact must be considered when the potential complications of arthroscopy are analyzed. In this chapter we shall consider the complications that may result from diagnostic and operative arthroscopic procedures on the knee.

Both the frequent and less common complications should be familiar to the arthroscopist. While the frequent complications are usually harmless and easy to treat, the less common ones can occasionally be life-threatening.

It is difficult to state an absolute complication rate due to the numerous factors that are involved. Arthroscopies either require a brief period of hospitalization or are done as outpatient procedures. Thus, the operator often does not have an opportunity to follow his patients, many of whom are subsequently seen and treated by private physicians. As a result, skin changes, effusions, recurrent pain, neuromas at incision sites, and even superficial infections are not seen by the surgeon performing the original arthroscopy, so a relatively large number of complications go undetected.

The nature of the patient population also influences the type and frequency of complications. Thus, patients treated at a trauma center show a relatively high incidence of fluid extravasation through acute capsuloligamentous ruptures and of postoperative hemarthrosis, whereas patients treated at an orthopedic hospital are more prone to irritative effusions and residual complaints since the population includes many older patients with chronic meniscal lesions and pronounced degenerative cartilage damage. The most comprehensive studies on complications rates in arthroscopy were published by Delee (1985) and Small (1986). While Delee reported on 118,590 arthroscopies with a complication rate of 0.78%, the second survey of the Complications Committee of the Arthroscopy Association of North America (Small 1986) covered 395,566 arthroscopies including 375,069 arthroscopies of the knee. There were 2215 complications reported, representing an overall complication rate of 0.56% (Table 12-1).

The problem with this most comprehensive survey to date lies in its retrospective nature. Most of the data are based on the memory of the surgeons. As Small (1986) himself points out, it is likely that survey respondents exaggerated the numbers of procedures performed and minimized the number of complications.

Of course, as new arthroscopic surgical procedures are developed, the technical difficulties mount, and the complication rates rise accordingly. Small (1986) reported a compli-

Table 12-1. Evaluation of 2215 complications in 395, 566 arthroscopies, after Small (1986)

Anesthetic complications	83
Instrument breakage	398
Ligament injuries	160
Femoral fractures	3
Nerve injuries	234
Vascular injuries	12
Infections	289
Thromboembolitic disease	752
Reflex sympathetic dystrophy	190
Miscellaneous	94

cation rate of 1.8% for surgical procedures on the anterior cruciate ligament and 2.4% for arthroscopic meniscal repairs.

The most recent study on complications in arthroscopic surgery covers a total of 10,262 procedures, 8791 of which were performed on the knee joint (Small 1988). Twenty-one of the most experienced arthroscopic surgeons in the U.S. participated in this *prospective* study. A total of 173 complications (1.68%) were recorded (Table 12-2). Iatrogenic cartilage injuries, however, were disregarded in this study. Looking at the complications rates for the individual procedures (Table 12-3), we find that complication rate is highest (7.17%) for lateral retinacular release. It is interesting to note that meniscal repair and meniscectomy have approximately the same incidence of complications (Table 12-3).

Table 12-2. Evaluation of 173 complications (=100%) in 10,262 arthroscopic operations, after Small (1988)

Hemarthrosis, hematoma	60.1%
Infection	12.1%
Thromboembolitic disease	6.9%
Anesthetic complications	6.4%
Instrument breakage	2.9%
Reflex sympathetic dystrophy	2.3%
Ligament injury	1.2%
Fracture	0.6%
Nerve injury	0.6%
Miscellaneous	6.9%

Table 12-3. Incidence of complications for specific arthroscopic procedures, after Small (1988)

Procedure	Incidence (in %)
Lateral retinacular release	7.17
ACL synthetic reconstruction	3.7
ACL allograft reconstruction	3.3
Synovectomy	3.12
Abrasion chondroplasty	1.89
Meniscal repairs (outside-in)	1.89
Medial meniscectomy	1.78
Plica excision	1.71
ACL autologous reconstruction	1.71
Chondroplasty	1.6
Medial meniscal repair	1.52
Lateral meniscectomy	1.1

Earlier studies were concerned mainly with diagnostic arthroscopies. Dick (1978) reviewed 3714 arthroscopies and observed no serious complications. Iatrogenic cartilage damage, with an incidence of 2%, was the most frequent complication reported.

A critical and differentiated review of over 2600 diagnostic and operative arthroscopies by Sherman (1986) indicated an overall complication rate of 8.2% (!). However, even minor wound healing problems, postoperative effusion, and hematomas at portal sites were classified as complications and recorded. By far the lowest complication rate was observed in purely diagnostic arthroscopy, while the highest rate was found in older patients (over age 50) with a tourniquet time in excess of 60 min.

A careful working technique, good arthroscopic visualization of the joint cavity, appropriate equipment, and adequate experience in arthroscopy are essential prerequisites for a low complication rate.

Kieser (1984) aptly described the evolution of the arthroscopist in terms of four stages of self-assessment:

I. Justified lack of confidence
II. Unjustified confidence
III. Justified confidence
IV. Unjustified lack of confidence

The enthusiastic beginner easily progresses to stage II, which is fraught with complications, although he imagines himself to be at stage III. By adopting a more realistic and critical attitude toward his own arthroscopic competence, the beginner can minimize the risk of iatrogenic trauma. A knowledge of these four stages can help to reduce the number of iatrogenic injuries, which are "more common than we care to admit" (Glinz).

A distinction is drawn between intraoperative and postoperative complications. The examiner should be able to recognize and treat intraoperative complications as soon as they occur. Postoperative complications arise after a latent period of hours, days, or even weeks.

12.1 Articular Cartilage Damage

Articular cartilage injuries by arthroscopic instruments are the most frequent complication of arthroscopy. They become less frequent as the experience level of the arthroscopist increases.

In a strict sense we may say that arthroscopy, even in experienced hands, invariably produces at least some degree of articular cartilage damage.

During video arthroscopy in a fluid medium, even superficial sites of cartilage exfoliation can appear quite large. Usually this is due to the magnifying effect of the arthroscope, and the lesion can be disregarded (see Fig. 11-7). In arthrotomies, on the other hand, most iatrogenic cartilage lesions are not detected during the procedure, but only when the patient again comes to arthroscopy for residual complaints. Most lesions occur at sites that are difficult or impossible to see in the arthrotomized knee (Fig. 12-1).

Video arthroscopy, by contrast, provides an immediate, unsparing, close-up view of the slightest technical deficiency in the operation. Cartilage lesions are visible for all to see, especially in fluid arthroscopy where cartilage tags do not lie flat, as they do in gas, but float in the intraarticular fluid.

Particular care must be exercised in the use of motorized instruments (cutter, burr, turbo cutter). A power cutting tip that slips from the meniscus or from the cartilage or bone area requiring treatment can do catastrophic damage to adjacent intact cartilage.

Mechanical instruments such as basket forceps, knives, scissors, and electrical cutting instruments can also produce deep cartilage lesions when used with improper technique in poorly accessible sites or under conditions of poor visibility (Fig. 12-2). The use of small instruments is recommended. The slightest contact of the electrosurgical instrument will leave brownish singe marks on the cartilage surface (Fig. 12-3), the color contrast causing the lesion to appear deeper and more extensive than it really is. The cartilage damage done by sharp cutting instruments is visible only when there is a defect with loss of cartilage substance. Isolated knife cuts in the cartilage are only briefly visible because the cut edges immediately reappose, similar to a cut in cheese. Cartilage injuries from mechanical

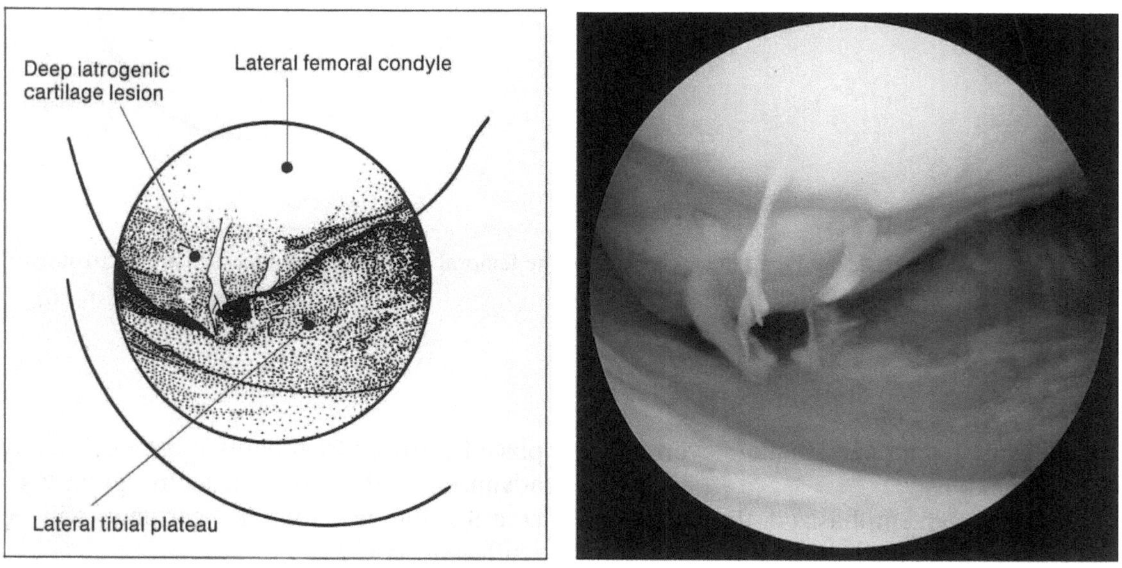

Fig. 12-1. Deep scoring of the articular cartilage on the lateral femoral condyle 6 months after open lateral meniscectomy. The patient underwent arthroscopy due to residual complaints

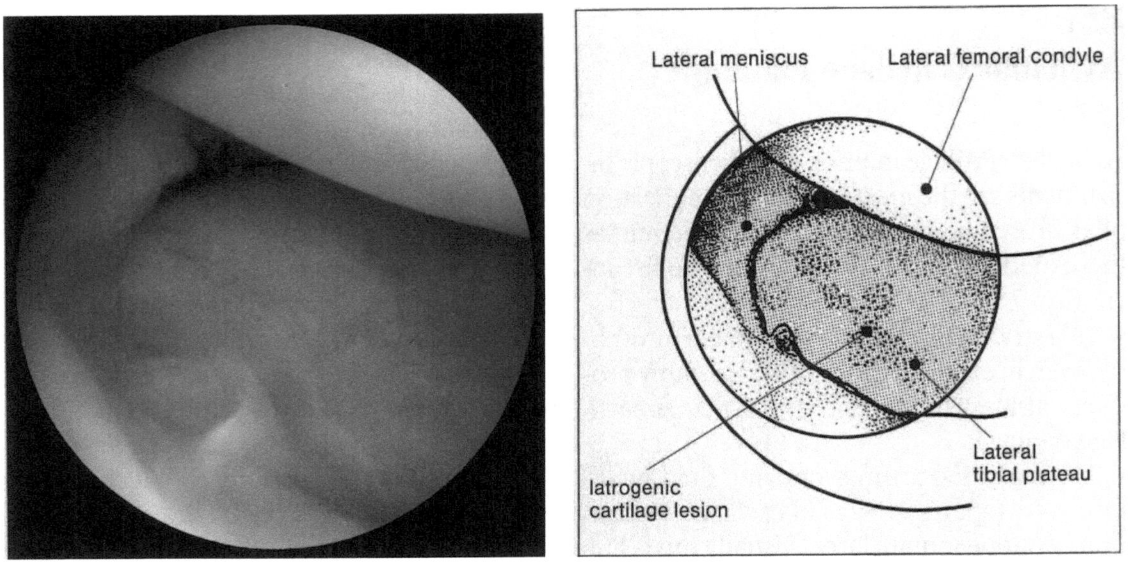

Fig. 12-2. Extensive cartilage lesions on the lateral tibial plateau 12 weeks after arthroscopic lateral meniscectomy. Arthroscopy was repeated due to recurrent effusions and persistent pain

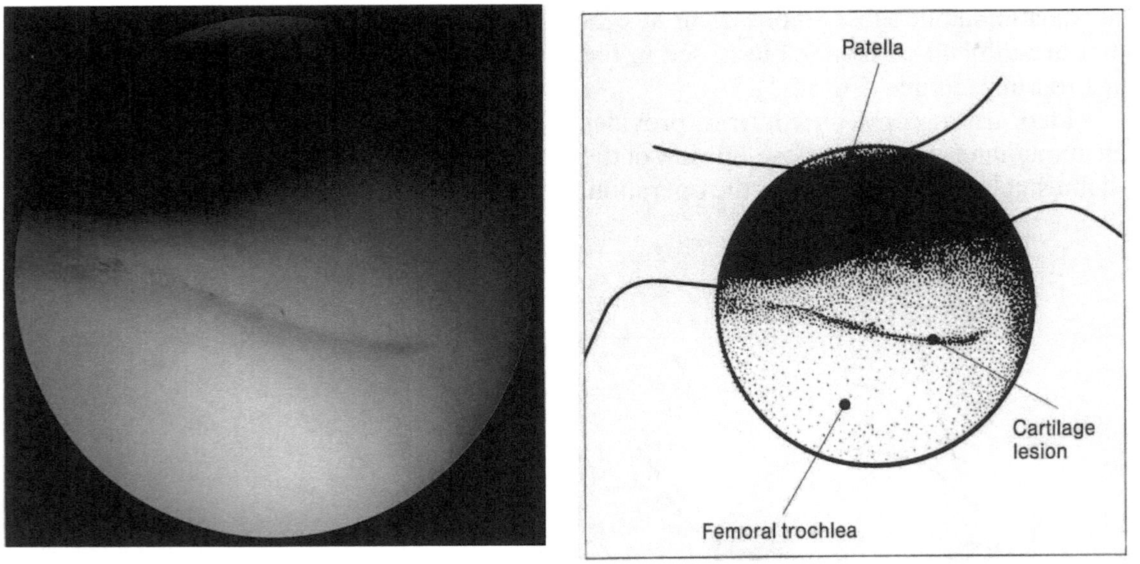

Fig. 12-3. Singed track left on the articular cartilage of the femoral trochlea by contact with an electrosurgical instrument used to resect a mediopatellar plica

knives tend to appear smaller, even when deep and extensive.

It should be emphasized that optimum placement of the instrument portal is one of the most important factors in the prevention of cartilage lesions. With an unfavorably placed portal, instruments must be forcibly advanced to the target structure, greatly increasing the risk that the cartilage will be scuffed or scored.

Even in diagnostic arthroscopy, significant cartilage damage can be caused by the

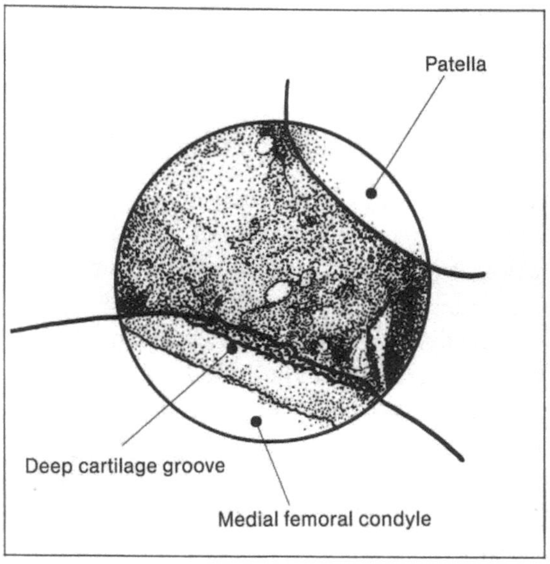

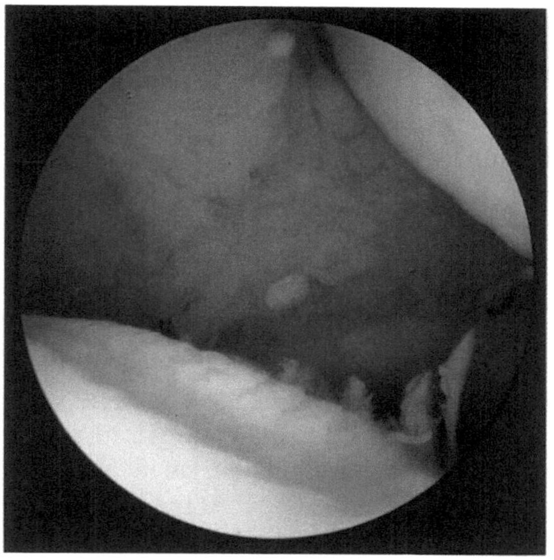

Fig. 12-4. Deep iatrogenic groove in the medial surface of the femoral trochlea following insertion of the arthroscopic sheath

telescope or by a projecting sheath (see Sect. 3.1.1). Insertion of the sheath represents a particularly dangerous phase. If the examiner forgets to exchange the blunt obturator for the sharp trocar, deep iatrogenic cartilage grooves can result (Fig. 12-4). For this reason and others, we have abandoned the use of a sharp trocar altogether (see Sect. 3.1.1).

In video arthroscopy, manipulating the arthroscope by the end of the video camera creates a very long extraarticular lever arm. This can cause the short, intraarticular portion of the scope to gouge out deep cartilage lesions even when minimal force is applied (see Fig. 7-7).

The following rules are helpful in avoiding damage to the articular cartilage:

- Perform all instrument maneuvers and operations under direct arthroscopic vision.
- Never move the sheath or instruments forcibly inside the joint.
- Change the angle of knee flexion slowly and carefully when an instrument is inside the joint.
- If the instrument portal is unfavorably located, do not hestiate to add a second, better portal.

12.2 Carrying Particles of the Incise Drape into the Joint

If an incise drape is used, the operator must be careful not to introduce small particles of the drape into the joint. This complication usually results from making too-small skin incisions directly through the adherent drape. The arthroscope or operating instrument may tear off small pieces of film and transport them into the intraarticular space.

This problem is avoided by cutting out a circular piece of drape material (about the size of a 50-cent piece) about the arthroscope and instrument portal sites before making the incisions.

Because an incise drape does not improve asepsis in arthroscopic procedures and can actually compromise it, we use this type of drape only if a major open or arthroscopic surgical procedure (e.g., ACL reconstruction) is planned for the same sitting. An incise drape is not required for purely diagnostic arthroscopy and for most arthroscopic operations.

12.3 Instrument Breakage

A complication of operative arthroscopy, the breakage of an arthroscopic operating instrument accounts for 18% of the overall complication rate (Small 1986).

We can understand the susceptibility of arthroscopic instruments to failure when we consider that their construction must meet conflicting demands. On the one hand, the instruments must be small enough to reach the target structures in the small articular compartments of the knee. At the same time, they must be stable and robust enough to cut or fragment hard tissues (meniscus, articular cartilage). Thus, arthroscopic instruments must combine an effective cutting action with a high mechanical strength and stability for their size.

An arthroscopic instrument used several times daily will inevitably undergo dulling and material fatigue. A possible consequence is failure of the instrument. The blades of cutting instruments are particularly susceptible to breakage. This has already prompted some manufacturers to design their instruments with built-in weak points to ensure that, when a designated load is reached, the blades will fracture in a way that prevents intraarticular loss of the broken piece.

If an instrument should break off inside the joint, the following procedure is recommended:

1. Remain calm and deliberate!!
2. Close the inflow and outflow lines. This will prevent fluid turbulence that might carry the broken piece to a difficult site.
3. Center the broken piece in the visual field.
4. Keep the knee stationary. Flexion or extension could cause the piece to slip suddenly into a posterior compartment, requiring additional time and effort for its location and retrievel.
5. Immobilize the broken piece with one or two percutaneous needles.
6. Grasp the broken piece with a grasping forceps. If the piece cannot be retrieved with this instrument or if the portal is unfavorably located, add a second portal and pass a second grasping instrument into the joint. The fragment can be transferred from the first forceps to the second for removal.

The use of a magnetic instrument (Golden Retriever, Accufex Co.) can facilitate the immobilization and extraction of an instrument fragment.

If, despite all efforts, the fragment is lost from the visual field, the hunt for it can be a very tedious process. The joint is thoroughly irrigated several times in an effort to bring the fragment out of hiding. It can be helpful to visualize both posterior recesses and suction them through the arthroscopic sheath. The suction may draw the fragment against the sheath, which can then be carefully retracted to a site where the fragment can be grasped and extracted through another portal.

If the lost fragment cannot be located arthroscopically, the knee is examined by image intensification fluoroscopy.

An effort should be made to retrieve the fragment arthroscopically, because an arthrotomy, no matter how extensive, cannot provide better visualization of the knee compartments. This especially applies to the posterior compartments–a favorite "hiding place" for broken instrument pieces – which would require an extremely wide arthrotomy for exposure. If the fragment slips again during the arthrotomy, it may be necessary to open the other side of the joint as well. Arthrotomy is a last-resort option, and it is better to leave the fragment in the joint until arthroscopic retrieval can be reattempted.

The regular cleaning, maintenance, and inspection of instruments can reduce the risk of instrument failure.

The following technical guidelines are helpful in avoiding instrument breakage:

- Always pass operating instruments into the joint with the blades closed.
- When moving an instrument within the joint, keep the blades closed and keep the instrument constantly in view. It is particularly dangerous to rotate an instrument with the blades open in the posterior com-

partments (e.g., to reach the posterior horn of the medial meniscus).
- In case of poor visualization, a foggy image, or a yellow-out or red-out (see Sect. 11.3 and 11.4), improve the image quality before doing anything else. If this cannot be done (e.g., because a tourniquet is not used), manipulate the instruments very slowly and carefully.
- Do not force instruments through bony spaces! Angled and curved instruments are at greatest risk when rotated in narrow spaces, even when the jaws are closed.

A knife blade that separates or breaks away from the knife handle while in the joint can be dangerous. The blade or fragment is extracted using the procedure described above.

12.4 Nerve Injuries

Small (1986) reports that nerve injuries account for 10% of all complications in arthroscopy. The peroneal nerve, femoral nerve, sciatic nerve, or saphenous nerve may be affected.

The nerves may be directly damaged by operating instruments. The infrapatellar branch of the saphenous nerve is particularly at risk; it may be stretched, partially divided, or transected during the placement of a medial instrument portal. A suture may be inadvertently tied over the nerve during suture placement for a meniscal repair. If absorbable suture material is used, symptoms should improve in about 3 months following absorption of the threads. Nerves that course posteriorly or posteromedially are susceptible to injury during meniscal repairs and during construction of a posteromedial or posterolateral portal.

Before an instrument portal is made, large veins are identified by transillumination (see Fig. 6-10) so that they can be avoided when the skin is incised. When a superficial vein is damaged, not only is vision obscured by the resultant hemorrhage, but the fine nerve fibers accompanying the vein are also severed. A painful neuroma may form at the site of the nerve section, compromising the outcome of the surgery.

The peroneal nerve, femoral nerve, and lateral femoral cutaneous nerve are susceptible to position-related injuries. When the patient is positioned supine, the peroneal nerve is vulnerable to pressure injury if the lateral post (see Fig. 4-1) is placed at the level of the joint line and a strong valgus stress is applied for a prolonged period to open the medial joint space.

The tourniquet time for arthroscopy should not exceed 120 min.

In patients with scant muscular development, paresthesias can occur after only a brief period of tourniquet inflation. These usually regress in the initial days following arthroscopy. However, the extent and location of a nerve injury cannot be accurately assessed until several days after the procedure.

Sherman (1986) noted a direct correlation between the duration of tourniquet use and the rate of postoperative complications: The longer the tourniquet time, the higher the complication rate.

12.5 Vascular Injuries

Serious vascular injuries are rare intra- and postoperative complications of arthroscopy. Only 12 vascular injuries were reported in more than 370,000 knee arthroscopies reviewed by the Arthroscopy Association (Small 1986).

There have been isolated reports of a false aneurysm of the inferior geniculate artery following a lateral incision (Manning 1987), and a false aneurysm of the popliteal artery has been described as a late complication (Beck 1986). Jeffries (1987) reported on two popliteal artery injuries that necessitated immediate vascular surgery. The arterial hemorrhage was noted immediately after tourniquet deflation. Both injuries were inflicted with a meniscotome during arthroscopic meniscectomy.

Some popliteal artery injuries may go unnoticed intraoperatively and in the immediate postoperative period, and several days may pass before symptoms appear.

Case report. A 55-year-old male with genu varum underwent arthroscopy for the planning of a corrective osteotomy. Sites of fraying on the posterior horn of the medial meniscus were removed arthroscopically with a basket forceps and knife. The knee became swollen after surgery, a suction drain yielding 1000 ml of bloody aspirate in the first 24 h. Swelling increased in subsequent days, especially in the popliteal fossa area, where a pulsatile mass with an audible bruit was noted on the 8th postoperative day. Digital subtraction angiography identified the mass as an arteriovenous aneurysm (Fig. 12-5). Operation disclosed a completely transected popliteal artery and an 8-mm elliptical hole in the popliteal vein.

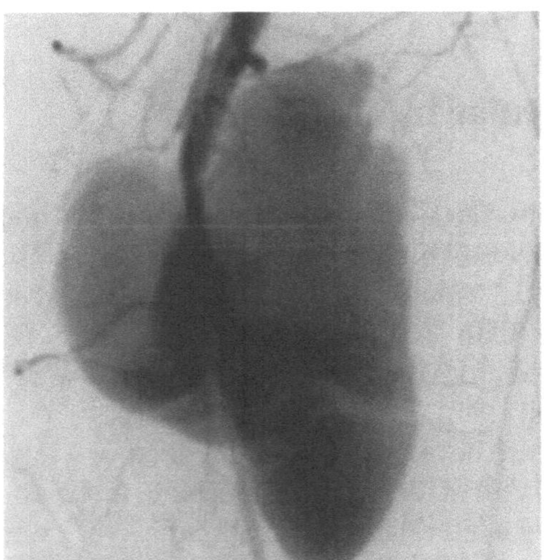

Fig. 12-5. Digital subtraction angiography demonstrates an arteriovenous aneurysm of the popliteal vessels 7 days after arthroscopic resection of the posterior horn of the medial meniscus

Major vascular injuries most commonly involve the popliteal artery, and most occur in association with arthroscopic procedures on the posterior horn of the medial meniscus. Thus, the surgeon must give particular attention to the close topographic relationship of this structure to the neurovascular bundle.

The key to avoiding this type of complication lies in the clear arthroscopic visualization of the posterior horn of the medial meniscus (see Sect. 11.8) so that surgery can be performed with optimum visibility.

A hard-to-see posterior meniscal segment can pose problems even for experienced arthroscopists, and surgeons are cautioned against cutting into the posterior horn with sharp knives that require pressure to exert their cutting action.

The vascular status of the limb should always be checked following arthroscopy. Massive drainage from the knee should raise suspicion of a vascular injury and prompt an immediate evaluation.

Preoperative evaluation of the pulses is especially important in elderly patients with circulatory problems. If blood circulation is impaired, this may be responsible for the patient's knee complaints or may pose a relative or even absolute contraindication to tourniquet usage during arthroscopy.

12.6 Ligament and Bone Injuries

Iatrogenic ligament injuries are a known but rare complication of knee arthroscopy. The application of an excessive valgus or varus strain to the knee can cause a ligament rupture, especially in elderly patients or patients with a preexisting capsuloligamentous injury. The collateral ligaments are particularly vulnerable when they are already partially torn or when the lateral or medial joint space is forcibly and abruptly stressed open during arthroscopy.

In arthroscopic arthrolyses, vision is so obscured by intraarticular adhesions that vigorous instrumentation can easily damage the medial or lateral capsule, the quadriceps tendon, or even the menisci. Blasier and Ciullo (1986) described one instance of quadriceps tendon rupture during an arthroscopic lateral retinacular release. Postoperatively there was an active extension deficit with suprapatellar pain, which finally was diagnosed as a severed quadriceps tendon one month after surgery.

The popliteus tendon is susceptible to injury during lateral meniscectomy. Additionally, an overextensive resection of meniscal tissue can lengthen the popliteal hiatus. If this divides the meniscal attachment to the popliteal hiatus, the isolated posterior horn of the lateral meniscus can become isolated and act like a pedunculated flap, causing intermittent locking. Thus, the surgeon must be particularly careful in this area when performing a lateral meniscectomy.

The medial meniscus is vulnerable to injury during suprameniscal portal placement. The percutaneous needle used to locate the portal can cause little damage, but if the knife used to incise the skin and capsule should slip, it can transect the entire meniscus. The best way to avoid this is to keep the cutting edge of the knife directed upward when the skin and capsule are incised (see Figs. 6-14 and 6-15).

Though it may seem unlikely, significant bone fractures have been reported in isolated cases as a complication of arthroscopy. Small (1986) notes that three femoral fractures were reported in the Arthroscopy Association survey.

12.7 Infection

Postoperative infection, the most feared complication of arthroscopy, has a reported incidence between 0.01% and 0.1% in the literature. The more than 370,000 knee arthroscopies reviewed by Small (1986) included 289 cases of infection (0.073%), 201 of which were deep infections (0.054%). This is substantially lower than the 2%–5% infection rate following arthrotomies.

It should be noted that 40%–80% of intraarticular knee infections are a result of percutaneous needle insertions and intraarticular injections. For example, intraarticular cortisone injections can cause such immune suppression that even a small number or organisms may be able to incite an intraarticular infection. If a joint infection develops after an injection or percutaneous aspiration (irritative effusion) in an elderly patient who has preexisting cartilage damage, the chances for successful treatment of this complication are reduced because symptoms are often misinterpreted or perhaps delayed or obscured by, say, the injection of steroids or local anesthetic.

Strict aseptic technique for all invasive procedures (aspiration, injection, arthroscopy) continues to be the best preventive measure against intraarticular infection.

In the very widely used technique of video arthroscopy, the camera is either soaked in disinfectant solution or wrapped in a sterile plastic sleeve. In the latter case the integrity of the plastic sleeve is routinely rechecked prior to operation. A particular trouble spot is the site where the sleeve attaches to the arthroscope, where small tears can form. If arthroscopy is performed without a video camera, the eyepiece of the scope is considered to be unsterile due to contact with the examiner's eye.

The most common causative organism of postarthroscopic knee infections is *Staphylococcus aureus*. Less common pathogens such as *Streptococcus pneumoniae, Staphylcoccus epidermidis, Haemophilus influenzae, Clostridium perfringens,* and *Neisseria gonorrhoeae* have also been isolated (Smith 1986, Berhang 1987).

Schonholtz (1986) reported on a hematogenous knee infection by *Moraxella osloensis*. Interestingly, the clinical picture was that of a joint infection, but bacterial smears prepared from aspirated fluid were sterile. Synovial biopsy was necessary to establish the diagnosis.

If an infection occurs despite all precautions, early arthroscopic intervention is of critical importance. An infection should be suspected following arthroscopy if the knee becomes erythematous, warm, swollen, and very tender to pressure after arthroscopy (the patient holds it in a flexed position). The joint is percutaneously aspirated under aseptic conditions. If the aspirated fluid is turbid, flocculent, or yellowish and putrid, copious arthroscopic irrigation of the entire joint cavity should be carried out at once.

If the patient also manifests systemic signs with fever, lymphangitis, leukocytosis, or an elevated sedimentation rate, the diagnosis of infection is virtually confirmed.

Regardless of which joint is affected, the management of joint infection consists of the following measures (Strobel, Pässler 1989):

1. *Protection and mechanical cleansing of the joint.* As in the surgical treatment of infection in general, the rule *"ubi pus, ibi evacua"* applies. The whole interior of the joint must be copiously irrigated, making certain that no compartments are missed (suprapatellar pouch, medial and lateral recesses, posterolateral and posteromedial corners). All fibrin tags and necrotic tissue particles must be washed from the joint to deprive microorganisms of vital culture media and prevent a recrudescence of the infection.
2. *Specific antibiotic therapy.* Unable to "do all the work" in an infected knee joint, antibiotics must be used in conjunction with the foregoing principle (evacuation of septic material) in order to cure infection and restore function. Systemic antibiotics, possibly combined with local antibiotic therapy (antibiotic-laden irrigating solution), play an adjunctive role to surgical treatment.
3. *Functional rehabilitation.* The primary goal of the treatment of joint infections should be to eradicate the infection with minimal trauma (e.g., by arthroscopic lavage and debridement) so that therapeutic exercises can be started as quickly as possible to preserve the motor function of the knee.

The decision between open or arthroscopic treatment of the infected knee joint will depend on the etiology of the infection. If the infection has resulted from open soft-tissue surgery, only the intraarticular space is accessible to arthroscopic treatment; infected soft tissues outside the joint will require separate debridement and suction irrigation.

With a clinically overt infection following knee arthroscopy or percutaneous aspiration or resulting from hematogenous spread, the joint can be treated by a purely arthroscopic procedure in suitable candidates.

The whole interior of the knee joint is copiously irrigated with up to 15–20 liters of irrigating solution. Even hard-to-reach sites in the joint are more accessible to arthroscopic irrigation than to irrigation through an arthrotomy wound. Moreover, arthroscopic irrigation delivers a greater amount of fluid through the joint than open lavage, so that a better irrigating effect is achieved in all compartments and recesses.

Fibrin deposits on cartilage surfaces are removed with a motorized instrument (shaver system) (Smith 1986). Hypertrophied or necrotic synovial tissue, which most commonly occurs in the suprapatellar pouch, is likewise removed. If the joint infection is far advanced, there will usually be a general synovitis that is best treated by synovectomy under antibiotic coverage.

Until the infecting organisms have been identified, a broad-spectrum systemic antibiotic (e. g., cephalosporins such as cefotaxime or cefuroxime) is given by intravenous injection. When the sensitivity report is obtained, the broad-spectrum antibiotic is changed, if necessary, to the most appropriate agent.

If local and general symptoms do not resolve with this therapy in 2 days, the joint should be reentered with the arthroscope and the irrigation and cleansing repeated.

Continuous suction irrigation through a loculated space such as the knee joint tends to create a "highway effect" in which fluid goes in one tube and out the other, following the shortest path between them. Areas distant from the "highway" are irrigated minimally, if at all. To prevent this effect, Jackson (1973) recommends a discontinuous suction irrigation in which the outflow tube is closed several times daily to allow maximum distention of the joint with irrigating fluid.

Knee infections following arthroscopy, percutaneous aspiration, intraarticular injection, or caused by hematogenous seeding can also be adequately treated without the use of suction irrigation. Smith (1986) treated 30 patients with a knee infection by arthroscopic irrigation and the removal of fibrin deposits, if present, combined with a 4–6 week course of antibiotic therapy. The results of this treatment were rated as good (less than 10° limitation of motion, no pain) or excellent (unlimited motion, no pain) in all cases.

Using a similar regimen, Ivey (1988) obtained good or excellent results in 91% of his 22 cases.

Following removal of the wound drains, intensive physical therapy is initiated. Only partial weight-bearing is permitted on the operated extremity for 4–6 weeks.

The prognosis of an intraarticular infection depends critically on prompt surgical intervention.

12.8 Compartment Syndrome

Compartment syndrome is a rare complication of knee arthroscopy. Isolated cases have been described by Noyes (1982), Peek (1984), and Bergström (1986).

If irrigating fluid extravasates from the joint during arthroscopy into the surrounding soft tissues and fascial compartments of the lower leg, the pressure within those compartments is elevated. The resulting vascular compression leads to ischemia and eventual necrosis of the enclosed muscles.

Fluid extravasation into the soft tissues of the knee and lower leg is a particular threat in extensive capsuloligamentous injuries where arthroscopy is performed at a high fluid pressure for a prolonged period of time. A massive, progressive swelling of the entire knee and lower leg should be considered a premonitory sign of compartment syndrome and should prompt immediate termination of the arthroscopic procedure. However, this complication is not easily recognized in its early stages due to the heavily wrapped and draped condition of the lower leg.

Even when the joint is intact, a very high intraarticular fluid pressure can cause rupture of the joint capsule, as Noyes and Spievack (1982) have demonstrated in cadaver experiments. They found that an intact knee capsule can rupture at a pressure of 294 cm H_2O. Intraarticular pressures of this magnitude can be reached during arthroscopy (Kohn 1988).

12.9 Hemarthrosis and Postoperative Effusion

Postoperative hemarthrosis is uncommon following diagnostic arthroscopy. However, iatrogenic injury of the infrapatellar fat pad or synovium during portal placement or during the arthroscopy itself can lead to the development of hemarthrosis.

Postoperative hemorrhage is more likely to follow operative arthroscopic procedures such as synovectomy, lateral retinacular release, or arthrolysis. Intraoperative bleeding that is noted during a lateral release can be controlled with a surgical instrument (e. g., electroknife) passed through an instrument portal.

With recurrent bouts of postoperative hemarthrosis, the possibility of a vascular injury or coagulation defect should be considered. The patient's coagulation status is tested by determining essential coagulation parameters: prothrombin time, partial thromboplastin time, bleeding time, platelet count.

To reduce bleeding, we inject a vasoconstrictor (e.g., epinephrine) postoperatively through the suction drain. This agent can be combined with a long-acting local anesthetic (e.g., carbostesin) for postoperative analgesia and can either be instilled directly through the arthroscopic sheath or injected through the intraarticular suction drain (dosage: 10 ml of

0.5% carbostesin with epinephrine diluted 1:200,000).

A mild postoperative irritative effusion is not a true complication. Recurrent effusions may signify residual intraarticular pathology such as unrecognized cartilage lesions, incompletely removed meniscal lesions, or residual joint instability.

Postoperatively we apply an elastic compression dressing to the knee. Ice bags are also applied to the knee during the initial hours after arthroscopy.

12.10 Thromboembolitic Complications

Thromboembolitic disease accounts for approximately one-third of all complications in arthroscopy. Even fatal pulmonary emboli have been reported (Small 1986). Between 0.1% and 0.2% of all arthroscopy patients are affected by thromboembolitic disease.

Although arthroscopy generally does not necessitate prolonged postoperative immobilization of the limb, all hospitalized patients are treated postoperatively with heparin (low dose, 3 x 5000 I.U. heparin calcium subcutaneously) unless a contraindication exists. Heparin can also be administered preoperatively by i.v. bolus injection (40 I.U./kg body weight) before the limb is exsanguinated. Preoperative heparin is contraindicated in patients who require the placement of an indwelling peridural catheter.

Postoperatively our patients wear a compression stocking on the healthy leg for thrombosis prophylaxis.

Due to the potentially disastrous effects of a deep leg or pelvic vein thrombosis or pulmonary embolism, even young overweight females who are heavy smokers or take oral contraceptives should receive appropriate antithrombotic treatment.

12.11 Synovial Fistula, Synovial Hernia

A suction drain left in the joint for more than 48 h, long skin incisions at the portal sites, frequent instrument changes through a single portal (often against tissue resistance), and skin incisions placed in the area of old scars predispose to the formation of a synovial fistula.

Every synovial fistula carries a significant risk of infection. It is, after all, an open communication with the extraarticular environment. When the presence of a synovial fistula is noted, the knee should be immobilized at once on a splint. The leg must be placed at rest to reduce intraarticular fluid production. When this is done, most synovial fistulas will heal without further treatment. Larger synovial fistulas or long-standing fistulas with an epithelialized tract are surgically excised. No matter whether the fistula is treated operatively or conservatively, antibiotic use is essential.

The instrument portals also form sites of predilection for synovial hernias. These lesions appear several weeks, or in some cases several days, after arthroscopy. The synovial membrane herniates into the subcutaneous tissue through the capsular incision made during construction of the instrument portal. Inspection of the site reveals a local, encapsulated, cystlike thickening. Treatment consists in extirpation of the lesion.

12.12 Reflex Sympathetic Dystrophy

The etiology of reflex sympathetic dystrophy (RSD) relates to a combination of endogenous (disposition, personality, mental disorders) and exogenous factors (traumatic or surgical insult, vascular disease). This syndrome is variously referred to in the literature as Sudeck's disease, causalgia, algodystrophy, and angiospasm. Approximately 10% of all cases involve the knee, which is the fourth most common site affected (Fig. 12-6). In the series reported by Small (1986), RSD accounted for 8.5% of complications.

Because arthroscopic diagnostic and operative procedures cause minimum joint trauma while permitting early mobilization with no significant period of immobility, one might assume that RSD has been eliminated as a complication of knee surgery. Thus it is important for the arthroscopic surgeon to consider this diagnosis when making the decision for surgery, and also in patients who have persistent postsurgical complaints.

Since the decision to perform arthroscopy is made more rapidly than the decision for ar-

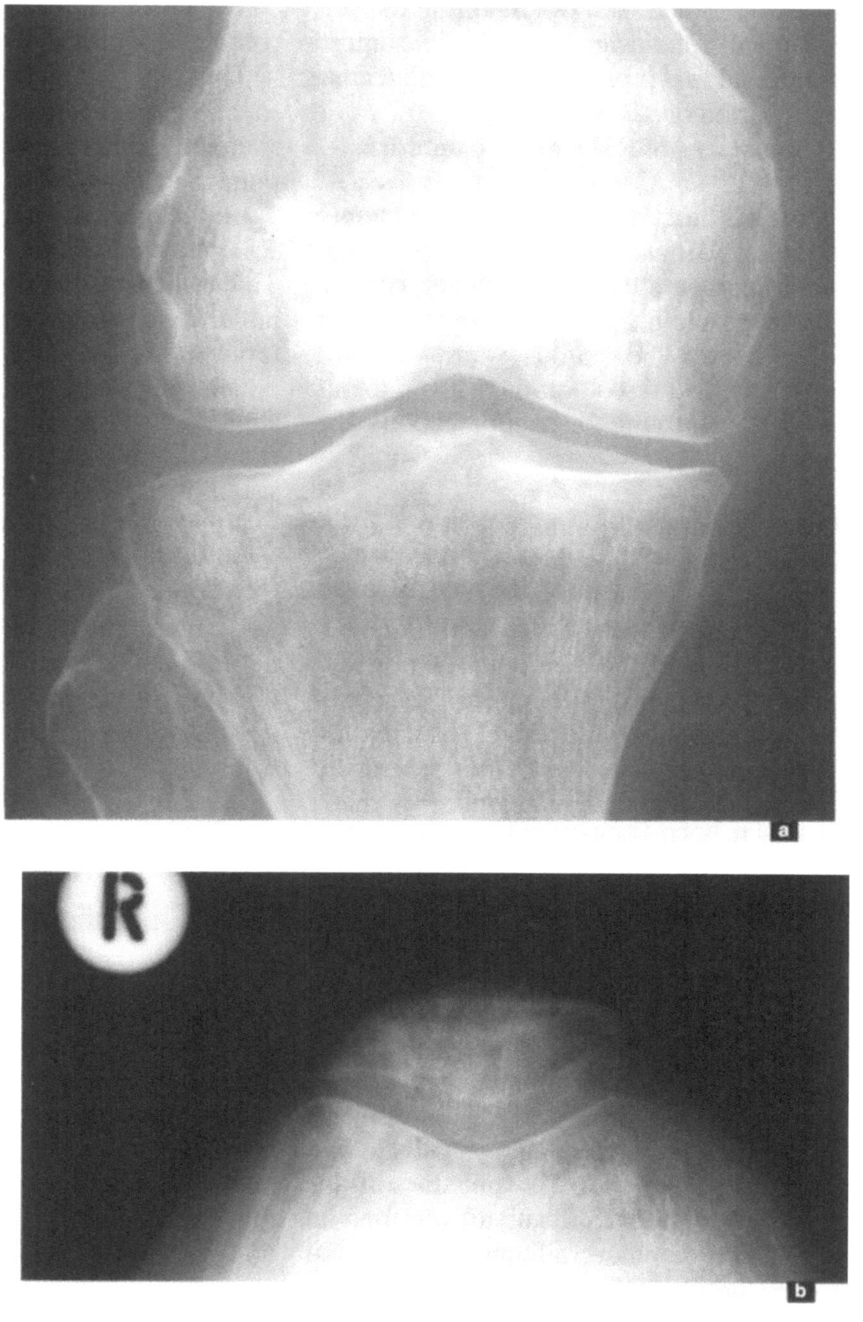

Fig. 12-6. a, b Reflex sympathetic dystrophy of the knee in a 41-year-old woman 8 weeks after arthroscopic medial meniscectomy. Radiographs show typical patchy decalcification

throtomy, the surgeon runs the risk of "walking into" RSD in patients who are arthroscopied for unexplained knee pain. It is known that even minor injuries such as sprains and contusions can precipitate RSD of the knee. Thus, both the soft-tissue envelope and the X-ray films should be closely scrutinized for evidence of RSD during the preoperative workup.

RSD should also be considered in cases where the patient shows initial marked improvement following arthroscopic surgery but then takes a progressive downhill course over a period of 3–4 weeks.

Three stages of RSD are recognized:

Stage I is the stage of acute inflammatory swelling. The main clinical features are spontaneous pain and local tenderness accompanied by swelling and function impairment of the knee. The skin is warm, doughy, and shows livid discoloration. Most patients describe a burning discomfort about the knee.

Stage II is marked by a regression of the diffuse soft-tissue swelling and contractures of the affected soft tissues (capsule, ligaments, muscles, subcutaneous tissue, skin). Pain becomes less intense, but tenderness to pressure and motion remains. The range of knee motion is diminished, and there is increasing muscular atrophy. X-rays at this stage may show the typical patchy marbling of periarticular bone (especially the patella) with a coarsening of the cancellous bone structure and sharpening of joint contours.

Inadequately treated or undiagnosed, the disease may progress to

Stage III. This is the end stage, characterized by restricted motion or complete ankylosis of the joint.

Since radiographic changes usually do not appear until stage II or III, while the soft-tissue signs are often difficult to interpret in stage I, a three-phase radionuclide scan has proven useful in suspected cases of RSD. Even in early cases, a perfusion deficit will be noted in the affected extremity.

In the three cases of postarthroscopic RSD observed by us, two patients had psychoautonomic factors (e.g., emotional stress) which evidently contributed to the onset of disease. Similar factors can occur in association with arthroscopic operations, as in the case of a competitive athlete whose team is in a critical situation and who feels a strong sense of urgency to return to action. One case of RSD occurred in a patient who underwent arthroscopy for a locked bucket-handle tear while his wife was about to deliver a child.

Thus, particular attention should be given to follow-up in patients who are in a stressful situation. It may even be appropriate to postpone the arthroscopic procedure.

The clinical and radiographic features of RSD may be seen in other disorders as well. This is illustrated by the case of a patient who underwent arthroscopic resection of the posterior horn of the medial meniscus. The patient did well for several weeks after the surgery, but then his condition began to deteriorate. Clinical and X-ray findings were consistent with RSD of the knee. Despite intensive therapy, the patient's symptoms did not improve, and X-rays finally demonstrated sites of bone erosion. The lesions were found to be metastatic to small-cell bronchial carcinoma. Thus, a repeat X-ray examination of the knee is recommended in cases where complaints persist or recur after surgery.

12.13 Skin Complications

Local skin irritation with slight redness about the portal sites is not unusual. Far less common are caustic lesions caused by disinfectants or burns caused by electrosurgical instruments. Forced movements of the leg in the holding fixture or excessive pressure against the lateral post can lead to hematoma formation in the affected skin areas.

12.14 Lost Tissue Fragments

In arthroscopic operations a tissue fragment such as a meniscal tag or bucket handle is frequently detached before it can be removed from the joint. When an attempt is made to extract the loose fragment through the instrument portal with a grasping instrument, the fragment may slip loose from the instrument while traversing the capsular incision and fall back into the joint cavity. It then becomes necessary to regrasp the fragment inside the joint. In other cases the fragment may slip or be scraped from the grasping instrument while in the subcutaneous tissue or before traversing the skin incision. Retrieval in this case can be particularly difficult if a small skin incision overlies a large capsular incision, so that a considerable amount of irrigating fluid has already leaked into the subcutaneous tissue. Blind "poking around" in the subcutaneous tissue rarely leads to recovery of the lost fragment. A better method is to transilluminate the soft tissues from inside the joint to determine the general location of the fragment. The subcutaneous fragment, which appears as a dark spot within the transilluminated area (see Fig. 6-10), can be easily removed in most cases by lengthening the skin incision.

If the fragment cannot be located, the procedure should be terminated and retrieval performed later, after sufficient time has elapsed for absorption of the subcutaneous fluid. Generally the subcutaneous fragment can be localized by palpation and removed through a small skin incision under local anesthesia.

Smaller fragments like those generated by a meniscectomy, the removal of an osteophyte, or chondroplasty with a coarse instrument can be carried by irrigating fluid into the subcutaneous tissue without the surgeon's awareness. Postoperatively, a small fragment can be felt in the area of the instrument portal. If the patient complains of pain, the tract of the instrument portal should be explored for debris.

12.15 Special Complications of Gas Arthroscopy

To date, two fatal pulmonary emboli have been described as complications of arthroscopy in gas (Grünwald 1988). Both patients had fresh bony injuries when the arthroscopy was performed (see Sect. 3.4.1).

We emphasize, therefore, that gas distention is contraindicated in the presence of an acute bony injury. Gas arthroscopy is also risky in knees with hemarthrosis, which can mask the presence of a radiographically invisible osseous injury.

Other reported complications of gas arthroscopy include pneumoscrotum (Henderson 1982) and pneumoperitoneum with severe acidosis (Lotmann 1987).

12.16 Arthroscopy of the "Wrong" Knee

One complication that should be mentioned is arthroscopy of the wrong knee, especially when one considers the potential legal ramifications. Routine checks should be incorporated into the preoperative preparations to ensure that "wrong-side surgery" cannot occur. At some centers the dorsum of the foot or the thigh is marked with waterproof ink on the eve or morning of surgery. The operative side should always be clearly indicated on the preoperative information sheet.

Prior to stability testing under general anesthesia, the operator should recheck the information sheet to confirm that the correct side is being prepared. We have had several close calls in which the wrong extremity was already fully draped and the patient intubated before the error was detected.

If several arthroscopies are performed in one day, it is convenient to schedule the procedures so that all the arthroscopies on one side (e.g., the right) are performed first, followed later in the day by arthroscopies on the opposite side. This eliminates the need to keep moving the arthroscopy cart from one side of the table to the other (see Sect. 4.5).

12.17 Other Rare Complications

There have been sporadic reports of very rare complications following arthroscopic procedures, most notably:

- a fistula between the prepatellar bursa and intraarticular space (Hadid 1984);
- osteomyelitis, meningococcal arthritis, bacteremia (Christopher 1982);
- herniation of the infrapatellar fat pad (Lindenbaum 1981);
- rupture of the semimembranosus bursa (Bunker 1984).

12.18 Late Complications

The recurrence of pain, swelling, or locking after arthroscopic surgery may be the result of inadequate treatment or a recurrence of disease. Common causes of residual complaints after arthroscopic surgery are:

- the inadequate treatment of meniscal lesions;
- the incomplete removal of loose bodies;
- severe articular cartilage disease.

In joints with extensive degenerative changes, chondromatosis, or multiple associated lesions, any of these factors may be responsible for a recurrence of complaints. In more than 10% of patients with associated lesions, even adequate arthroscopic treatment will not provide significant relief of complaints (Löhnert 1985).

13 Patient Information

Providing the patient with necessary information about his condition and the proposed arthroscopic procedure not only establishes a basis of trust between the patient and physician but also avoids misunderstandings that could ultimately lead to litigation. Particular attention should be given to the patient interview, therefore.

Many patients have misconceptions about what will happen during arthroscopy. Some regard arthroscopy as a "drop in" procedure that is over with quickly and may be repeated as often as desired. Moreover, euphoric press reports have helped to foster the belief that arthroscopic surgery can work miracles and often effects a total cure. This attitude is just as unfounded as an irrational fear of the procedure.

13.1 Selecting Patients for Arthroscopy

In most cases a patient is selected for arthroscopy, and his expectations assessed, at the time of the initial clinical examination in an office setting or ambulatory facility.

The examiner explains to the patient why an arthroscopic examination and operation is being recommended (diagnostic evaluation or treatment planning; see Chap. 2).

If arthroscopic surgery is deemed necessary, the advantages of this method are discussed: shorter period of immobilization, faster rehabilitation, shorter hospital stay or outpatient procedure less morbidity.

If arthroscopy is to be done as an inpatient procedure, the hospital stay will probably range from 2 to 10 days, depending on the operation.

The length of hospitalization is predictable for most procedures. However, the arthroscopist should not allow himself to be pressured in terms of meeting a deadline or an expected outcome. If the patient will consent to arthroscopy only if he has 100% assurance that he can return to work or athletic competition 10 days after the procedure, then surgery should be withheld until the patient adopts a more realistic attitude. Usually it is enough to point out that the extent of pathologic changes cannot be accurately predicted prior to arthroscopy, yet the extent of pathology will critically influence the success of the procedure and the length of hospitalization and convalescence.

Since expectations vary among different individuals, an effort is made to convey to the patient the various possibilities of an arthroscopic operation and the chances for success. It should be pointed out that more than 10% of knee patients do not experience a significant improvement of their symptoms. Especially in patients with degenerative joint changes, unreasonably high expectations should be discouraged. On the other hand, patients who have had knee problems for some years are those most likely to benefit from the significant pain relief that arthroscopic surgery can provide. This differs from the attitude of athletes and acutely injured patients who may be disappointed with anything short of a total cure. An effort should also be made to foster realistic expectations in patients with a torn anterior cruciate ligament.

13.2 Preoperative Patient Conduct

Once the patient has elected to undergo an arthroscopic procedure, a date is set for the inpatient or outpatient surgery. Since arthroscopy is not an emergency procedure, age-related operative risks and serious coexisting disorders should either be excluded or taken into account when planning the procedure. Any coexisting disease, even a banal one such as a cold, influenza, or sore tonsils, is sufficient grounds for postponement of surgery. The same applies to skin infections (pimples) or unhealed abrasions about the knee.

On the morning of surgery the skin about the knee is shaved, and the patient is allowed nothing by mouth.

Video arthroscopy is almost unique among surgical procedures in that it allows the patient to witness the diagnostic and therapeutic actions of the surgeon on the monitor. Often this will give the patient his first real understanding of his condition and will help him to realize that there may be sequelae and residual complaints. Of course, this is possible only if regional or local anesthesia is used.

General anesthesia is recommended for anxious or uncooperative patients. It is also advised when the patient might otherwise have to witness the "fumblings" of an inexperienced arthroscopist. The patient will still have the opportunity to view the major preoperative (e.g., meniscus flap) and postoperative findings (e.g., a stable residual meniscal rim) on videotape after the operation.

Many centers offer patients the option of purchasing a videotape of their arthroscopy, which they can play on their home videocassette recorder.

13.3 Preoperative Interview

Having explained the goal of the arthroscopy to the patient in the first consultation, the examiner conducts a final preoperative interview for the purpose of answering the patient's questions. Communication is assisted by a knee model, which is used to show the patient which structures are presumed to be injured and how they are to be treated.

The arthroscopic treatment options for the diagnosed condition are explained to the patient *in terms that he can understand.*

Meniscal Injuries. It is possible to remove the entire meniscus arthroscopically, but it is preferable to remove only the part that is actually torn. Once the piece has been removed, it may be necessary to perform another arthroscopy in a few months or years if the residual meniscus left by the first arthroscopy becomes severely damaged. This does not mean that negligence was committed in the first operation. The purpose, rather, is to leave some functioning meniscal tissue in the knee for as long as possible so that it can help protect the joint. With a recent injury, it may be possible to repair the torn meniscus with sutures.

Articular Cartilage Lesions. Lesions of the articular cartilage can be treated arthroscopically. Special motorized instruments similar to a small electric shaver are used to cut off small bits of cartilage and simultaneously remove them from the joint by suction. If the cartilage is merely softened, removal of the softened areas will lead to further general weakening of the cartilage. Therefore we do not remove cartilage that is softened or slightly frayed. We only remove undermined areas or large cartilage tags that have a fibery consistency. When this kind of damage is seen, we look for the possible cause, which may be an angular limb deformity or a lateralized patella.

If an area is found to be denuded of cartilage, the exposed bone can be freshened with a motorized burr to stimulate the formation of fibrocartilage. Here it must be emphasized that this "replacement cartilage" does not have the same stability as normal articular cartilage. Following this procedure (subchondral abrasion), weight must be kept off the leg for approximately 10 weeks. The patient must be informed of this preoperatively and decide whether he wishes the surgeon to do a subchondral abrasion if a cartilage defect is found. Some patients may find the prolonged convalescence unacceptable for personal or occupational reasons.

Removal of a Loose Body. The patient is told that a loose body in the knee sometimes cannot be located by arthroscopy, even if the fragment is visible on X-rays. Not every object that appears "loose" on X-rays is actually mobile and intraarticular. Typical examples are fragments broken from the medial patellar facet by a dislocating patella. While X-rays show fragments lying medial to the patella, arthroscopy usually shows only tearing or hemorrhage in the medial retinaculum. If the dislocation is old, arthroscopy may show no abnormalities at all. The "loose" bodies appearing next to the medial patellar facet on X-rays actually lie outside the synovium in the subcutaneous tissue. A tibial bony avulsion of the posterior cruciate ligament or a fabella also can be mistaken for a loose body in the posterior compartment. It is not uncommon for rounded or target-shaped calcifications of the posterior capsule in degenerative joint disease to prompt the X-ray diagnosis of a "loose body."

Division or Removal of the Mediopatellar Plica. A hypertrophied medial synovial plica may be responsible for unexplained complaints on the medial and anteromedial side of the knee (see Fig. 8-40). The offending plica can be removed arthroscopically. A bloody joint effusion may develop following the resection of a medial plica very close to the capsule wall.

Lesions of the Synovial Membrane. If the patient's symptoms are caused by intraarticular adhesions or pathologic changes in the synovial lining of the knee, these can be removed arthroscopically. In patients with rheumatoid disease, removal of the entire synovial membrane is often beneficial. However, a prognosis regarding the improvement of joint function cannot be offered prior to surgery.

Rupture of the Anterior Cruciate Ligament. Management of the torn anterior cruciate ligament is perhaps one of the most difficult therapeutic decisions to be made. Treatment depends on the location and age of the tear and on associated lesions, and options range from conservative to operative. Before surgery is performed, it should be determined whether the patient is willing or able to accept the 6–12 month rehabilitation period necessary for an autologous reconstruction of the anterior cruciate ligament. The patient is informed that the ligament and surrounding structures must be examined arthroscopically before treatment can be planned. Often the degree of injury to intraarticular structures cannot be accurately assessed before arthroscopy.

Since many patients desire the shortest possible rehabilitation for occupational reasons, the patient should state prior to arthroscopy whether the surgeon may proceed with open surgery (arthrotomy) in case disease is found that cannot be treated by arthroscopy alone.

The surgeon who is acquiring his initial experience in arthroscopic surgery should always keep open the option of arthrotomy. In this regard, patients find it reassuring when they are told that the late results of arthrotomy are comparable to those of arthroscopy.

If a patient expressly refuses open surgery, the less experienced arthroscopist who doubts his ability to carry the operation to completion should limit the procedure to a diagnostic arthroscopy and then refer the patient to an experienced arthroscopist for the operative procedure itself.

The diagnosis and the proposed procedure are entered on the preoperative information sheet. Note is also made of patient risk factors that might increase the complication rate or compound the difficulty of postoperative care (e.g., diabetes mellitus, chronic circulatory problems, cortisone medication).

The percentages stated in the literature on the incidence of complications about which the patient must be informed range between 1% and 3%. These figures are for general orientation only and are not legally binding. Thus, the complications that are most frequent and most threatening to the patient are listed on the information sheet even if some occur with frequencies well below 1%. One such complication is infection, whose incidence is less than 0.5%. Effusion or hemarthrosis can occur after some arthroscopies. During medial portal placement the infrapatellar branch of the saphenous nerve may be stretched, partially divided, or completely transected resulting in an area of numbness on the anteromedial aspect of the knee. It is possible that the complaints which brought the patient to arthroscopy will persist in the same or altered form. Persistent pain or a reduction of knee motion are uncommon after arthroscopic procedures but should nevertheless be mentioned.

Finally the completed information sheet is signed by the operating physician and by the patient.

13.4 Postoperative Consultation

Following completion of the arthroscopic procedure, the surgeon explains to the patient what was found and the type of postoperative care that will be required. Three basic postoperative care regimens are offered depending on the nature of the procedure:

First Regimen
- Diagnostic arthroscopy
- Meniscectomy
- Excision of a mediopatellar plica
- Removal of a loose body
- Chondral debridement:

Weight bearing is permitted after swelling subsides. As a precaution, forearm crutches are used for 3–7 days to reduce pressure on the knee, and nonsteroidal antirheumatics are given. Sport may be resumed according to the results of isokinetic tests (Cybex, Akron).

Second Regimen
Associated capsuloligamentous injuries
- Meniscal repair:

A 0° Mecron splint is worn for 6 weeks.

Weeks 1 and 2:	0°–0°–80° passive motion with floor contact.
Weeks 3 and 4:	0°–2°–80° active motion with partial weight bearing.
Weeks 5 and 6:	0°–0°–90° active motion with full weight bearing.

Third Regimen
- Lateral release:

Patellar restraint bandage (e.g., Juzo) is worn for 3 months.

At 3 weeks electrostimulation of the vastus medialis muscle is started and continued for 8 weeks, accompanied by appropriate physical therapy.

In addition to the special measures outlined above, the patient should cool the operated knee with an ice bag several times daily for about 10–20 min, starting on the first day. The patient should also start regular quadriceps tightening exercises on the first day, tensing the muscle group for 5–10 seconds at a time.

Outpatient follow-up visits are scheduled for 1 week, 2 weeks, and 6 weeks after surgery. These examinations may be conducted by the referring orthopedist or family doctor, or they may be done in the hospital-based ambulatory unit. The wound sutures are removed at 2 weeks.

Before signing out, the patient is given written discharge instructions that include information on what types of sport he may engage in and what types he should avoid or participate in to a limited degree.

Patients who have severe cartilage lesions and/or degenerative changes but have only mild clinical complaints should be educated about the eventual fate of their knee. Because the articular cartilage cannot regenerate or be replaced by other cartilage, it is essential to protect the cartilage that remains. This is difficult for many patients to understand. We find it helpful to compare the residual cartilage to a worn automobile tire that has only a few millimeters of tread left. Once it is stipulated that this worn set of tires, like the cartilage in the knee joint, cannot be replaced, it becomes clear that the life of the tires can be greatly extended if the driver does not screech the tires when pulling out, avoids quick stops, and does not make high-speed turns. The damaged knee cartilage should be protected in similar fashion. For example, the patient should avoid sports that are highly stressful to the knee, such as alpine skiing, soccer, football, basketball, volleyball, and tennis. Usually this will be no problem for patients who are not athletically inclined. The patient is encouraged to participate in "knee-friendly" activities such as swimming (backstroke), cycling, and walking on level ground. Patients are discouraged from giving up sports altogether.

On the day of discharge, the patient is urged to contact his family doctor or the hospital at once if any problems or complications arise. He is alerted to the signs of thrombosis and told to present immediately if he notices a combination of deep calf pain and swelling. If severe pain occurs, if the oral temperature rises above 38° C, or if the knee becomes grossly swollen, the patient should telephone the hospital or his surgeon without delay. Mild knee swelling is normal, however, and does not require medical attention.

14 Documentation

Given the panoply of normal and pathologic findings that are encountered in diagnostic and operative arthroscopy, the accurate documentation of findings is a necessity. When the procedure is completed, the surgeon no longer has the opportunity to obtain or check findings, so he must rely on a written record (operation report, documentation sheet) that is supplemented if possible by photographic or video documentation. Arthroscopic findings are generally acquired in a very short time, i.e., within a few minutes, so the documentation method must be fast, thorough, and reproducible.

Because multiple arthroscopies are often performed in succession, it is difficult for the surgeon to remember, after the fifth arthroscopy, the condition of the lateral meniscus in the first patient. Unless a finding is documented shortly after the procedure, it is likely to be forgotten. In patients with persistent complaints or requiring a second procedure, critical information may be lacking. In the case of a legal dispute, major problems will arise if documentation is poor or fragmentary.

The basic advantage of diagnostic and operative arthroscopy–earlier discharge–places high demands on documentation, which must ensure a rapid, flawless flow of information among the surgeon, ward physician, nurses, physiotherapist, and family doctor. The routinely dictated operative report often does not reach the ward until the patient is about to be discharged or has already gone home.

14.1 Written Documentation

14.1.1 Operation Report

The operation report continues to be the most proven and useful form of surgical documentation. The length of the operation report varies greatly from one examiner to the next, ranging from a few lines to multiple single-spaced typewritten pages. On the one hand, it is not sufficient to say, for example, that "a bucket-handle tear of the medial meniscus with an intact lateral meniscus" was found and treated by "excision of the bucket handle." But on the other hand, it wastes time and places a needless burden on the clerical staff to detail the findings and the operative procedure at epic length. One typewritten page is usually sufficient to describe the normal and pathologic findings and the operative measures that were performed.

Kieser (quoted in Hempfling 1987) notes that the operation report should be legible and a pleasure to read (no illegible handwriting or computer-readable forms). The surgeon should not use abbreviations that are known to only a small circle of colleagues. He should indicate any areas of the joint that he was unable to see, and he should note any problems he had visualizing specific anatomic structures so that this information will be available for any subsequent procedure that is performed.

The following points are covered in the operation report:

- History: Give a brief description of the antecedent history to document the indication for arthroscopy. For example: The patient sustained an external rotation injury 5 days ago while playing soccer. A tense effusion was aspirated the next day by the family doctor, yielding blood. The patient was referred for arthroscopy to determine the source of the hemarthrosis.
- Clinical findings: Mention significant clinical findings such as a positive Lachman test or intraarticular effusion.
- Results of examination under anesthesia (see Chap. 5).
- Positioning parameters: supine, use of tourniquet or exsanguination; indicate tourniquet pressure (e.g., 400 mm Hg).
- Arthroscope portal: high anterolateral, low anterolateral. Describe any effusion that was aspirated. Indicate the distention medium, e.g., nonelectrolytic solution (purisole), Ringer's lactate, NaCl.
- Examination procedure: Indicate normal and pathologic findings, following the sequence used in the examination (see Table 8-1): retropatellar cartilage, suprapatellar pouch (superior plica, synovitis?), lateral recess (epicondylar area, popliteal hiatus, popliteus tendon, Outerbridge ridge), femoropatellar joint (femoropatellar contact, lateralization?), anteromedial capsule (mediopatellar plica, synovitis?), medial compartment (condition of articular cartilage, medial meniscus, posterior horn of medial meniscus), intercondylar area (infrapatellar plica, anterior cruciate ligament, posterior horn of medial meniscus, posterior cruciate ligament, infrapatellar fat pad), lateral compartment (lateral meniscus, articular cartilage, popliteal hiatus), posterolateral recess.
- Instrument portal: State the location of the instrument portal. If special portals were used (e.g., posteromedial), state their indication.
- Operative measures that were performed: Indicate the operative procedure and the instruments used (e.g., motorized instruments, electrocautery, basket forceps, suction punch).
- Completion of arthroscopy: Note placement of suction drain, skin suture, instillation of local anesthetic, application of elastic compressive bandage, use of a cast or splint.
- Postoperative procedure: Explain postoperative measures in detail, especially if a documentation sheet did not accompany the patient to the ward (see Sect. 14.1.2).
- Specimens submitted for histologic examination: Biopsies taken intraoperatively or tissues removed from the joint are sent for histologic examination. The pathologist should know the site from which each specimen originated.

14.1.2 Documentation Sheets

To speed the flow of information between the surgeon and aftercare unit, the arthroscopist should fill out a standard documentation sheet at the conclusion of the procedure, before the patient has left the operating suite. Boxes are marked on the sheet to indicate the anesthetic technique, the result of the examination under anesthesia, the irrigating solution, the portal sites, the principal arthroscopic findings and treatment measures, and the postoperative orders. A blank is available for writing in the diagnosis. It is helpful to have diagrams of the knee already printed on the sheet so that lesions of the articular cartilage or menisci can be drawn together with the extent of therapeutic measures (e.g., the extent of a meniscectomy).

This simple worksheet documenting the pathologic findings and therapeutic measures conveys to the ward physician, nurses, and physical therapists a fast, clear impression of the postoperative status of the joint. It is particularly important to specify the program of postoperative care. It must be known whether full weight bearing is allowed or whether partial weight bearing is to be enforced for a specified period. The permitted ranges of active and passive motion are also indicated.

It should additionally be noted whether the procedure has been documented photographically or on videotape. If a video record has been made, the sheet should indicate the number of the videocassette on which the findings are recorded.

We have had good results with the use of standard documentation sheets at our centers. Though it takes little time to fill out, the sheet greatly clarifies the course of postoperative treatment for attending physicians, nurses, and physiotherapists. Use of this sheet eliminates staff confusion, and its potentially distressful effect on the patient, regarding the conduct of postoperative care.

Numerous attempts have been made to develop comprehensive, often multi-page documentation forms and to promote them for routine clinical use. Certainly such forms are advantageous in that they compel the examiner to make an accurate record of all findings and provide an excellent source of research data. For routine clinical work, however, the disadvantages of lengthy forms often outweigh their practical value. On the one hand, they cannot replace the operation report; on the other, filling out a multi-page form can be tedious and time-consuming. In extreme cases 8 minutes might be needed to perform the arthroscopy while 10 minutes are needed to complete the forms. Another drawback relates to individual differences in the willingness of surgeons to fill out multi-page forms conscientously, especially if the forms are thought to be of little practical use.

Every operator can create his own documentation sheet that meets the essential requirement of such a document: that it be convenient to use under routine clinical conditions. Sometimes less is more, i.e., it is much better to fill out a one-page sheet conscientously than to fill out a very scientific-looking, multi-page document superficially or haphazardly.

It should be added, however, that comprehensive, multi-page documentation forms can be quite useful when it comes to special inquiries. In this case data should be entered by marking boxes so that the forms can be computer-read and evaluated.

Klein's Documentation Sheet for Arthroscopic Surgery

The arthroscopic worksheet developed by Wilhelm Klein in 1987 is a clinically proven documentation system that can be computer-evaluated. The worksheet consists of two pages: The first page contains blank spaces for identifying data and numerous fill-in boxes for documenting the history, clinical findings, arthroscopic findings, arthroscopic surgical measures, and postoperative care. Abbreviations used on the sheet are keyed on the left side of the page. The second page contains schematic anatomic diagrams on which pathologic findings and therapeutic measures can be drawn. The first row of diagrams is for preoperating findings, the second for postoperative findings.

Each sheet has two carbonless write-through copies attached; one copy (blue) is for the next attending physician and the second (yellow) is for the operator. The original (white) sheet is sent to the ward and is placed with the patient's chart or records.

The data entered on the sheet can be read into a computer and evaluated. The computer software, also developed by Klein, is menu-controlled and guides the user through the program. A knowledge of programming is unnecessary.

SFA Arthroscopy Protocol

The Foundation for the Promotion of Arthroscopy (SFA) has developed an arthroscopy protocol which strikes a balance between the needs for practice-oriented and scientific documentation. The preoperative findings and the results of stability testing under general anesthesia are entered in boxes on the first page. The diagnosis and treatment are written in by hand. Schematic diagrams are provided for sketching the findings and the therapeutic measures that were performed. Postoperative care is also prescribed. Pages 2 and 3 are for the more precise documentation of findings and treatment. The findings (page 2) and therapeutic measures are marked in boxes in checklist fashion. Thus, the form satisfies the need for the rapid conveyance of arthroscopic findings and treatment and is consistent with the requirements of computer-assisted evaluation.

14.2 Photographic and Video Documentation

Even the most comprehensive operation report or documentation sheet cannot convey the visual findings of arthroscopy as well as a picture. The adage that "one picture is worth a thousand words" is especially true in arthroscopy. Routine documentation of findings on still photographs or videotape is an excellent way to ensure that findings of interest are permanently recorded.

There is a tendency for beginners to record too much. But as experience is gained, the volume of photographed and taped material will quickly dwindle to a manageable scale.

The arthroscopic surgeon is under no legal or ethical obligation to make a visual record of his procedures. At present the use of photodocumentation is left entirely to the discretion of the operator. In practice, however, this omission frequently results in the situation of a patient returning for a second arthroscopy because the initial findings were inadequately documented, or because no documentation was made or can be located. If adequate photographic or videotape records are available from the diagnostic arthroscopy, it will be far easier for the next attending physician to review quickly the initial intraarticular findings.

14.2.1 Photographic Documentation

Direct Photography

By far the best color fidelity is provided by still photography with a camera coupled directly to the eyepice of the arthroscope. Adapters are available to fit the standard, interchangeable lenses of single-lens reflex (SLR) cameras. The 24 x 36 mm image format is adequately utilized by a moderately priced 135-mm telephoto lens, although a more elegant solution is to use a special zoom lens of the type produced by Storz.

Modern electronic cameras require no more than a 150-watt light source whose color temperature corresponds to that of artificial light. However, indoor film rated at 160 ASA is not sensitive enough for arthroscopic photography, and commercially available 400-ASA film is barely adequate. The xenon light source delivers more power (300 W) at a daylight color temperature but still is only a compromise. The best solution is to use a flash generator that has variable intensity levels and an attachment for TTL metering (Fig. 14-1).

Even with a flash generator, however, large intraarticular spaces such as the suprapatellar pouch or blood-soaked tissues may not be adequately lit. Sufficient exposure can still be obtained in these cases by "fooling" the automatic exposure control. For example, a camera loaded with 200-ASA film can produce a brighter image of the suprapatellar pouch if the film speed adjustment on the camera is set to 100 ASA. This causes the flash control to emit more light, which is reflected from the joint onto the more sensitive film. Similarly, a 200 ASA setting should be selected when 400 ASA film is used. Many cameras have a special manual control for this "creative exposure" work.

Because direct arthroscopic photography invariably compromises asepsis to some degree, it does not appear suitable for routine documentation.

The operator cannot simultaneously aim the camera and trip the shutter with the nonsterile hand while controlling the arthroscope with the other hand. Consequently, the arthroscopic procedure must be interrupted while the photograph is taken. A telescope with a video camera attached must be removed and set aside while a different scope is inserted. Then the operative area is draped with two large, transparent sheets, leaving the eyepiece of the scope uncovered so that the camera can be coupled to it (Fig. 14-2).

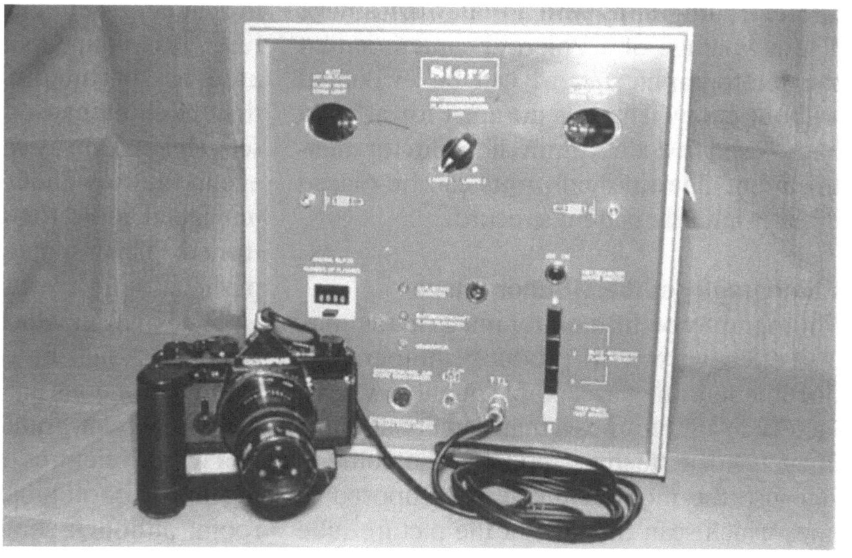

Fig. 14-1. Flash generator (Storz) connected to a single-lens reflex camera with motor drive

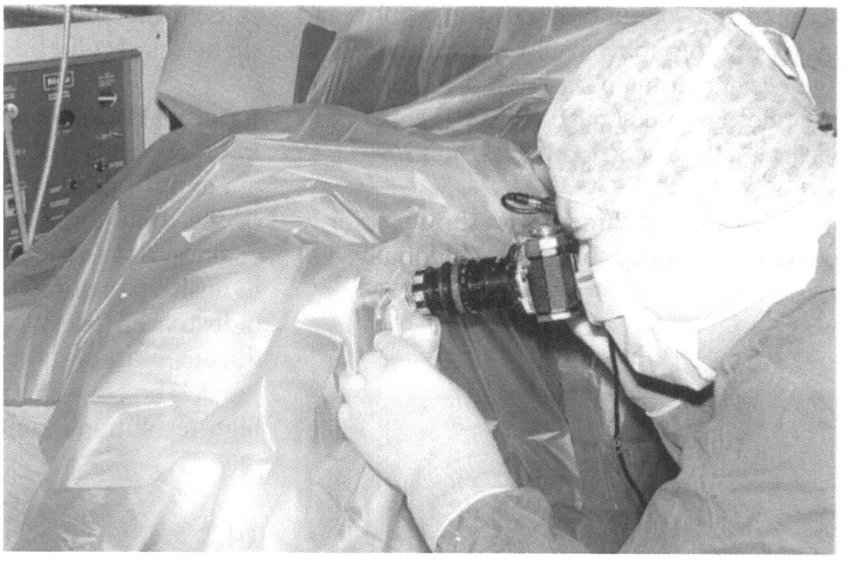

Fig. 14-2. Photographic documentation of the arthroscopic image. The operative area is draped with two large plastic sheets to preserve asepsis

After the pictures have been taken, the special drapes are removed, the cable attachments are disconnected by a sterile assistant, and the telescope is removed from the sheath. The operator must then regown and reglove before proceeding with the arthroscopy.

It should be added that an arthroscopist used to working from the screen must readjust to looking directly through the scope (smaller image, color changes, different orientation) when camera-to-eyepiece photography is used.

With the advent and increasing utilization of video arthroscopy, operators are relying less and less on the direct photodocumentation of intraarticular findings. Nevertheless, direct photography with an SLR camera does offer the advantage of a superb image quality that is unsurpassed by any other method, and it is recommended for those who require optimum image quality for special purposes. Nearly all the arthroscopic views presented in this book were photographed directly through the arthroscopic eyepiece with an SLR camera.

Direct Photography with a Polaroid Camera
The advantage of a Polaroid camera is that the photographic record can be evaluated without delay. There is no need for a "data back" used to code 35-mm slide film for identification. The finished prints can be placed directly into the patient's record.

Photography of the Monitor Image
Photography of the monitor image is a simple, cost-effective way to produce photographic documentation of acceptable quality. A satisfactory result requires a high-quality monitor image and a steady tripod for the camera. Because the monitor image is composed of lines which scan the face of the picture tube several times per second, the shutter speed must be longer than one complete image cycle. A "normal" exposure time of, say, 1/125 sec like that commonly used in hobby and travel photography would fall within an image cycle, causing a dark band to appear on the photographic image (Fig. 14-3). This limits the shutter speed to not less than 1/8 to 1/15 sec.

When an SLR camera with shutter priority is used, the shutter speed is set manually, and the camera automatically selects the aperture. But if an aperture-priority system is used, an aperture must be set which ensures that the shutter speed will be no less than 1/15 sec. This is done by capturing the monitor image in the viewfinder and watching the shutter speed indicator as the aperture ring is turned. This is quickly and easily accomplished.

The room in which the monitor is photographed should be completely darkened to avoid extraneous light and reflections on the monitor screen. Sometimes it is more convenient to take pictures from a videotape recording than to photograph "live" in the operating room, although some quality will be sacrificed.

We have had good results with commercially available 200 or 400 ASA slide film. Because these films are balanced for daylight, a slight loss of color fidelity will be experienced.

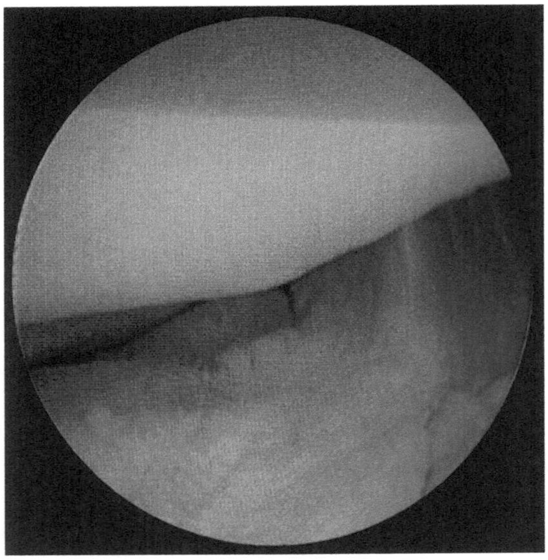

Fig. 14-3. The dark band at the top of the picture and the lined pattern result from photographing the monitor image at too fast a shutter speed (1/60 sec). The lateral triangle is depicted

External Photodocumentation Unit
In practice it can be difficult to keep the camera and tripod accurately positioned in front of the monitor. The slightest change in the position of the camera or monitor can result in unsharp pictures. To answer this problem, industry has developed a separate photodocumentation unit consisting of a large "sealed box" which houses the camera and a high-resolution monitor (Fig. 14-4).

14.2.2 Video Documentation

With the widespread use of video arthroscopy, it is only natural that videotape recorders have become a mainstay in the documentation of findings. Connected to the video output of the monitor, the video recorder provides a safe and reliable documention method.

Depending on quality requirements, the examiner may choose between the semiprofessional 3/4-inch Umatic system or the standard 1/2-inch "home" video system (VHS). If very high quality is desired, a Umatic video recorder should be purchased. Umatic video-

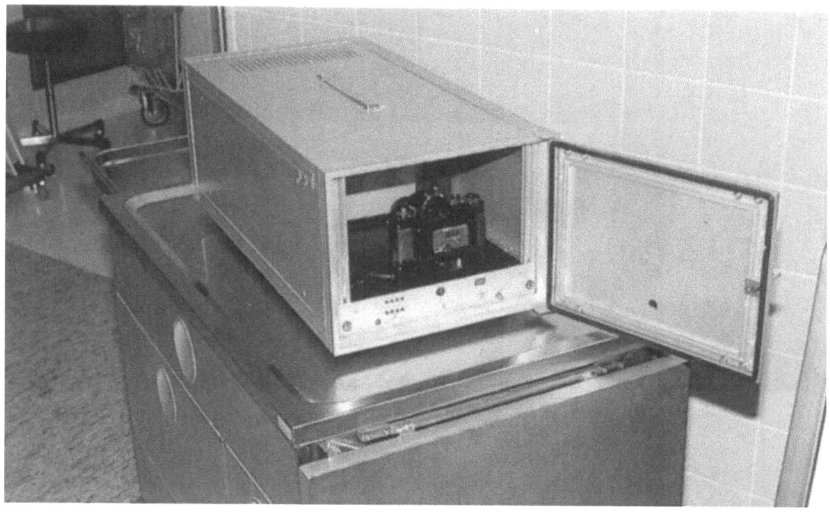

Fig. 14-4. External photodocumentation unit

cassettes are expensive but guarantee exceptional quality even when the tapes are edited for special presentations or patient information. The time counters (minutes and seconds) built into some Umatic recorders are particularly helpful for cataloging cases and make it easy to locate specific segments.

If a 1/2-inch system is used, a VHS recorder is recommended since that format is far more widely used than Beta. The patient can be offered a cassette of "his arthroscopy" to take home.

Video documentation of the entire arthroscopy from the first minute to the last is appropriate only if unusual pathology is present or a special operative procedure is applied. The routine documentation of every arthroscopy on Umatic or VHS cassettes is not only very costly (videocassettes, filing space) but also makes it difficult to catalog individual video sequences. Moreover, a stack of unedited videotapes is unlikely to be of much practical use.

A major disadvantage of video documentation lies in the difficulty of retrieving a particular finding or operative sequence. Besides a video recorder and monitor, considerable time is required to locate the desired segment. A videocassette cannot be "clipped" to the patient's file as a standard document.

Videotape is unsurpassed for documenting the conduct of special operative techniques. This makes it an ideal medium for instructional presentations in arthroscopic courses and workshops.

14.2.3 Video Printers

Video printers are devices for making a permanent record of the monitor image at a specific moment in time. Similar to a video recorder in design, these devices reproduce the monitor image in the form of a black-and-white or color picture, depending on the type of equipment used.

The black-and-white video printer (e.g., Mitsubishi P/61E) generates a picture with a resolution of 640 dots by 576 lines in 64 shades of gray. Approximately 17 sec is needed to print out one 100 x 74 mm black-and-white picture. If multiple copies of a "critical finding" are desired (e.g., for hospital files, for the patient, and for the patient's personal physician), they are easily produced. The cable of the video printer plugs into the video output of the monitor.

Color documentation is available with color video printers such as the Mitsubishi CP/100E (Fig. 14-5). Printout of a color picture, which has a resolution of 640 dots times 580 lines in 64 shades of color, takes about 70–80 sec. The thermal transfer printer works

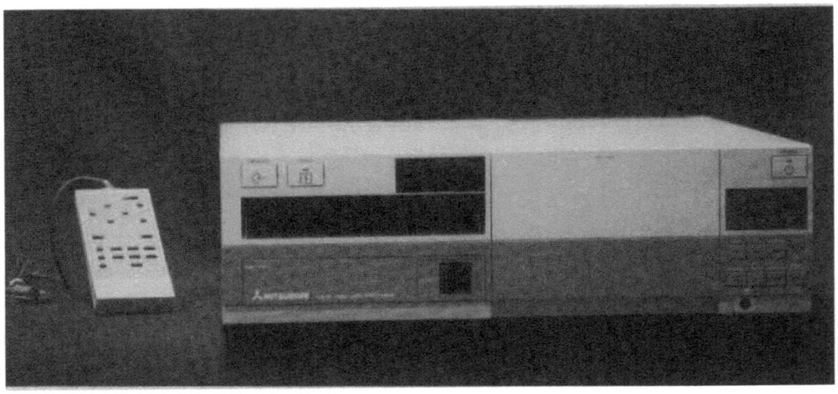

Fig. 14-5. Mitsubishi CP/100E color video printer

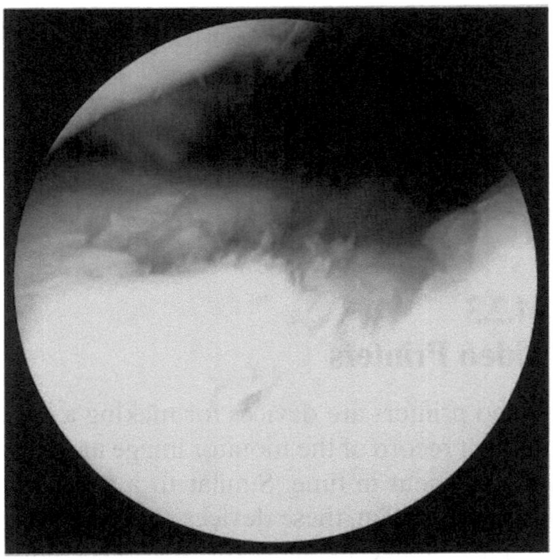

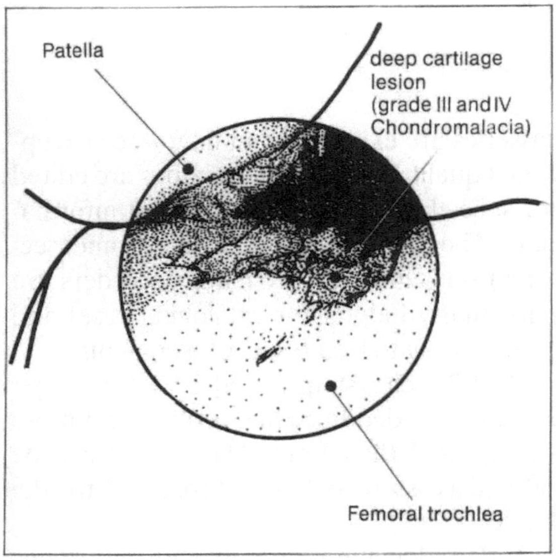

Fig. 14-6. Video-printer documentation of extensive, deep cartilage lesions on the femoral trochlea of a 54-year-old man with severe retropatellar pain. Note the marked fibrillation of the retropatellar cartilage

by the sublimation principle, meaning that an instantaneous color video image of photographic quality (Fig. 14-6) is produced from the three primary colors and printed out using a contact printing process.

During arthroscopy the video printer may be operated by OR personnel or by the surgeon himself using a wired remote control. This control can be wrapped in a sterile plastic sleeve like the video camera (see Fig. 4-12).

When findings are documented with a video printer, arthroscopy does not have to be interrupted when pictures are made. The operator can check the quality of the picture at once to determine whether the documentation is adequate (Fig. 14-6). There are no problems of sterile technique.

15
Training in Arthroscopy

The widespread use of arthroscopy and arthroscopic surgery has led to a growing need for training opportunities in the field.

Diagnostic arthroscopy and arthroscopic surgery can be learned by reading textbooks, attending courses and workshops, and by observing an experienced arthroscopist at work. Perhaps the poorest way to learn arthroscopy is to buy and read a textbook, order the necessary equipment, and carry out the producure on a patient. Such attempts at self-teaching will quickly meet with insurmountable problems. It is doubtful, moreover, that every physician can become fully competent in arthroscopic surgery. Color blindness, slowness of accommodation, poor spatial recognition, and lack of motor skills are factors cited by Miller (1985) that can cause extreme difficulty in learning arthroscopic surgery. A "heave-ho mentality" can be another stumbling block to learning the arthroscopic technique.

The beginner requires a great deal of inner calm, composure, and *time* to deal with the problems that he must face while learning the arthroscopic technique.

The aspiring arthroscopist should not be told that he must perform 100 (200, 300, or 500) arthroscopic examinations before attempting his first arthroscopic operation. The level of competence that is achieved at a given stage depends primarily on individual motor skills and the quality of instruction. The self-trained learner, even if possessed of excellent manual skills, will progress more slowly than one who is guided through the procedure by an experienced teacher. Arthroscopy, even more than most other forms of surgery, consists of a thousand small details. Considering the fact that even a slight error in positioning the fiberoptic cable can quickly lead to loss of orientation, one can appreciate the value of having an expert in attendance who can correct mistakes as they are made.

For the student who possesses an adequate basic knowledge of anatomy and diagnosis, the path to becoming an "arthroscopist" might consist of the following stages:

15.1
Attending an Arthroscopic Course or Workshop

For one who has no experience in arthroscopy and does not know a colleague who regularly practices it, attending an arthroscopic course or workshop can provide an excellent introduction to this "new technique." Through lectures and especially through the hands-on practice on training models that is frequently offered, the attendee can become familiar with the instruments that are employed.

In some courses and workshops, arthroscopic procedures can be performed on cadaveric knees under the supervision of an experienced instructor. A no less important reason to attend an arthroscopic workshop is the opportunity to meet with experienced arthroscopists and inquire whether subsequent visits with them might be arranged.

Almost every arthroscopic course or workshop includes exhibits by manufacturers who demonstrate the latest developments in equipment and instrumentation. Before buying a complete system, however, the beginner should seek the advice of an experienced arthroscopist. Industry representatives may tend to gloss over the weaknesses of their own products.

Both beginning and advanced courses in arthroscopy are available. The beginning courses focus on basic principles. The novice is more interested in the "ABC's" of arthroscopy than in what instruments are best for meniscal repairs or what kind of shaver head is best for a synovectomy. The advanced practitioner, on the other hand, will profit more from discussions on special indications and operative techniques.

15.2 Practice on a Knee Model

In settings where arthroscopic equipment is already available, the beginner can practice arthroscopic procedures on a training model of the knee, which can be either purchased or obtained on loan from manufacturers. These models contain access ports through which the arthroscope and instruments can be inserted to inspect and probe the "joint cavity" and perform operative procedures on simulated intraarticular structures.

While practice on a knee model cannot replace experience in live patients, it does permit the learner to rehearse and master the most important basic principles of arthroscopic technique either on his own or, preferably, under the guidance of a qualified instructor (Fig. 15-1). Specific exercises that can be done on training models include familiarization with the examination procedure, correct positioning of the light post, handling of the camera, visualization of the probing hook within the arthroscopic field, and the probing of intraarticular structures. Such exercises are helpful in facilitating the beginner's "first attempt" in a patient's knee.

The skin and muscular shell of the model are easily opened to allow replacement of the menisci, cruciate ligaments, collateral ligaments, patella, and infrapatellar fat pad. The menisci are available in intact or predamaged forms (e.g., with a longitudinal tear). The advanced learner can perform various procedures on these menisci using a variety of instruments.

The following training sequence on the model has proven effective:

1. Orientation
2. Standard examination procedure
3. Selective visualization of designated structures
4. Triangulation and selective probing

Once the trainee has become oriented within the knee, he may commence the standard ex-

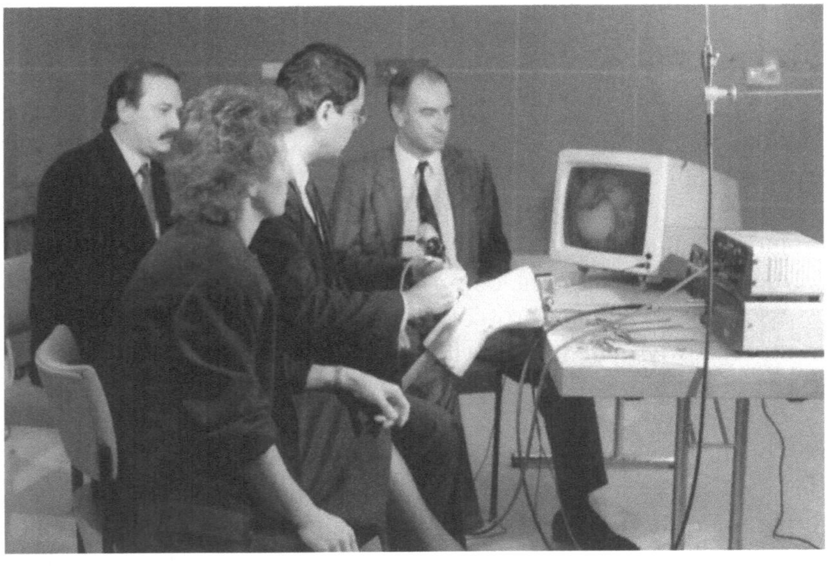

Fig. 15-1. Arthroscopy is practiced on a plastic knee model under the supervision of an instructor

amination procedure (see Sect. 8-1). Most trainees will forget one or more parts of the diagnostic sequence or will attempt to inspect structures without rotating the light post to the required position. Since the change from "traditional arthroscopy" to video arthroscopy can be difficult, it is recommended that a video system be used during work on the model.

Once the examination routine has been mastered, the trainee attempts to demonstrate specific structures chosen by himself or by the supervising colleague. This exercise always begins with insertion of the arthroscope. After the first three steps have been mastered, the tip of the probing hook is visualized (triangulation principle, see Fig. 7-18), and the intraarticular structures are probed. The trainee applies the rendezvous technique (see Sect. 7.7) as he attempts to reach different portions of the joint. The lateral compartment of the model knee is easily inspected by stressing open the lateral joint space.

Once arthroscopy of the knee has been learned, the arthroscopy of other large joints can be attempted (shoulder, elbow, ankle), always beginning with practice on a plastic training model.

Table 15-1. Progression of skills in arthroscopy

1. Diagnostic examination
2. Placement of the instrument portal, triangulation principle, use of the probe
3. Synovial biopsy
4. Chondroplasty (e.g., of the patella and medial femoral condyle)
5. Removal of loose bodies
6. Resection of medial meniscal flap tears
7. Resection of bucket-handle tears of both menisci
8. Resection of posterior horn tears of both menisci
9. Treatment of discoid menisci
10. Lateral retinacular release
11. Arthrolysis
12. Internal fixation of loose osteochondral fragments
13. Meniscal repairs
14. Repair or reconstruction of the anterior cruciate ligament
15. Diagnostic and operative arthroscopy of other joints (shoulder, elbow, ankle, wrist)

15.3 Visiting an Experienced Arthroscopist

Visiting an experienced arthroscopist and participating in arthroscopic operations can be a very valuable learning experience. The initial stage is a period of observation only in which the novice observes the individual steps of arthroscopy starting with positioning, draping, arthroscope insertion, and placement of the instrument portals and culminating with operative arthroscopic procedures.

In the second stage the beginner acquires his first experience by assisting the arthroscopist. He holds the patient's leg and may guide the camera or palpate selected sites with the probing hook. This second stage can be shortened by appropriate preparation that includes practice on a training model.

The third stage is that of independent arthroscopy. The learner inserts the arthroscope himself, follows the standard routine for diagnostic inspection of the joint, con-

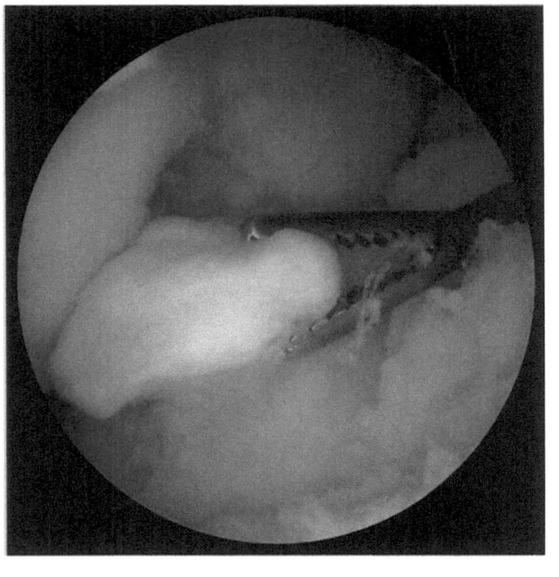

Fig. 15-2. Grasping forceps remove a joint mouse in a patient with a 10-year history of osteochondritis dissecans

structs the instrument portal, and probes the joint cavity. Even at this stage it is prudent to maintain contact with the senior arthroscopist. There are always opportunities to pick up new hints, tricks, and techniques that can enhance one's knowledge and skill.

Some hospitals and arthroscopy units offer practical operative courses for this purpose on a regular basis, in which theoretical and practical exercises are conducted in small group settings.

The progression of skills in arthroscopy is a continuous process which takes place as the arthroscopist grows in knowledge and experience. The progression outlined in Table 15-1 is for orientation only. Experienced arthroscopists know, for example, that a posterior horn tear of the medial meniscus can be extremely difficult to treat operatively, especially in a joint with minimum valgus laxity, while the removal of a loose body or a meniscal flap or bucket-handle tear can be accomplished in only a few minutes (Fig. 15-2).

For the practitioner of arthroscopy, continuing education is the key to ensuring that his practice will keep pace with new trends and scientific discoveries. For example, while arthroscopic reconstruction of the anterior cruciate ligament and meniscal repairs were still widely ridiculed a few years ago, today increasing numbers of operators are embracing these techniques.

16
Spectrum of Arthroscopic Surgery

In May of 1955, the Tokyo surgeon Watanabe removed a pedunculated tumor from the suprapatellar pouch of the knee under arthroscopic vision. In 1961 he performed the first arthroscopic removal of an intraarticular loose body, and in 1962 he gained worldwide acclaim by performing the first successful arthroscopic resection of a meniscal flap tear. Meniscal tears are among the most common knee injuries, and until a few years ago meniscectomies were at the focal point of arthroscopic interest.

Today, due in large part to ongoing refinements in arthroscopic instrumentation, virtually all intraarticular lesions can be treated arthroscopically. As more experience is gained, new arthroscopic operating techniques and modifications are continually being developed, and there is no end in sight.

16.1 Advantages and Disadvantages of Arthroscopic Surgery

The growth of arthroscopic surgery in recent years would not have been possible were it not for the fundamental advantages of arthroscopic surgery over traditional open techniques of operation. Whereas an open meniscectomy, for example, usually requires several days or perhaps weeks of hospitalization, an arthroscopic meniscectomy requires only a short hospital stay or can even be done as an outpatient procedure.

A few hospitals have their own arthroscopic surgical departments. Some ambulatory units for arthroscopic surgery are freestanding and autonomous; others are hospital-sponsored and -controlled.

When it comes to deciding between open or arthroscopic surgery, the criteria used in selecting a treatment method (morbidity, length of hospital stay, complication rate, rehabilitation time) clearly favor arthroscopic surgery. The advantages and disadvantages of the two modalities are important considerations in the decision-making process.

The main advantages of open surgery are that it is technically simpler than arthroscopy and does not require special operating instruments. Its numerous disadvantages are listed in Table 16-1.

Arthroscopy, on the other hand, requires a specialized instrument set. The operating technique is complex, and less experienced surgeons often require more time to complete an operation than if open surgery were used. If greater instrument access is needed, this generally cannot be accomplished as readily in arthroscopic surgery as in an open operation. However, these disadvantages and initial problems in arthroscopic surgery contrast with a number of fundamental avantages (Table 16-2).

Table 16-1. Disadvantages of open knee operations

- Longer hospital stay
- Higher morbidity
- Longer rehabilitation
- More time off the job
- Disturbance of proprioception
- Higher complication rate
- Limited ability to control the depth of resection (e.g., in meniscectomies)

Table 16-2. Advantages of arthroscopic operations

- Low morbidity
- Short hospital stay or outpatient treatment
- Early return to work
- Rapid return to athletic fitness
- Little or no disturbance of proprioception
- Cosmetically favorable scars
- Ability to detect associated injuries
- Ability to operate under vision in hard-to-reach sites

As experience is gained, less time is needed to perform arthroscopic procedures. The case load of seasoned arthroscopic surgeons is limited essentially by anesthesia induction, patient preparation and positioning, skin preparation, and preparation and layout of the arthroscopic equipment and surgical instruments.

16.2 Arthroscopic Surgical Instruments

In addition to the basic equipment for arthroscopy (see Chap. 3) and video system components, every arthroscopic operation requires special surgical instruments that are designed to meet a variety of demands (Table 16-3).

Instruments for arthroscopic surgery may be mechanical, motorized, or electrosurgical. Mechanical instruments are classified by shape as straight, curved, or angled.

The basic surgical instruments are of the straight type. In curved instruments the shaft is curved to the right, left, or upward, the jaws of the instrument following the curvature of the shaft. In angled instruments, the jaws are angled to the right, left, up, or down relative to the shaft.

Both mechanical and motorized instruments must be sufficiently stable to prevent instrument breakage resulting in fragment loss within the joint. Some instruments have a built-in weak point to ensure that breakage occurs outside the joint.

The punch is the most frequently used mechanical instrument in arthroscopic surgery. With a motorized system (shaver system), tissue pieces can be simultaneously divided, fragmented, and aspirated from the joint. Various shaver attachments can be used (syn-

Table 16-3. Requirements of an instrument for arthroscopic surgery

- Small dimensions
- High stability
- Good cutting or grasping function
- Ease and comfort of use
- Favorable price

Table 16-4. Spectrum of arthroscopic operations

- Meniscus
  - Partial meniscectomy
  - Subtotal meniscectomy
  - Total meniscectomy
  - Repair
- Anterior cruciate ligament
  - Repair (partial rupture)
  - Repair (complete rupture)
  - Alloplastic reconstruction
- Articular cartilage
  - Shaving
  - Subchondral abrasion chondroplasty
  - Pridie drill holes
- Loose bodies and osteochondral fragments
  - Removal
  - Internal fixation
- Osteochondritis dissecans
  - Inversion plasty
- Lateral release
- Synovium
  - Biopsy
  - Partial synovectomy
  - Total synovectomy
- Excision of mediopatellar plica
- Metallic implant removal
- Plication of medial retinaculum
- Arthrolysis
- Tumor removal
- Empyema therapy
  - Lavage
  - Debridement (removal of fibrin deposits)

ovial resector, Rosenberg resector, meniscus cutter, round burr, turbo cutter) depending on the structure that is treated.

Technical advances have made it possible to apply the traditional electrosurgical principles of general surgery to arthroscopic procedures. This requires the use of a nonelectrolytic irritating solution (e.g., purisole) and grounding of the patient with a neutral electrode. The cutting portion of the instrument is designed much like a probing hook and has an insulated shaft. The electrocautery is advantageous over a mechanical knife in that it is immune to dulling, it reduces postoperative bleeding by the coagulation of small vessels, and its use is easily learned. The palpating probe of diagnostic arthroscopy in effect becomes a cutting probe for operative arthroscopy.

New instruments for arthroscopic surgery are constantly being developed and marketed by industry. Some of these instruments are so specific in their design that they can be used only for certain arthroscopic operations.

Laser technology is also being applied to selected tasks in arthroscopic surgery, but at present laser instruments have not reached a stage of development where they can be recommended for routine clinical use.

16.3 Arthroscopic Surgery

In closing, we direct our attention to the types of knee operation that can be performed using arthroscopic techniques (Table 16-4). For a detailed discussion of these procedures, the reader is referred to textbooks of arthroscopsurgery (see Bibliography) and to the selected surgical topics in the Bibliography.

References

17.1 Textbooks of Evaluation of the Knee Joint

Hackenbruch, W., Henche, H. R.: Diagnostik und Therapie von Kapselbandläsionen am Kniegelenk. Eular Verlag, Berne, 1981

Muhr, G., Wagner, M.: Kapsel-Band-Verletzungen des Kniegelenkes – Diagnostikfibel. Springer, Berlin Heidelberg New York, 1981

Müller, W.: Das Knie. Form, Funktion und ligamentäre Wiederherstellungschirurgie. Springer, Berlin Heidelberg New York, 1982

Strobel, M., Stedtfeld, H.-W.: Diagnostik des verletzten Kniegelenkes. Hans Marseille Verlag, Munich, 1988

Strobel, M., Stedtfeld, H.-W.: Diagnostic Evaluation of the knee. Springer, Berlin Heidelberg New York, 1990

17.2 Textbooks of Diagnostic Arthroscopy and Arthroscopic Surgery

Casscells, S. W.: Arthroscopy: Diagnostic and surgical practice. Lea and Febiger, Philadelphia, 1984

Chassaing, V., Parier, J.: Arthroskopie des Kniegelenkes, Diagnostik und operative Therapie. Deutscher Ärzte – Verlag, Cologne, 1988

Dandy, D. J.: Arthroscopy surgery of the knee. Churchill-Livingstone, Edinburgh, 1981

Dandy, D. J.: Arthroscopy of the knee: a diagnostic colour atlas. Gower Medical Publishing, London, 1984

Glinz, W.: Diagnostische Arthroskopie und arthroskopische Operationen am Kniegelenk. 2nd edn. Verlag Hans Huber, Berne, 1987

Henche, H. R., Holder, J.: Die Arthroskopie des Kniegelenks. Springer, Berlin Heidelberg New York, 1988

Hofer, H. (Ed.): Fortschritte in der Arthroskopie. Ferdinand Enke – Verlag, Stuttgart, 1985

Jackson, R. W., Dandy, D. J.: Arthroscopy of the knee. Grune & Stratton, New York, 1976

Johnson, L. L.: Arthroscopic surgery: principles and practice. C. V. Mosby Company, St. Louis, 1986

Klein, W., Huth, Th. F.: Arthroskopie und Histologie von Kniegelenkserkrankungen. Schattauer Verlag, Stuttgart, 1980

Löhnert, J., Raunest, J.: Arthroskopische Chirurgie des Kniegelenkes. Regensberg & Biermann, Münster, 1985

Müller, W., Hackenbruch, W. (eds.): Surgery and Arthroscopy of the knee. Springer, Berlin Heidelberg New York, 1988

Parisien, J. S. (ed.): Arthroscopic surgery. McGraw-Hill Book Company, New York 1988

Schonholtz, G. J.: An atlas of arthroscopic surgery of the knee. C. C. Thomas, Springfield Illinois, 1988

Schonholtz, G. J.: Arthroscopic surgery of the shoulder, elbow and ankle. C. C. Thomas, Springfield, Illinois, 1986

Schonholtz, G. J.: An atlas of arthroscopic surgery of the knee. C. C. Thomas, Springfield, Illinois, 1988

Shahriaree, H.: O'Connor's textbook of arthroscopic surgery. J. B. Lippincott Company, Philadelphia, 1984

Tiling, Th. (ed.): Arthroskopische Meniskuschirurgie. Ferdinand Enke- Verlag, Stuttgart, 1986

Trickey, E. L., Hertel, P. (eds.): Surgery and arthroscopy of the knee. Springer, Berlin Heidelberg, New York, 1986

Watanabe, M., Takeda, S., Ikeuchi, H.: Atlas of arthroscopy. 2. Auflage. Springer, Berlin Heidelberg, New York, 1970

Watanabe, M. (ed.) Arthroscopy of small joints. Igaku-Shoin, Tokyo New York, 1985

17.3 Development of Arthroscopy

Bircher, E.: Die Arthroendoskopie. Zbl. Chir. 48: 1460–1461 (1921)

Bircher, E.: Die Binnenverletzung des Kniegelenkes und ihre Diagnose. Schweiz. med. Wschr. 6: 921 (1923)

Bircher, E.: Beitrag zur Pathologie (Arthrotis deformans) und Diagnose der Meniskusverletzungen (Arthroendoskopie). Bruns Beitr. klin. Chir. 127: 239-250 (1921)

Bozzini, P.: Lichtleiter, eine Erfindung zur Anschauung innerer Theile und Krankheiten nebst der Abbildung. In: Hufeland, C. (ed.): Journal der practischen Wundarzneykunst. Berlin 24: 107–124 (1806)

Bozzini, P.: Der Lichtleiter. Verlag der Landesindustrie – Comtoirs Weimar, 1807

Bruck, J.: Das Urethroskop Galvanisches Glühlicht. Breslau, 1867

BURMAN, M. S.: Arthroscopy or the direct visualisation of joints. An experimental cadaver study. J. Bone Joint Surg. (Am.) 13: 669–695 (1931)
BURMAN, M. S., FINKELSTEIN, H., MAYER, L.: Arthroscopy of the knee joint. J. Bone Joint Surg. (Am.) 16: 255–268 (1934)
BURMAN, M. S., SUTRO, C. J.: Arthroscopy by fluorescence: An experimental study. Arch. phys. Ther. 16: 423 (1935)
BURMAN, M. S., MAYER, L.: Arthroscopic examination of the knee joint. Arch. Surg. 32: 846–874 (1936)
DONNER, K.: Geschichte der Arthroskopie. In: BLAUTH, W., DONNER, K. (eds.): Arthroskopie des Kniegelenkes. Georg Thieme Verlag, Stuttgart, 1979
FINKELSTEIN, H., MAYER, L.: The arthroscope, a new method of examining joints. J. Bone Joint Surg. (Am.) 13: 583 - 588 (1931)
HELLER, D.: Eugen Bircher - Arzt, Militär, Politiker. Ein Beitrag zur Zeitgeschichte. Verlag Neue Züürcher Zeitung, Zürich, 1988
HURTER, E.: L'arthroscopie. Rev. Chir. orthop. 41: 763–766 (1955)
IINO, S.: Normal arthroscopic findings of the knee joint in adult cadavers. J. Jap. orthop. Ass. 14: 467–523 (1939)
JACKSON, R. W.: Memories of the early days of arthroscopy: 1965–1975. The formative years. Arthroscopy 3: 1–3 (1987)
JOYCE, J. J.: History of the Arthroscopic Association of North America. Its origin and growth. Arthroscopy 3: 265–268 (1987)
KAWASHIMA, W.: Arthrocopy of the tuberculous knee in its early stage. J. Jap. orthop. Ass. 18: 651–655 (1943)
KREUSCHER, P. H.: Semilunar cartilage disease: a plea for early recognition by means of the arthroscope and the early treatment of this condition. Illinois med. J. 47: 290–292 (1925)
LEITER, F.: Zur Geschichte der Elektro-Endoskopie in Wien. Wien med. Wochenschr. 76: 1143 (1926)
MAYER, L., BURMANN, M. S.: Arthroscopy in the diagnosis of meniscal lesions of the knee joint. Amer. J. Surg. 43: 501–511 (1939)
OHNSORGE, J.: Farbphotographie des Kniegelenksinnenraumes über ein neues Glasfiberendoskop. Langenbecks Arch. klin. Chir. 325: 965–967 (1969)
SOMMER, R.: Die Endoskopie des Kniegelenkes. Zbl. Chir. 64: 1692–1697 (1937)
TAKAGI, K.: Practical experiences using Takagi's arthroscope. J. Jap. orthop. Ass. 8: 132 (1933)
TAKAGI, K.: The arthroscope. J. Jap. orthop. Ass. 14: 359–441 (1939)
TAGAKI, K.: The classic: Arthroscope. Clin. Orthop. 167: 6–8 (1982)
VAUBEL, E.: Die Endoskopie des Kniegelenkes. Zeitschr. Rheumaforsch. 1: 210 - 213 (1938)
WATANABE, M., TAKEDA, S.: On the popularization of arthroscopy. J. Jap. orthop. Ass. 27: 258 (1953)
WATANABE, M.: The development and present status of the arthroscope. J. Jap. med. Instr. 25: 11 (1954)
WATANABE, M., TAKEDA, S.: The number 21 arthroscope. J. Jap. orthop. Ass. 34: 1041 (1960)
WATANABE, M.: Arthroscopic diagnosis of the internal derangements of the knee joint. J. Jap. orthop. Ass. 42: 993–1002 (1968)
WATANABE, M.: Memories of the early days of arthroscopy. Arthroscopy 2: 209–214 (1986)
WILKE, K. H.: Endoskopie des Kniegelenkes an der Leiche. Brunœs Beitr. klin. Chir. 169: 75–83 (1939)

17.4 Diagnostic Arthroscopy and General Arthroscopic Surgery

ALM, A., GILLQUIST, J., LILJEDAHL, S. O.: The diagnostic value of arthroscopy of the knee joint. Injury 5: 319–324 (1974)
ANGEL, K. R., HALL, D. J.: Anterior cruciate ligament injury in children and adolescents. Arthroscopy 5: 197–200 (1989)
ANGEL, K. R., HALL, D. J.: The role of arthroscopy in children and adolescents. Arthroscopy 5: 192–196 (1989)
BACH, B. R., WARREN, R. F.: „Empty wall" and „vertical strut" signs of ACL insufficiency. Arthroscopy 5: 137–140 (1989)
BARBER, F. A.: Penetrating knee injuries: the nail gun. Arthroscopy 5: 172–175 (1989)
BARRACK, R. L., SKINNER, H. B., BRUNET, M. E., HADDAD, R. J.: Functional performance of the knee after intraarticular anaesthesia. Am. J. Sports Med. 11: 258–261 (1983)
BARRONIAN, A. D., ZOLTAN, J. D., BUCON, K. A.: Magnetic resonance imaging of the knee: correlation with arthroscopy. Arthroscopy 5: 187–191 (1989)
BEHFAR, A. S., REFIOR, H. J.: Arthroskopie des kindlichen Kniegelenkes. Z. Orthop. 124: 751–754 (1986)
BELLIER, G., DUPONT, J. Y., LARRAIN, M., CAUDRON, C., CARLIOZ, H.: Lateral discoid menisci in children. Arthroscopy 5: 52–56 (1989)
BERGSTRÖM, R., GILLQUIST, J., LYSHOLM, J., HAMBERG, P.: Arthroscopy of the knee in children. J. Pediatr. Orthop. 4: 542–545 (1984)
BERGSTRÖM, R., GILLQUIST, J.: The use of an infusion pump in arthroscopy. Arthroscopy 2: 41–45 (1986)
BERMAN, J. M.: Arthroscopy update. Auxiliary portal for assessing patellofemoral alignment.
Orthop. Rev. 19: 819–820 (1990)
BERNER, W., TSCHERNE, H.: Videotechnik bei der Arthroskopie. Unfallheilkunde 85: 441–443 (1982)
BLEULER, P., GANZONI, N.: Arthroskopische Kniediagnostik an der nichtspezialisierten chirurgischen Abteilung. Helv. chir. Acta 45: 13–16 (1978)
BOMBERG, B. C., MCGINTY, J. B.: Acute hemarthrosis of the knee: indications for diagnostic arthroscopy. Arthroscopy 6: 221–225 (1990)
BRENNER, H.: Was kostet arthroskopisches Operieren ? Arthroskopie 1: 143- 147 (1988)
BRIEF, L. P.: Arthroscopy, self education and humility. Arthroscopy 2: 88- 89 (1986)
BROWN, M. F., DANDY, D. J.: Intra-articular ganglia in the knee. Arthroscopy 6: 322–323 (1990)
BRÜHLMANN-KELLER, H., KIESER, C., ZULLIG, R.: Arthrographie und Arthroskopie in der Meniskusdiag-

nostik. Eine prospektive Blindstudie zum Vergleich ihrer Leistung und Ökonomie. Unfallchirurg 89: 547–550 (1986)

Buckley, J. R., Hood, G.M., Macrae, W.: Arthroscopy under local anaesthesia. J. Bone Joint Surg. (Br.) 71: 126–127 (1989)

Bühler, U., Kieser, C.: Endoskopische Veränderungen im Kniegelenk nach Meniskektomie. Zschr. Unfallmed. Berufskrankh. 2: 133–137 (1978)

Burstein, D. B., Fischer, D. A.: Isolated rupture of the popliteus tendon in a professional athlete. Arthroscopy 6: 238–241 (1990)

Casscells, S. W.: Arthroscopy of the knee joint: A review of 150 cases. J. Bone Joint Surg. (Am.) 53: 287–298 (1971)

Casscells, S. W.: The place of arthroscopy in the diagnosis and treatment of internal derangement of the knee; an analysis of 1.000 cases. Clin. Orthop. 151: 135–142 (1980)

Casscells S. W.: Outerbridge's ridges. Arthroscopy 6: 253 (1990)

Chandler, E. J.: 35-Millimeter photograph from Video. Arthroscopy 1: 268- 269 (1985)

Contzen, H.: Indikationen für die Arthroskopie des Kniegelenkes. Unfallchir. 4: 150–152 (1978)

Dandy, D. J., Jackson, R. W.: The impact of arthroscopy on the management of disorders of the knee. J. Bone Joint Surg. (Br.) 57: 346–348 (1975)

Dandy, D. J., Jackson, R. W.: The diagnosis of problems after meniscectomy. J. Bone Joint Surg. (Br.) 57: 349–352 (1975)

Dandy, D. J., Flanagan, J. P., Steenmeyer, V.: Arthroscopy and the management of the ruptured acl. Clin. Orthop. 167: 43–49 (1982)

Dandy, D. J.: Arthroscopy in the treatment of young patients with anterior knee pain. Orthop. Clin. North Am. 17: 221–229 (1986)

Dandy, D. J.: Arthroscopy in other countries: presidential guest lecture. Arthroscopy 6: 248–251 (1990)

DeHaven, K. E.: Diagnosis of acute knee injuries with haemarthrosis. Am. J. Sports Med. 9: 9–14 (1980)

Dorfmann, H., Dreyfus, P.: Arthroskopie des Kniegelenkes. Münch. Med. Wschr. 13: 611–614 (1972)

Eichenauer, M., Mostegl, A., Agreiter, H.: Korrelation zwischen klinischem, arthrographischem und arthroskopischem Befund bei Meniskusläsionen. Chirurg 57: 719–722 (1986)

Eriksson, E., Sebik, A.: Comparison between transpatellar tendon and lateral approach to the knee during arthroscopy. Am. J. Sports Med. 8: 100- 105 (1980)

Eriksson, E., Sebik, A.: Arthroscopy and arthroscopic surgery in a gas versus a fluid medium. Orthop. Clin. North Am. 13: 293–298 (1982)

Eriksson, E., Haggmark, T., Saartok, T., Sebik, A., Ortengren, B.: Knee arthroscopy with local anaesthesia in ambulatory patients. Methods, results and patient compliance. Orthopedics 9: 186–188 (1986)

Farid, F., Weber, H., Heide, H., Lörinz, W.: Der Stellenwert der transarthroskopischen Synoviadialyse bei hartnäckigen Ergüssen verschiedener Genese und differentialdiagnostischem Wert der Synoviaflüssigkeitsanalyse. Pp. 189–192 In: Hofer, H. (ed.): Fortschritte in der Arthroskopie. Ferdinand Enke – Verlag, Stuttgart, 1985

Finsterbush, A., Frankl, U., Matan, Y., Mann, G.: Secondary damage to the knee after isolated injury of the anterior cruciate ligament. Am. J. Sports Med. 18: 475–479 (1990)

Franke, J.: Die Arthroskopie des Kniegelenkes. Zbl. Chir. 106: 201–206 (1981)

Fraser, K.: Theatre nursing. Arthroscopy. Nurs. Stand. 5: 49 (1990)

Fruensgaard, S., Johannsen, H. V.: Incomplete ruptures of the anterior cruciate ligament. J. Bone Joint Surg. (Br.) 71: 526–530 (1989)

DeHaven, K. E., Collins, H. R.: Diagnosis of internal derangements of the knee. The role of arthroscopy. J. Bone Joint Surg. (Am.) 57: 802–810 (1975)

Fullerton, L. R.: Knee arthroscopy in the military population: An analysis of 600 knee arthroscopies. Arthroscopy 2: 259–261 (1986)

Gächter, A., Rosetto, M.: Verteilung der Relevanz der Knorpelschädigung am Knie. Pp. 31–36 In: Hofer, H. (ed.): Fortschritte in der Arthroskopie. Ferdinand Enke – Verlag, Stuttgart, 1985

Gaudernak, T.: Der posttraumatische Hämarthros des Kniegelenkes – Arthroskopische Abklärung der Ursache. Unfallchirurgie 8: 159–169 (1982)

Gillies, H., Seligson, D.: Precision in the diagnosis of meniscal lesions: A comparison of clinical evaluation, arthrography and arthroscopy. J. Bone Joint Surg. (Am.) 61: 343–346 (1979)

Gillquist, J, Hagberg, G.: A new modification of the technique of arthroscopy of the knee joint. Acta chir. Scand. 142: 123–130 (1976)

Gillquist, J, Hagberg, G., Oretorp, N.: Arthroscopy in acute injuries of the knee joint. Acta Orthop. Scand. 48: 190–196 (1977)

Gillquist, J, Hagberg, G.: Findings at arthroscopy and arthrography in knee injuries. Acta Orthop. Scand. 49: 398–401 (1978)

Glinz, W.: Diagnostische Bedeutung der Arthroskopie bei Präarthrosen des Kniegelenkes. Z. Unfallmed. Berufkrankh. 67: 260–266 (1974)

Glinz, W.: Die Arthroskopie bei Meniskusverletzungen. Z. Unfallmed. Berufkrankh. 69: 106–115 (1976)

Glinz, W.: Arthroskopische Diagnostik der traumatischen Knorpelläsionen am Kniegelenk. Hefte Unfallheilk. 129: 242–246 (1977)

Glinz, W.: Diagnostische Arthroskopie und arthroskopische Operation: Erfahrungen bei 500 Kniearthroskopien. Helv. Chir. Acta 46: 25–32 (1979)

Glinz, W.: Indikationen zur Arthroskopie nach Verletzungen des Kniegelenkes. Z. Unfallmed. Berufskrankh. 75: 133–139 (1982)

Glinz, W.: Indikationen zur Arthroskopie. Dtsch. Med. Wschr. 17: 669–670 (1983)

Glinz, W.: Arthroskopie in der Kinderchirurgie. Z. Kinderchir. 39: Suppl. 1: 15–16 (1984)

Glinz, W.: Arthroskopie – Die stille Revolution. Pp. 1–5 In: Hofer, H. (ed.): Fortschritte in der Arthroskopie. Ferdinand Enke – Verlag, Stuttgart, 1985

Glinz, W., Ricklin, R., Frei, E.: Die partielle vordere Kreuzbandruptur. Pp. 173–176 In: Hofer, H. (ed.):

Fortschritte in der Arthroskopie. Ferdinand Enke - Verlag, Stuttgart, 1985

Glotzer, W., Benedetto, K. P.: Indikation und Technik der Arthroskopie. ZFA 58: 1594–1596 (1982)

Gronert, H. J., Stewin, J.: Möglichkeiten und Grenzen der Arthroskopie beim frischen traumatischen Kniebinnenschaden. Unfallheilk. 83: 108–114 (1980)

Haage, H., Watanabe, M.: Arthrographie und Arthroskopie. Betrachtungen über die Wertigkeit der Methoden. Z. Orthop. 111: 178–183 (1973)

Hansen, H., Thomsen, P. B., Dyreborg, E.: Arthroscopy of the knee. An analysis of 588 consecutive knee arthroscopies. Acta Orthop. Scand. 54: 24- 28 (1983)

Haus, J., Behfar, A. S., Refior, H. J.: Arthroskopische Erfahrungen zur diagnostischen und therapeutischen Wertung von Knorpelschäden des Femoropatellargelenks. Pp. 41–43 In: Hofer, H. (ed.): Fortschritte in der Arthroskopie. Ferdinand Enke - Verlag, Stuttgart, 1985

Hempfling, H.: Die kombinierte endoskopisch-radiologische Untersuchung des Kniegelenkes. Z. Orthop. 120: 874–876 (1982)

Hempfling, H.: Wann welches Arthroskop? Dtsch. Med. Wschr. 112: 437–439 (1987)

Henche, H. R.: Indikation, Technik und Resultate der Arthroskopie nach Traumatisierung des Kniegelenkes. Orthopädie 3: 178–183 (1974)

Henche, H. R.: Indikation und Technik der Arthroskopie des Kniegelenkes. Orthop. Praxis 12: 165–167 (1976)

Henche, H. R.: Indikationen zur Arthroskopie. Schweiz. Rundschau Med. 68: 190–192 (1979)

Henche, H. R.: Arthroskopische Diagnostik des posttraumatischen Kniegelenksschadens. Chirurg 50: 612–617 (1979)

Henche, H. R.: Beinhalterung zur Erleichterung der arthroskopischen Untersuchung des Kniegelenkes. Chirurg 53: 747 (1982)

Hertel, E.: Arthroskopische Diagnostik von Kniegelenksveränderungen. Orthop. Praxis 14: 201–204 (1978)

Hertel, E.: Der Wert der arthroskopischen Diagnostik von Kniegelenksveränderungen. Orthop. Praxis 15: 446 (1979)

Hirschowitz, D.: Clinical assessment, arthrography, arthroscopy and arthrotomy in the diagnosis of internal derangements of the knee. J. Bone Joint Surg. (Br.) 58: 367 (1976)

Hörster, G., Theermann, R.: Vergleichende Meniskusdiagnostik mittels Arthrographie und Arthroskopie. Pp. 23–27 In: Tiling, T. (ed.): Arthroskopische Meniskuschirurgie. Ferdinand Enke - Verlag, Stuttgart, 1976

Howe J. G., Wertheimer C., Johnson R. J., Nichols C. E., Pope M. H., Beynnon B.: Arthroscopic strain gauge measurement of the normal anterior cruciate ligament. Arthroscopy 6: 198–204 (1990)

Hsu, R. W.: The study of Maquet dome high tibial osteotomy. Arthroscopic-assisted analysis. Clin. Orthop. 243: 280–285 (1989)

Huang, T. L., Rieger, R. W., Barmada, R., Ray, R. D.: Correlation of arthroscopy with other diagnostic modalities. Orthop. Clin. North Am. 10: 523–534 (1979)

Ikeuchi, H.: Supplementary study of arthroscopic anatomy on the knee joint. Part I: Plicae, ligaments and tendons. J. Jap. Orthop. Ass. 52: 1–10 (1978)

Ikeuchi, H.: Supplementary study of arthroscopic anatomy on the knee joint. Part II: Menisci. J. Jap. Orthop. Ass. 52: 11–24 (1978)

Jackson, R. W., Abe, J.: The role of arthroscopy in the management of disorders of the knee. J. Bone Joint Surg. (Br.) 54: 310–322 (1972)

Jackson, R. W.: The role of arthroscopy in the management of the arthritic knee. Clin. Orthop. 110: 28–35 (1974)

Jackson, R. W., Dehaven, K.E.: Arthroscopy of the knee. Clin. Orthop. 107: 87–92 (1975)

Jackson, D. W.: Videoarthroscopy: A permanent medical record. Am. J. Sports Med. 6: 213–216 (1978)

Jackson, D. W., Ovadia, D. N.: Videoarthroscopy: present and future developments. Arthroscopy 1: 108–115 (1985)

Johnson, L. L., Becker, R. L.: Arthroscopy, technique and the role of the assistant. Orthop. Rev. 9: 31–43 (1976)

Johnson, L. L.: Impact of diagnostic arthroscopy on the clinical judgement of an experienced arthroscopist. Clin. Orthop. 167: 75–83 (1982)

Johnson, L. L., Shneider, D., Austin, M. D., Goodman, F. G., Bullock, J. M., Debruin, J. A.: Two percent glutaraldehyde: A desinfection in arthroscopy and arthroscopic surgery. J. Bone Joint Surg. (Am.) 64: 237–239 (1982)

Jones, J. R., Allum, R. L.: Acute traumatic haemarthrosis of the knee: expectant treatment or arthroscopy? Ann. R. Coll. Surg. Engl. 71: 40–43 (1989)

Juhl, M., Boe, S.: Arthroscopy in children with special emphasis on meniscal lesions. Injury 17: 171–173 (1986)

Juhl, M., Krebs, B.: Arthroscopy and synovial hemangioma or giant cell tumour of the knee. Arch. Orthop. Trauma. Surg. 108: 250–252 (1989)

Kaempfe, F., D'Amato, C.: An unusual intra-articular ganglion of the knee with interosseous extension. A case report. J. Bone Joint Surg. (Am.) 71: 773–775 (1989)

Kerschbaumer, F., Agreiter, Z., Eichenauer, M.: Die Chondropathia patellae - arthroskopische Diagnostik und klinischer Verlauf. Pp. 37–40 In: Hofer, H. (ed.): Fortschritte in der Arthroskopie. Ferdinand Enke - Verlag, Stuttgart, 1985

Kieser, C., Rüttimann, A.: Die Arthroskopie des Kniegelenkes. Schweiz. Med. Wschr. 106: 1631–1637 (1976)

Kohn, D., Aigner, R.: Entscheidungen vor, während und nach der Kniegelenksarthroskopie. Fortschr. Med. 103: 317–320 (1985)

Kohn, D., Bruckl, R., Lobenhoffer, P.: Kurze technische Mitteilung: Videotechnik und Sterilität bei der Arthroskopie. Z. Orthop. 123: 897–898 (1985)

Kohn, D.: Arthroscopy in acute injuries of anterior cruciate deficient knees: Fresh and old intraarticular lesions. Arthroscopy 2: 98–102 (1986)

Kohn, D., Siebert, W., Bardenheuer, H.: Der intraartikuläre Druck bei der Kniegelenksarthroskopie.

Eine experimentelle und klinische Studie. Arthroskopie 1: 94–99 (1988)

KOHN, D., MÜNCH, E. O.: Der pathologische arthroskopische Befund im Patellofemoralgelenk und seine klinische Bedeutung. Orthop. Praxis 24: 145- 147 (1988)

KÖPPE, W., FENGLER, F., NUSCHENPICKEL, H.: Erste Erfahrungen mit der Arthroskopie des Kniegelenkes im gasförmigen Medium. Beitr. Orthop. Traumatol. 31: 622–626 (1984)

KORN, M. W., SPITZER, R. M., ROBINSON, K. E.: Is there still a role for knee arthrography? Arthroscopy 1: 40–43 (1985)

KREMPEN, J. F., SILVER, R. A., HADLEY, J.: The use of a peritoneal catheter for the irrigation system in arthroscopy: A better system for accurate diagnosis. Clin. Orthop. 128: 214–215 (1977)

KRONER, K., FRUENSGAARD, S.: Synovial venous hemangioma of the knee joint. Arch. Orthop. Trauma. Surg. 108: 253–254 (1989)

LEHRBERGER, K., ROSENMEYER, B.: Stellenwert der arthroskopischen Diagnostik bei der Patellaluxation und -subluxation. Pp. 63–71 In: HOFER, H. (ed.): Fortschritte in der Arthroskopie. Ferdinand Enke – Verlag, Stuttgart, 1985

LEWICKY, R. T., ABESHAUS, M. M.: Simplified technique for posterior knee arthroscopy. Am. J. Sports Med. 10: 22–23 (1982)

LINDBERG, U., HAMBERG, P., LYSHOLM, J., GILLQUIST, J.: Arthroscopic examination of the patellofemoral joint using a central, one-portal technique. Orthop. Clin. North Am. 17: 263–268 (1986)

LINDBERG, U., LYSHOLM, J., GILLQUIST, J.: The correlation between arthroscopic findings and the patellofemoral pain syndrome. Arthroscopy 2: 103–107 (1986)

LINDBLAD, S.: Arthroscopic and synovial correlates of pain in osteoarthritis. Semin. Arthritis. Rheum. 18: 91–93 (1989)

LINDBLAD, S., WREDMARK, T.: Traumatic synovitis analysed by arthroscopy and immunohistopathology. Br. J. Rheumatol. 29: 422–425 (1990)

LYSHOLM, J., GILLQUIST, J.: Arthroscopic examination of the posterior cruciate ligament. J. Bone Joint Surg. (Am.) 63: 363–366 (1981)

MARIANI, P. P.: Indications in diagnostic arthroscopy of the knee. Ital. J. Orthop. Traumatol. 8: 337–343 (1982)

MCGINTY, J. B., FRIEDMAN, P. A.: Arthroscopy of the knee. Clin. Orthop. 121: 173–180 (1976)

MCGINTY, J. B., MATZA, R. A.: Arthroscopy of the knee. Evaluation of on outpatient procedure under local anaesthesia. J. Bone Joint Surg. (Am.) 60: 787–789 (1978)

MCGINTY, J. B.: Arthroscopy: A technique or a subspecialty? Arthroscopy 3: 292–294 (1987)

MENAPACE, C.: Die arthroskopische Meniskusdiagnostik. Pp. 10–22 In: TILING, T. (ed.): Arthroskopische Meniskuschirurgie. Ferdinand Enke – Verlag, Stuttgart, 1985

MENNET, P.: Möglichkeiten und Grenzen der Kniearthroskopie. Schweiz. Med. Wschr. 101: 1591 (1971)

MEYERS, J. F., PIERRE, R. K. S., SUTTER, S., CASPARI, R. B., WHIPPLE, T. L.: Arthroscopic evaluation of anterior cruciate ligament reconstruction. Arthroscopy 2: 155–161 (1986)

MITAL, M. A., KARLIN, L. I.: Diagnostic arthroscopy in sport injuries. Orthop. Clin. 11: 771–785 (1980)

MORGAN, C. D.: Fluid delivery systems for arthroscopy. Arthroscopy 3: 288- 291 (1987)

NOLE, R., MUNSON, N. M., FULKERSON, J. P.: Bupivacaine and saline effects on articular cartilage. Arthroscopy 1: 123–127 (1985)

NORWOOD, L. A., SHIELDS, C. L., RUSSO, J.: Arthroscopy of the lateral meniscus in knees with normal arthrograms. Am. J. Sports Med. 5: 271–274 (1977)

NOYES, F. R., BASSETT, R. W., GROOD, E. S., BUTLER, D. L.: Arthroscopy in acute traumatic haemarthrosis of the knee. Incidence of anterior cruciate tears and other injuries. J. Bone Joint Surg. (Am.) 62: 687–695 (1980)

NOYES, F. R., STABLER, C. L.: A system for grading articular cartilage lesions at arthroscopy. Am. J. Sports Med. 17: 505–513 (1989)

O'CONNOR, R. L.: Arthroscopy in the diagnosis and treatment of acute ligament injuries of the knee. J. Bone Joint Surg. (Am.) 56: 333–337 (1974)

OEHLER, W. D., JANKA, P.: Arthroskopische Diagnostik und therapeutische Konsequenzen beim Hämarthros des Kniegelenkes. Unfallchir. 8: 96–98 (1982)

OGILVIE-HARRIS, D. J., BAUER, M., COREY, P.: Prostaglandin inhibition and the rate of recovery after arthroscopic meniscectomy. A randomised double-blind prospective study. J. Bone Joint Surg. (Br.) 67: 567–571 (1985)

OHNSORGE, J.: Die Arthroskopie des Kniegelenkes. Fortschr. Endoskopie 2: 29–34 (1970)

ORETORP, N., ELMERSON, S.: Arthroscopy and irrigation control. Arthroscopy 2: 46–50 (1986)

PAAR, O., SCHNEIDER, B.: Vergleichende klinische und arthroskopische Untersuchung des Kniegelenkes bei Chondromalacia patellae. Aktuel-Traumatol. 19: 142–6 (1989)

PAGNAMENTA, M., KIESER, C.: Die Resultate der arthroskopischen Untersuchung unklarer Kniegelenksergüsse. Schweiz. Med. Wschr. 112: 1369–1375 (1982)

PALEY, D., JACKSON, R. W.: Synovial haemangioma of the knee joint: diagnosis by arthroscopy. Arthroscopy 2: 174–177 (1986)

PATEL, D.: Proximal approaches to arthroscopic surgery of the knee. Am. J. Sports Med. 9: 296–303 (1981)

PATEL, D.: Superior lateral-medial approach to arthroscopic meniscectomy. Orthop. Clin. North Am. 13: 299–305 (1982)

PEVEY, J. K.: Outpatient arthroscopy of the knee under local anaesthesia. Am. J. Sports Med. 6: 122–127 (1978)

POTTS, H., NOBLE, J.: Arthroscopic surgery in the very young. J. Bone Joint Surg. Br. 71: 541 (1989)

REAGAN, B. F., MCINERNY, V. K., TREADWELL, B. V., ZARINS, B., MANKIN, H. J.: Irrigation solutions for arthroscopy. A metabolic study. J. Bone Joint Surg. (Am.) 65: 629–631 (1983)

RUFFIN, M. T., HUNTER, R. E.: Arthroscopy in the geri-

atric patient. Acute injuries and chronic joint diseases. J. Am. Geriatr. Soc. 37: 977–979 (1989)
RUSHTON, N., DANDY, D. J., NAYLOR, C. P. E.: The clinical, arthroscopic and histological findings after replacement of the ACL with carbon-fibre. J. Bone Joint Surg. (Br.) 65: 308–309 (1983)
SCHEURER, I., REHN, J.: Die Technik der Arthroskopie mit Lachgasfüllung. Unfallheilk. 81: 661–663 (1978)
SELESNICK, F. H., NOBLE, A. B., BACHMAN, B. C., STEINBERG, F. L.: Internal derangement of the knee: Diagnosis by arthrography, arthroscopy and arthrotomie. Clin. Orthop. 198: 26–30 (1985)
SMITH, J. B.: „Retrospectopic" arthroscopy. Arthroscopy 1: 17–21 (1985)
SPERNER, G., BENEDETTO, K. P., GLÖTZER, W.: Die Wertigkeit der Arthroskopie nach traumatischer Patellaluxation. Sportverletzung Sportschaden 2: 20–23 (1988)
STALDER, J.: Arthroscopy should not become a victim of its own success. Rev. Med. Suisse Romande. 109: 539–544 (1989)
STAMM, F., GLINZ, W.: Die Arthroskopie des Kniegelenkes bei der akuten Sportverletzung und beim chronischen Sportschaden. Med. u. Sport 24: 13–16 (1984)
STAUBLI, U., BIRRE, S.: The popliteus tendon and its fascicles at the popliteal hiatus: gross anatomy and functional arthroscopic evaluation with and without anterior cruciate ligament deficiency. Arthroscopy 6: 209–220 (1990)
STEINBRÜCK, K., WIEHMANN, J.-C.: Untersuchung des Kniegelenks. Wertigkeit klinischer Befunde unter arthroskopischer Kontrolle. Z. Orthop. 126: 289-295 (1988)
STOTHER, I. G.: Arthroscopy. Injury. 21: 283–286 (1990)
SUMAN, R. K., STOTHER, I. G., ILLINGWORTH, G.: Diagnostic arthroscopy of knee in children. J. Bone Joint Surg. (Br.) 66: 535–537 (1984)
SWEENEY, H. J.: Teaching arthroscopic surgery at the residency level. Orthop. Clin. North Am. 13: 255–261 (1982)
TAMM, J.: Ergebnisse und Aussagewert der Arthroskopie am Kniegelenk. Unfallchir. 4: 153–156 (1978)
TUBBS, N.: Injured ligaments of the knee. Injury 21: 291–293 (1990)
TURBA, J. E., GANGL, P.: Acute gout arthritis precipitated by arthroscopy. A case report. Am. J. Sports Med. 14: 420–421 (1986)
WATANABE, M.: Arthroscopy: The present state. Clin. Orthop. 10: 503–521 (1979)
WALZ, G., HEMPFLING, H.: Die Akut-Arthroskopie bei klinisch stabilem Knie mit Hämarthros. Deutsch. med. Wochenschr. 110: 1692–1695 (1985)
WENTZENSEN, A., WELLER, S.: Arthroskopische Untersuchungen von gestielten autologen Sehnentransplantaten zum Ersatz des vorderen Kreuzbandes. Chirurg 53: 225–228 (1982)
WHIPPLE, T. L., BASSETT, F. H.: Arthroscopic examination of the knee: Polypuncture technique with percutaneous intra-articular manipulation. J. Bone Joint Surg. (Am.) 60: 444–453 (1978)
WREDMARK, T., LUNDH, R.: Arthroscopy under local anaesthesia using controlled pressure irrigation with prilocaine. J. Bone Joint Surg. (Br.) 64: 583–585 (1982)
WITTNER B., MULLER FARBER J.: Die Arthroskopie nach kindlichen Kniegelenkverletzungen--ein hilfreiches oder überflüssiges diagnostisches Verfahren? Aktuel. Traumatol. 19: 139–141 (1989)
WRUHS, O.: Die Arthroskopie. Orthop. Praxis 9: 75–78 (1972)
WRUHS, O.: Die Arthroskopie des Kniegelenkes. Z. Orthop. 111: 664–665 (1973)
WRUHS, O.: Endoskopisch fanDFbare Veränderungen des Femur-Patellargelenkes. Z. Orthop. 111: 525–526 (1973)
WRUHS, O.: Arthroskopische Befunde bei Vorverlagerung der Tuberositas tibiae. Hefte Unfallheilk. 127: 46–57 (1975)
ZIV, I., CARROLL, N. C.: The role of arthroscopy in children. J. Pediatr. Orthop. 2: 243–247 (1983)
ZOLLINGER, H.: Indikation und Aussage der Gelenkendoskopie bei der Chondropathia patellae. Z. Orthop. 115: 617 (1977)
ZAK, K., BARTSCH, H.: Arthroskopie und arthroskopische Operation in Lokalanästhesie – Anwendung und Grenzen. Orthop. Praxis 24: 52–54 (1988)
ZARINS, B.: Arthroscopic surgery in a sports medicine practice. Orthop. Clin. North Am. 13: 415–421 (1982)

17.5 Anaesthesia, Analgesia

BUCKLEY, J. R., HOOD, G. M., MACRAE, W.: Arthroscopy under local anaesthesia. J. Bone Joint Surg. (Br.) 71: 126–127 (1989)
BUCKLEY, J. R.: Operative arthroscopy under local anaesthetic. J. R. Coll. Surg. Edinb. 34: 82–87 (1989)
BUTTERWORTH, J. F., CARNES, R. S., SAMUEL, M. P., JANEWAY, D., POEHLING, G. G.: Effect of adrenaline on plasma concentrations of bupivacaine following intra-articular injection of bupivacaine for knee arthroscopy. Br. J. Anaesth. 65: 537–539 (1990)
CHIRWA, S. S., MACLEOD, B. A., DAY, B.: Intraarticular bupivacaine (Marcaine) after arthroscopic meniscectomy: a randomized double-blind controlled study. Arthroscopy 5: 33–35 (1989)
CLAEYS, M. A., HANDELBERG, F., CASTELEYN, P. P.: Deep sedation for arthroscopic knee surgery. Acta. Orthop. Belg. 55: 53–57 (1989)
DAHL, M. R., DASTA, J. F., ZUELZER, W., MCSWEENEY, T. D.: Lidocaine local anesthesia for arthroscopic knee surgery. Anesth. Analg. 71: 670–674 (1990)
FULKERSON, J. P., FOLCIK, M. A.: Analgesia following arthroscopic surgery: Comparison of diflunisal and acetaminophen with codeine. Arthroscopy 2: 108–110 (1986)
KHOURY, G. F., STEIN, C., GARLAND, D. E.: Intra-articular morphine for pain after knee arthroscopy. Lancet 336: 874 (1990)
MARTIN, R. C., BROWN, D. E., ZELL, B. K., LICHTMAN, D. M.: Diagnostic and operative arthroscopy of the

knee under local anesthesia with parenteral medication. Am. J. Sports Med. 17: 436–439 (1989)
McLoughlin, C., McKinney, M. S., Fee, J. P., Boules, Z.: Diclofenac for day-care arthroscopy surgery: comparison with a standard opioid therapy. Br. J. Anaesth. 65: 620–623 (1990)
Steelman, V. M.: Intraoperative music therapy. Effects on anxiety, blood pressure. Aorn J 52: 1026–1034 (1990)
White, A. P., Laurent, S., Wilkinson, D. J.: Intra-articular and subcutaneous prilocaine with adrenaline for pain relief in day case arthroscopy of the knee joint. Ann. R. Coll. Surg. Engl. 72: 350–352 (1990)
Yacobucci, G. N., Bruce, R., Conahan, T. J., Kitz, D. S., Torg, J. S.: Arthroscopic surgery of the knee under local anesthesia. Arthroscopy 6: 311–314 (1990)
Zuurmond, W. W., Van Leeuwen, L., Helmers, J. H.: Recovery from fixed-dose midazolam-induced anaesthesia and antagonism with flumazenil for outpatient arthroscopy. Acta. Anaesthesiol. Scand. 33: 160–163 (1989)

17.6 Special Arthroscopic Surgery

17.6.1 Instrumentation

Balduini, F. C., Peff, T. C., Torg, J. C.: Application of electrothermal energy in arthroscopy. Arthroscopy 1: 259–263 (1985)
Bauer, M., Jackson, R. W.: Intra-articular pressure in the knee during routine arthroscopy. Arthroscopy 2: 198–199 (1986)
Bergström, R., Gillquist, J.: The use of an infusion pump in arthoscopy. Arthroscopy 2: 41–45 (1986)
Bert, J. M.: Use of 1.5% glycine as nonconductive fluid medium for arthroscopic electrosurgery. Arthroscopy 3: 248–252 (1987)
Besser, M. I. B., Stahl, S.: Arthroscopic surgery performed under local anesthesia as an outpatient procedure. Arch. Orthop. Trauma. Surg. 105: 296–297 (1986)
Buess, G., Eitenmüller, J., Theiss, R., Hildebrand, E., Hutterer, F.: Meniskusresektion mit Diathermie, Optimierung der Instrumentenisolation mit Keramikbeschichtung. Pp. 197–205 In: Hofer, H. (ed.): Fortschritte in der Arthroskopie. Ferdinand Enke – Verlag, Stuttgart, 1985
Dehaven, K.: Principles of triangulation for arthroscopic surgery. Orthop. Clin. North Am. 13: 329–336 (1982)
Dobson, P. J.: Electrosurgical arthroscopic meniscectomy: new instrumentation and technique. J. Bone Joint Surg. (Br.) 69: 162 (1987)
Dolk, T., Augustini, B. G: Elevated position of suction outflow during arthroscopic motorized surgery: an experimental study. Arthroscopy 5: 97–100 (1989)
Dolk, T., Augustini, B. G.: Elevated position of the irrigation outflow during arthroscopy: an experimental study. Arthroscopy 5: 93–96 (1989)
Eichhorn, J., Kolditz, D., Krämer, J.: Vorteile der Hochfrequenzchirurgie bei der Meniskektomie. Pp. 43–49 In: Hofer, H. (ed.): Fortschritte in der Arthroskopie. Ferdinand Enke – Verlag, Stuttgart, 1985
Ewing, J. W., Noe, D. A., Kitaoka, H. B., Askew, M. J.: Intraarticular pressures during arthroscopic knee surgery. Arthroscopy 2: 264–269 (1986)
Haupt, P. R., Duspiva, W.: Flüssigkeitspumpen zur kontinuierlichen Gelenkspülung bei der Arthroskopie. Aktuel. Traumatol. 14: 106–107 (1984)
Johnson, J. C, Pierson, R. H., Bach, B. R.: A suture „retractor": a technical aid for bucket-handle meniscal resections. Arthroscopy 6: 327–328 (1990)
Johnson, L. L.: Creating the proper environment for arthroscopic surgery. Orthop. Clin. North Am. 13: 283–292 (1982)
Kolditz, D., Krämer, J., Eichhorn, J.: Die Technik der Elektroresektion bei arthroskopischen Kniegelenksoperationen. Pp. 244–248 In: Hofer, H. (ed.): Fortschritte in der Arthroskopie. Ferdinand Enke – Verlag, Stuttgart, 1985
Lidge, R. T.: Leg holders in arthroscopic surgery. Orthopedics 7: 1043 (1984)
Parisien, J. P., Dzenis, P.: Development of modern arthroscopic techniques, fundamentals of endoscopes, basic equipment for diagnosis and surgery. Pp. 47–67 In: Parisien, J. S. (ed.): Arthroscopic surgery. McGraw-Hill Book Company, New York 1988
Powell, J., Glasgow, M. M. S.: Arthroscopic electrosurgery of the knee. J. Bone Joint Surg. (Br.) 69: 849 (1987)
Rand, J. A., Gaffey, T. A.: Effect of electrocautery on fresh human articular cartilage. Arthroscopy 1: 242–246 (1985)
Schosheim, P. M., Caspari, R. B.: Evaluation of electrosurgical meniscectomy in rabbits. Arthroscopy 2: 71–76 (1986)
Schretzmair, N. A., Colberg, H.: Beinlagerungsgerät zur Erleichterung von Arthroskopie und Arthrotomie am Kniegelenk. Sportverletzung Sportschaden 2: 24–25 (1988)
Smith, C. F., Johansen, W.E., Vangsness, C.T., Sutter, L.V., Marshall, G.J.: The carbon dioxide laser. A potential tool for orthopedic surgery. Clin. Orthop. 242: 43–50 (1989)
Wittenberg, H.-R., Müller, K.-M.: Untersuchungen über das Schneideverhalten von Knorpelfräsen bei Gonarthrose. Arthroskopie 1: 138–142 (1988)

17.6.2 Meniscectomy

Aglietti, P., Buzzi, R., Pisaneschi, A.: Results of partial arthroscopic meniscectomies in anterior cruciate ligament deficient knees. Pp. 358–359 In: Müller, W., Hackenbruch, W. (eds.): Surgery and Arthroscopy of the knee. Springer, Berlin Heidelberg New York, 1988
Bergström, R., Hamberg, P., Lysholm, J., Gillquist, J.: Comparison of open and endoscopic meniscectomy. Clin. Orthop. 184: 133–136 (1984)
Benedetto, K. P., Glötzer, W., Sperner, G.: Die ar-

throskopische Meniskusteilresektion. Akt. Traumatol. 16: 21–25 (1986)
Berner, W.: Die arthroskopische Meniskusresektion. Unfallheilk. 86: 241–245 (1983)
Boe, S., Hansen, H.: Arthroscopic partial meniscectomy in patients aged over 50. J. Bone Joint Surg. (Br.) 68: 707 (1986)
Boszotta, H., Wendrinsky, R., Ohrenberger, G., Sauer, G.: Die arthroskopische Operation in einem Krankenhaus der Regelversorgung. Ergebnisse nach 227 arthroskopischen Meniskektomien. Unfallchirurg 91: 91- 95 (1988)
Calvisi, V., Preite, R., Romanini, L.: Cystic degeneration of the external meniscus. Part 2: Arthroscopic meniscectomy. Ital. J. Orthop. Traumatol. 15: 33–41 (1989)
Carson, W. R.: Arthroscopic meniscectomy. Orthop. Clin. North Am. 10: 619- 627 (1971)
Dandy, D. J.: Early results of closed partial meniscectomy. Brit. med. J. 1: 1099–1101 (1978)
Dandy, D. J.: The bucket handle meniscal tear: A technique detaching the posterior segment first. Orthop. Clin. North Am. 13: 369–385 (1982)
Durand, A., Richards, C. L., Malouin, F.: Strength recovery and muscle activation of the knee extensor and flexor muscles after arthroscopic meniscectomy. A pilot study. Clin. Orthop. 262: 210–226 (1991)
Eastwood, D. M.: The failures of arthroscopic partial meniscectomy. Injury 16: 587–590 (1985)
Ferkel, R. D., Davis, J. R., Friedman, M. J., Fox, J. M., Del Pizzo, W., Snyder, S. J., Berasi, C. C.: Arthroscopic partial medial meniscectomy. An analysis of unsatisfactory results. Arthroscopy 1: 44–52 (1985)
Georgoulis, A, Lais, E., Hertel, P.: Arthroscopic meniscectomy on patients with untreated rupture of the anterior cruciate ligament. Pp. 360 – 365 In: Müller, W., Hackenbruch, W. (eds.): Surgery and Arthroscopy of the knee. Springer, Berlin Heidelberg New York, 1988
Genelin, F., Obrist, J., Kropfl, A., Zirknitzer, J.: Vergleichende Untersuchung zwischen arthroskopischen und offenen Meniskusoperationen. Unfallchirurgie 15: 133–135 (1989)
Gillquist, J., Hamberg, P., Lysholm, J.: Endoscopic partial and total meniscectomy. A comparative study. Acta Orthop. Scand. 53: 975–979 (1982)
Gillquist, J., Oretorp, N.: The technique of endoscopic total meniscectomy. Orthop. Clin. North Am. 13: 363–367 (1982)
Gillquist, J., Oretorp, N.: Arthroscopic partial meniscectomy. Technique and long term results. Clin. Orthop. 167: 29–33 (1982)
Glinz, W.: Arthroskopische partielle Meniskektomie. Helv. chir. Acta 47: 115–119 (1980)
Glinz, W., Ghafier, M.: Arthroskopische Meniskusresektion: Resultate 1 – 7Jahre nach der Operation. Pp. 61–71 In: Tiling, T. (ed.): Arthroskopische Meniskuschirurgie. Ferdinand Enke – Verlag, Stuttgart, 1986
Glötzer, W., Benedetto, K.P.: Die arthroskopische Meniskusresektion. Pp. 35- 42 In: Tiling, T. (ed.): Arthroskopische Meniskuschirurgie. Ferdinand Enke – Verlag, Stuttgart, 1986
Guhl, F. J.: Excision of flap tears. Orthop. Clin. North Am. 13: 387–397 (1982)
Hamberg, P., Gillquist, J., Lysholm, J., Oberg, B.: The effect of diagnostic and operative arthroscopy and open meniscectomy on muscle strength in the tigh. Am. J. Sports Med. 11: 289–292 (1983)
Hamberg, P., Gillquist, J., Lysholm, J.: A comparison between arthroscopic meniscectomy and modified open meniscectomy. J. Bone Joint Surg. (Br.) 66: 189–192 (1984)
Hanley, S. T., Warren, R. F.: Arthroscopic meniscectomy in the anterior cruciate ligament – deficient knee. Arthroscopy 3: 59–65 (1987)
Hayashi, L. K., Yamaga, D. M., Ida, K., Miura, T.: Arthroscopic meniscectomy for discoid lateral meniscus in children. J. Bone Joint Surg. (Am.) 70: 1495–1499 (1988)
Hede, A., Hejgaard, N., Lasrsen, E.: Partial or total open meniscectomy? a prospective randomized study. Int. Orthop. 10: 105–108 (1986)
Hershman, E. B., Nisonson, B.: Arthroscopic meniscectomy: A follow-up report. Am. J. Sports Med. 11: 253–257 (1983)
Holder, J.: Endoskopische Operationstechnik am Meniskus. Arthroskopie 1: 38–44 (1988)
Ikeuchi, H.: Arthroscopic treatment of the discoid lateral meniscus. Clin. Orthop. 167: 19–28 (1982)
Inoue, K., Mikanagi, K., Morita, H., Mamiki, T.: CO_2 Laser meniscectomy und Arthroscopy. Pp. 349 In: Müller, W., Hackenbruch, W. (eds.): Surgery and Arthroscopy of the knee. Springer, Berlin Heidelberg New York, 1988
Jackson, R. W., Dandy, D. J.: Partial meniscectomy. J. Bone Joint Surg. (Br.) 58: 142 (1976)
Jackson, R. W., Rouse, D. W.: The results of partial arthroscopic meniscectomy in patients over 40 years of age. J. Bone Joint Surg. (Br.) 64: 481–485 (1982)
Kelley, M. J.: Meniscal trauma and surgical intervention. A review of literature. J. Sports Med. Phys. Fitness. 30: 297–306 (1990)
Kentsch, A.: Zur arthroskopischen Behandlung des schwierigen Innenmeniskus. Arthroskopie 1: 51–52 (1988)
Klein, J., Tiling, T., Roeddecker, K.: Vergleichende Untersuchung zur arthroskopischen Meniskektomie unter Wasser und unter Gas. Pp. 50–53 In: Tiling, T. (ed.): Arthroskopische Meniskuschirurgie. Ferdinand Enke – Verlag, Stuttgart, 1986
Klein, W., Schulitz, K. P.: Arthroscopic meniscectomy. Arch. Orthop. Trauma. Surg. 101: 231–237 (1983)
Krämer, J., Rosenthal, A., Moraldo, M., Müller, K. M.: Elektroresektion des Meniskus. Arthroskopie 1: 45–49 (1988)
Kundinger, R., Heller, G., Wuschech, H.: Die arthroskopische Meniskuschirurgie. Zbl. Chir. 111: 1497–1502 (1986)
Löhnert, J., Raunest, J.: Die partielle arthroskopische Meniskusresektion. Chirurg 55: 474–479 (1982)
Löhnert, J., Raunest, J.: Arthroskopische Meniskusresektion und offene Meniskektomie – eine vergleichende Studie. Chirurg 57: 723–727 (1986)
Löhnert, J.: Arthroskopische Meniskuschirurgie. Arthroskopie 1: 25–37 (1988)

LYSHOLM, J., GILLQUIST, J.: Endoscopic meniscectomy. Int. Orthop. 5: 265–270 (1981)

LYSHOLM, J., GILLQUIST, J.: Arthroscopic meniscectomy in athletes. Am. J. Sports Med. 11: 436–438 (1983)

MARSHALL, S., LEVAS, M. G., HARRAH, A.: Simple arthroscopic partial meniscectomy associated with anterior cruciate deficient knees. Arthroscopy 1: 22–27 (1985)

MARTENS, M. A., BACKAERT, M., HEYMAN, E., MULIER, J. C.: Partial arthroscopic meniscectomy versus total open meniscectomy. Arch. Orthop. Trauma. Surg. 105: 31–35 (1986)

McBRIDE, G. G., CONSTINE, R. M., HOFMANN, A. A., CARSON, R. W.: Arthroscopic partial medial meniscectomy in older patient. J. Bone Joint Surg. (Am.) 66: 547–551 (1984)

McGINTY, J. B., GEUSS, L. F., MARVIN, R. A.: Partial or total meniscectomy. J. Bone Joint Surg. (Am.) 66: 547–551 (1977)

METCALF, R. W.: The torn medial meniscus. Pp. 93–110 In: PARISIEN, J. S. (ed.): Arthroscopic surgery. McGraw-Hill Book Company, New York, 1988

MILLER, G. K., DRENNAN, D. B., MAYLAHN, D. J.: The effect of technique on histology of arthoscopic partial meniscectomy with electrosurgery. Arthroscopy 3: 36–44 (1987)

NORTHMORE-BALL, M. D., DANDY, D. J.: Long-term results of arthroscopic partial meniscectomy. Clin. Orthop. 167: 34–42 (1982)

NORTHMORE-BALL, M. D., DANDY, D. J., JACKSON, R. W.: Arthroscopic, open partial and total meniscectomy. J. Bone Joint Surg. (Br.) 65: 400–404 (1983)

PATEL, D., PARISIEN, J. S.: The torn lateral meniscus. Pp. 111–123 In: PARISIEN, J. S. (ed.): Arthroscopic surgery. McGraw-Hill Book Company, New York 1988

PETTRONE, F. A.: Meniscectomy: Arthrotomy versus arthroscopy. Am. J. Sports Med. 10: 355–359 (1982)

RAND, J. A.: Arthroscopic management of degenerative meniscus tears in patients with degenerative arthritis. Arthroscopy 1: 253–258 (1985)

RAUNEST, J., LÖHNERT, J.: Langzeitergebnisse nach 450 arthroskopischen Meniskusresektionen. Orthop. Praxis 2: 110 (1986)

REIKERAS O.: Arthroscopic resection of meniscal flaps of the knee. Acta. Orthop. Scand. 60: 28–29 (1989)

SARAGAGLIA, D., TOURNE, Y., CHAMSEDDINE, A., BUTEL, J.: Les sutures meniscales associees a la refection du ligament croise anterieur. Resultats compares des sutures des lesions recentes et chroniques: 102 cas. Rev. Chir. Orthop. 76: 170–176 (1990)

SIMPSON, D. A., THOMAS, N. P., AICHROTH, P. M.: Open and closed meniscectomy. A comparative analysis. J. Bone Joint Surg. (Br.) 68: 301–304 (1986)

SPRAGUE, N. F.: The bucket-handle tear: technique using two incisions. Orthop. Clin. North Am. 13: 337–348 (1982)

STOFFEL, D., GLINZ, W., RICKLIN, T., FREI, E.: Rearthroskopie nach arthroskopischer Meniskusresektion. Pp. 86–89 In: TILING, T. (ed.): Arthroskopische Meniskuschirurgie. Ferdinand Enke – Verlag, Stuttgart, 1986

TREGONNING, J. A. R.: Closed partial meniscectomy. J. Bone Joint Surg. (Br.) 65: 378–382 (1983)

VANDERMEER, R. D., CUNNINGHAM, F. K.: Arthroscopic treatment of the discoid lateral meniscus: results of long-term follow-up. Arthroscopy 5: 101–109 (1989)

WEISS, C. B., LUNDBERG, M., HAMBERG, P., DEHAVEN, K. E., GILLQUIST, J.: Non-operative treatment of meniscal tears. J. Bone Joint Surg. Am. 71: 811–22 (1989)

WHIPPLE, T. L., CASPARI, R. B., MEYERS, J. F.: Laser energy in arthroscopic meniscectomy. Orthopedics 6: 1165–1169 (1983)

WHIPPLE, T. L., CASPARI, R. B., MEYERS, J. F.: Arthroscopic meniscectomy. An interim report at three to four years after operation. Clin. Orthop. 183: 105–114 (1984)

WHIPPLE, T. L.: Arthroscopic medial meniscectomy. Operative techniques and problems. Orthopedics 8: 109–114 (1985)

17.6.3 Meniscus refixation

BARATZ, M. E., REHAK, D. C., FU, F. H., RUDERT, M. J.: Peripheral tears of the meniscus. The effect of open versus arthroscopic repair on intraarticular contact stresses in the human knee. Am. J. Sports Med. 16: 1–6 (1988)

BARBER, F. A., STONE, R. G.: Meniscal repair – an arthroscopic technique. J. Bone Joint Surg. (Br.) 67: 39–41 (1985)

BARBER, F. A.: Meniscus repair: results of an arthroscopic technique. Arthroscopy 3: 25–30 (1987)

CASSIDY, R. E., SHAFFER, A. J.: Repair of peripheral meniscus tears – a preliminary report. Am. J. Sports Med. 9: 209–214 (1981)

CLANCY, W. G., GRAF, B. K.: Arthroscopic meniscal repair. Orthopedics 6: 1125–1129 (1983)

DEFRERE, J., FRANCKART, A., BASSLEER, R.: Meniscus repair by arthroscopy. Pp. 306–316 In: MÜLLER, W., HACKENBRUCH, W. (eds.): Surgery and Arthroscopy of the knee. Springer, Berlin Heidelberg New York, 1988

DEHAVEN, K. E.: Meniscus repair – open versus arthroscopic. Arthroscopy 1: 173–174 (1985)

DISTEFANO, V., BIZZLE, B.: A technique of arthroscopic meniscoplasty. Orthopedics 6: 1135–1140 (1983)

DUSTMANN, H. O., GODOLIAS, G.: Indikation, Technik und Ergebnisse der offenen und arthroskopischen Meniskusfixation. Orthop. Praxis 2: 131–137 (1986)

HACKENBRUCH, W., BAUMGARTNER, R., MÜLLER, W.: Arthroskopische Meniskusnaht und funktionelle Nachbehandlung. Pp. 206–210 In: HOFER, H. (ed.): Fortschritte in der Arthroskopie. Ferdinand Enke – Verlag, Stuttgart, 1985

HACKENBRUCH, W., BAUMGARTNER, R., MÜLLER, W., MENDELIN, R.: Meniskusrefixation. Unfallchirurg 90: 73–78 (1987)

HAMBERG, P., GILLQUIST, J., LYSHOLM, J.: Suture of new and old peripheral meniscus tears. J. Bone Joint Surg. (Am.) 65: 193–197 (1983)

HENNING, C. E.: Arthroscopic repair of meniscus tears. Orthopedics 6: 1130- 1132 (1983)

HERTEL, P., LAIS, E.: Is meniscus refixation sensible? Beitr. Orthop. Traumatol. 36: 28–32 (1989)

JAKOB, R. P., STÄUBLI, H. U.: Indikation, instrumentelle Technik und Ergebnisse der arthroskopischen Meniskusrefixation. Pp. 157–166 In: HOFER, H. (ed.): Fortschritte in der Arthroskopie. Ferdinand Enke - Verlag, Stuttgart, 1985

KARPF, P. M., SAGSTETTER, C., AIGNER, R., RUPP, N.: Erfahrungen mit der Meniskusnaht. Unfallchirurg 88: 15–19 (1985)

KEENE, G. C. R., PATERSON, R. S.: Arthroscopic menisceal suture. J. Bone Joint Surg. (Br.) 69: 162 (1987)

KOHN, D.: Offene oder arthroskopische Meniskusnaht? - eine experimentelle Studie. Orthop. Praxis 24: 305–308 (1988)

KUENDIGER, R., WUSCHECH, H. HELLER, G.: Indikation und Technik der arthroskopischen Meniskusrefixation. Zbl. Chir. 111: 1056–1060 (1986)

LANDSIEDL, F.: Verbesserte Outside-In-Technik der arthroskopischen Meniskusnaht. Arthroskopie 1: 190–191 (1988)

LEE, W. K. C., MAGUIRE, M.G.: A new technique for arthroscopic menisceal repair. J. Bone Joint Surg. (Br.) 71: 166 (1989)

MARSHALL, S. C.: Combined arthroscopic-open repair of meniscal injuries. Pp. 317–327 In: MÜLLER, W., HACKENBRUCH, W. (eds.): Surgery and Arthroscopy of the knee. Springer, Berlin Heidelberg New York, 1988

MILLER, D. B.: Arthroscopic meniscus repair. Am. J. Sports Med. 16: 315–320 (1988)

MORGAN, C. D., CASSCELLS, S. W.: Arthroscopic meniscus repair: A save approach to the posterior horns. Arthroscopy 2: 3–12 (1986)

ROSENBERG, T., SCOTT, S., PAULOS, L.: Arthroscopic surgery: Repair of peripheral detachment of the meniscus. Contemp. Orthop. 10: 43–50 (1985)

ROSENBERG, T., SCOTT, S., COWARD, D. B., DUNBAR, W. H., EWING, W., JOHNSON, L. L., PAULOS, L.: Arthroscopic meniscal repair evaluated with repeat arthroscopy. Arthroscopy 2: 14–20 (1986)

SCHMID, A., SCHMID, F., TILING, T.: Elektronenmikroskopische Befunde am Meniskus nach Naht. Pp. 125–133 In: Tiling, T. (ed.): Arthroskopische Meniskuschirurgie. Ferdinand Enke - Verlag, Stuttgart, 1986

SCOTT, G. A., JOLLY, B. L., HENNING, C. E.: Combined posterior incision and arthroscopic intraarticular repair of the meniscus. An examination of factors affecting healing. J. Bone Joint Surg. (Am.) 68: 847–861 (1986)

STONE, R. G., MILLER, G. A.: A technique of arthroscopic suture of torn menisci. Arthroscopy 1: 226–232 (1985)

STONE, R. G., BARBER, F.: Meniscus repair, an arthroscopic technique. J. Bone Joint Surg. (Br.) 67: 39–41 (1985)

STONE, R. G., VAN WINKEL, G. N.: Arthroscopic review of meniscal repair: Assessment of healing parameters. Arthroscopy 2: 77–81 (1986)

STONE, R. G.: Meniscal repair. Pp. 189–197 In: PARISIEN, J. S. (ed.): Arthroscopic surgery. McGraw-Hill Book Company, New York, 1988

VAN ARKEL, E. R., VAN DE WEIJER, H. T.: Arthroscopic suturing of the meniscus. Ned. Tijdschr. Geneeskd. 134: 2299–2301 (1990)

WARREN, R. F.: Arthroscopic meniscus repair. Arthroscopy 1: 170–172 (1985)

WARREN, R. F., HANLEY, S., BACH, B.R.: Chronic anterior cruciate ligament injury. Pp. 125–133 In: PARISIEN, J. S. (ed.): Arthroscopic surgery. McGraw-Hill Book Company, New York, 1988

WIRTH, C. J.: Meniscus repair. Clin. Orthop. 157: 153–160 (1981)

WIRTH, C. J., RODRIGUEZ, M., MILACHOWSKI, K. A.: Meniskusnaht - Meniskusersatz. Georg Thieme Verlag, Stuttgart, 1988

WUSCHECH, H., KUNDIGER, R., HELLER, G.: Indikation und Technik der arthroskopischen Meniskusrefixation. Zbl. Chir. 111: 1056–1063 (1986)

17.6.4 Degenerative cartilage lesions, Osteochondritis

BERT, J. M., MASCHKA, K.: The arthroscopic treatment of unicompartmental gonarthrosis: a five-year follow-up study of abrasion arthroplasty plus arthroscopic debridement and arthroscopic debridement alone. Arthroscopy 5: 25–32 (1989)

CASSCELLS, S.W.: What, if any, are the indications for arthroscopic debridement of the osteoarthritic knee? Arthroscopy 6: 169–170 (1990)

CHANG, R. W., FALCONER, J., STULBERG, S. D., ARNOLD, W. J., DYER, A. R.: Prerandomization: an alternative to classic randomization. The effects on recruitment in a controlled trial of arthroscopy for osteoarthrosis of the knee. J. Bone Joint Surg (Am.) 72: 1451–1455 (1990)

DANDY, D. J.: Abrasion chondroplasty. Arthroscopy 2: 51–53 (1986)

GUHL, J. F.: Arthroscopic treatment of osteochondritis dissecans. Clin. Orthop. 167: 65–67 (1982)

EICHHORN, J., STROBEL, M.: Erweiterte Indikationen zur Arthroskopie. Pp. 151–155 In: CHASSAING, V., PARIER, J.: Arthroskopie des Kniegelenkes - Diagnostik und operative Therapie. Deutscher Ärzte - Verlag, Cologne, (1988)

FEDERICO, D. J., LYNCH, J. K., JOKL, P.: Osteochondritis dissecans of the knee: a historical review of etiology and treatment. Arthroscopy 6: 190–197 (1990)

HOMMINGA, G. N., BULSTRA, S. K., BOUWMEESTER, P. S., VAN DER LINDEN, A. J..: Perichondral grafting for cartilage lesions of the knee. J. Bone Joint Surg. (Br.) 72: 1003–1007 (1990)

HUBBARD, M. J. S.: Arthroscopic surgery for chondral flaps in the knee. J. Bone Joint Surg. (Br.) 69: 794–796 (1987)

JOHNSON, L. L.: Arthroscopic abrasion arthroplasty historical and pathologic perspective: Present status. Arthroscopy 2: 54–69 (1986)

JOHNSON L. L., UITVLUGT G., AUSTIN M. D., DETRISAC D. A., JOHNSON C.: Osteochondritis dissecans of the

knee: arthroscopic compression screw fixation. Arthroscopy 6: 179–189 (1990)
KLEIN, W.: Die maschinelle arthroskopische Chirurgie der Gonarthrose. Indikation, Technik, Nachuntersuchungsergebnisse. Arthroskopie 1: 109–115 (1988)
MILLER, K. G., MAYLAHN, D. J., DRENNAN, D. B.: Treatment of idiopathic osteonecrosis of the medial femoral condyle with arthroscopic debridement. Arthroscopy 2: 21 (1986)
OGILIVIE-HARRIS, D. J., JACKSON, R. W.: The arthroscopic treatment of chondromalacia patellae. J. Bone Joint Surg. (Br.) 66: 660–665 (1984)
RAE, P. J., NOBLE, J.: Arthroscopic drilling of osteochondral lesions of the knee. J. Bone Joint Surg. (Br.) 71: 534 (1989)
ROSENTHAL, A., EICHHORN, J., NITZSCHKE, E.: Ergebnisse der arthroskopischen Chirurgie der Gonarthrose. Arthroskopie 1: 116–123 (1988)
SCHMID, A., SCHMID, F., TILING, T.: Electron microscope findings after cartilage shaving. Pp. 426 – 432 In: MÜLLER, W., HACKENBRUCH, W. (eds.): Surgery and Arthroscopy of the knee. Springer, Berlin Heidelberg New York, 1988
SCHMIDT, H., HASSE, E.: Arthroscopic surgical treatment of circumscribed cartilage damage with spongiolization or Pridie drilling. Beitr. Orthop. Traumatol. 36: 35–37 (1989)
SCHONHOLTZ, G., LING, B.: Arthroscopic chondroplasty of the patella. Arthroscopy 1: 92–96 (1985)
SCHONHOLTZ, G. J.: Arthroscopic debridement of the knee joint. Orthop. Clin. North. Am. 20: 257–263 (1989)
SPRAGUE, N. F.: Arthroscopic debridement for degenerative knee joint disease. Clin. Orthop. 160: 118–123 (1981)
WHIPPLE, T. L.: Osteoarthritis and chondromalacia. Pp. 135–145. In: PARISIEN, J.S. (ed.): Arthroscopic surgery. McGraw-Hill Book Company, New York 1988
WIEDEL, J. D.: Arthroscopy in steroid induced osteonecrosis of the knee. Arthroscopy 1: 68–69 (1985)

17.6.5 Removal of Loose Bodies

CHANDLER, E. J.: Loose bodies. Pp. 227–236 In: SHAHRIAREE, H.: O'Connor's textbook of arthroscopic surgery. J. B. Lippincott Comp., Philadelphia, 1984
COOLICAN, M. R., DANDY, D. J.: Arthroscopic management of synovial chondromatosis of the knee. Findings and results in 18 cases. J. Bone Joint Surg. (Br.) 71: 498–500 (1989)
DANDY, D. J., O'CAROLL, P. F.: The removal of loose bodies from the knee under arthroscopic control. J. Bone Joint Surg. (Br.) 64: 473–474 (1982)
EICHHORN, J., KRÄMER, J.: Praktische Tips zum arthroskopischen Operieren. Arthroskopie 1: 50 (1988)
JOYCE, J. J.: Osteochondral loose bodies, foreign bodies, osteochondritis dissecans. Pp. 173–188. In: PARISIEN, J.S. (ed.): Arthroscopic surgery. McGraw-Hill Book Company, New York, 1988
KAY, P. R., FREEMONT, A. J., DAVIES, D. R.: The aetiology of multiple loose bodies. Snow storm knee. J. Bone Joint Surg. (Br.) 71: 501–504 (1989)
McGINTY, J. B.: Arthroscopic removal of loose bodies. Orthop. Clin. North Am. 13: 313–318 (1982)

17.6.6 Plica syndrome (shelf syndrome)

ANDERSEN, E., POULSEN, T. D.: Plica mediopatellaris – arthroscopic resection under local anaesthesia. Arch. Orthop. Trauma. Surg. 106: 18–19 (1986)
BARBER, F. A.: Fenestrated medial patella plica. Arthroscopy 3: 253–257 (1987)
BROOM, M. J., FULKERSON, J. P.: The plica syndrome: A new perspective. Orthop. Clin. North Am. 17: 279–281 (1986)
HANSEN, H., BOE, S.: The pathological plica in the knee. Results after arthroscopic resection. Arch. Orthop. Trauma. Surg. 108: 282–4 (1989)
HARDAKER, W. T., WHIPPLE, T. L., BASSETT, F. H.: Diagnosis and treatment of the plica syndrome of the knee. J. Bone Joint Surg. (Am.) 62: 221 (1980)
HEMPFLING, H.: Systematik der Plicae im oberen Recessus. Pp. 81–85 In: HOFER, H. (ed.): Fortschritte in der Arthroskopie. Ferdinand Enke – Verlag, Stuttgart, 1985
HUGHSTON, J. C., STONE, M., ANDREWS, J. R.: The suprapatellar plica: Its role in internal derangement of the knee. J. Bone Joint Surg. (Am.) 55: 1318 (1973)
JACKSON, R. W., MARSHALL, D. J., FUJISAWA, Y.: The pathologic medial shelf. Orthop. Clin. North Am. 13: 307–312 (1982)
JOHANSEN, O.: Rupture of the medio-patellar plica. One of the many causes of anterior knee pain. Tidsskr. Nor. Laegeforen. 109: 1069–1070 (1989)
KOHN, D., BRÜCKL, R.: Die Mehrfachdurchtrennung der Plica synovialis mediopatellaris unter arthroskopischer Sicht – Nachuntersuchungsergebnisse. Pp. 96–101 In: HOFER, H. (ed.): Fortschritte in der Arthroskopie. Ferdinand Enke – Verlag, Stuttgart, 1985
KOSHINO, T., OKAMOTO, R.: Resection of painfull shelf (plica synovialis mediopatellaris) under arthroscopy. Arthroscopy 1: 136–141 (1985)
KLEIN, W., SCHULITZ, K. P., HUTH, F.: Die „Plica-Krankheit" des Kniegelenkes. Dtsch. Med. Wschr. 104: 1261–1264 (1979)
KLEIN, W.: The medial shelf of the knee: A follow-up study. Arch. Orthop. Trauma. Surg. 102: 67–72 (1983)
LÖHNERT, J., RAUNEST, J.: Das Plica-Syndrom des Kniegelenkes. Orthop. Praxis 22: 126–130 (1985)
MORALDO, M., SCHLEBERGER, R.: Besteht ein Zusammenhang zwischen der pathologischen Plica mediopatellaris und dem Krankheitsbild der Chondropathia patellae? Orthop. Praxis 24: 77–78 (1988)
MUNZINGER, U., RUCKSTUHL, J., SCHERRER, H., GSCHWEND, N.: Internal derangement of the knee joint

due to pathologic synovial folds: The mediopatellar plica syndrome. Clin. Orthop. 155: 59–63 (1981)
Muse, G. L., Grana, W. A., Hollingsworth, S.: Arthroscopic treatment of medial shelf syndrome. Arthroscopy 1: 63–67 (1985)
Nottage, W. M., Sprague, N. F., Auerbach, B. J., Shahriaree, H.: The medial patellar plica syndrome. Am. J. Sports Med. 11: 211–214 (1983)
Ogata, S., Uhthoff, H. K: The development of synovial plicae in human knee joints: an embryologic study. Arthroscopy 6: 315–321 (1990)
Older, J., Hanspal, R., Cardoso, T.: The medial shelf: An anatomical, clinical and pathological study. Pp. 82–86 In: Trickey, E.L., Hertel, P. (eds.): Surgery and arthroscopy of the knee. Springer, Berlin Heidelberg New York, 1986
Patel, D.: Arthroscopy of the plicae: Synovial folds and their significance. Am. J. Sports Med. 6: 217–225 (1978)
Patel, D.: Plica as a cause of anterior knee pain. Orthop. Clin. North Am. 17: 273–277 (1986)
Pipkin, G.: Knee injuries: the role of the suprapatellar plica and suprapatellar bursa in simulating internal derangement. Clin. Orthop. 74: 161 (1971)
Reider, B., Marshall, J. L., Warren, R. F.: Persistant vertical septum in the human knee joint. J. Bone Joint Surg. (Am.) 63: 1185–1187 (1981)
Richmond, J. C., McGinty, J. B.: Segmental arthroscopic resection of the hypertrophic mediopatellar plica. Clin. Orthop. 178: 185–189 (1983)
Sakakibara, J.: Arthroscopic study in Iino's band (plica synovialis mediopatellaris). J. Jap. Orthop. Ass. 50: 513–522 (1976)
Vaughan-Lane, T., Dandy, D. J.: The synovial shelf syndrome. J. Bone Joint Surg. (Br.) 64: 475–476 (1982)

17.6.7 Fibroarthrolysis

Delpizzo, W., Fox, J. M., Friedman, M., Snyder, S., Terkel, R.: Operative arthroscopy for the treatment of arthrofibrosis of the knee. Contemp. Orthop. 10: 67 (1985)
Jackson, D. W., Schaefer, R. K.: Cyclops syndrome: loss of extension following intra-articular anterior cruciate ligament reconstruction. Arthroscopy 6: 171–178 (1990)
O'Connor, R. L.: Intra-articular adhesions and fibrous ankylosis of the knee. Pp. 289–298 In: Shahriaree, H. (ed.): O'Connor's textbook of arthroscopic surgery. J.B. Lippincott Company, Philadelphia, 1984
Parisien, J. S.: The stiff knee. Pp. 163–171 In: Parisien, J. S. (ed.): Arthroscopic surgery. McGraw-Hill Book Company, New York, 1988
Sprague, N., O'Connor, R. L., Fox, J. M.: Arthroscopic treatment of postoperative knee fibroarthrosis. Clin. Orthop. 166: 165 (1982)

17.5.8 Therapy of Empyema

Ivey, M., Clark, R.: Arthroscopic debridement of the knee for septic arthritis. Clin. Orthop. 199: 201 (1985)
Ivey, M.: The infected knee. Pp. 155–161 In: Parisien, J.S. (ed.): Arthroscopic surgery. McGraw-Hill Book Company, New York 1988
Jackson, R. W.: The septic knee – arthroscopic treatment. Arthroscopy 1: 194–197 (1985)
Jackson, R. W., Parsons, C. J.: Distension – irrigation treatment of major joint sepsis. Clin. Orthop. 96: 160–163 (1973)
Jarrett, M. P., Grossmann, L., Sadler, A. H., Grayzel, A. L.: The role of arthroscopy in the treatment of septic arthritis. Arthritis Rheum. 24: 737- 739 (1981)
Montgomery, S. C., Campbell, J.: Septic arthritis following arthroscopy and intra-articular steroids. J. Bone Joint Surg. (Br.) 71: 540 (1989)
Nottage, W. M.: Arthroscopic management of the septic knee. Pp. 299–302 In: Shahriaree, H. (ed.): O'Connor's textbook of arthroscopic surgery. J. B. Lippincott Company, Philadelphia, 1984
Parisien, J. S.: Arthroscopic management of pyarthrosis. An overview. Bull. Hosp. Jt. Dis. Orthop. Inst. 47:52–57 (1987)
Schonholtz, G. J., Scott, W. O.: Moraxella septic arthritis of the knee joint. case report. Arthroscopy 2:96–97 (1986)
Smith, M. J.: Arthroscopic treatment of the septic knee. Arthroscopy 2:30–34 (1987)
Stanitski, C. L., Harvell, J. C, Fu, F. H.: Arthroscopy in acute septic knees. Management in pediatric patients. Clin. Orthop. 241: 209–212 (1989)
Strobel, M., Pässler, H.: Zur Behandlung der intraartikulären Infektion des Kniegelenkes. Chir. Praxis 41: 73–78 (1989)
Thiery, J. A.: Arthroscopic drainage in septic arthritides of the knee: a multicenter study. Arthroscopy. 5: 65–69 (1989)

17.6.9 Suturing and Reconstruction of the Anterior Cruciate Ligament

Bahuaud, J., Rebour, J., Mayer, J., Besse, D., Mautalen, F., Baspeyre, H.: Reconstruction of the anterior and posterior cruciate ligaments of the knee under arthroscopy. First results. Pp. 204–212 In: Müller, W., Hackenbruch, W. (eds.): Surgery and Arthroscopy of the knee. Springer, Berlin Heidelberg New York, 1988
Bartlett, E. C.: Arthroscopic repair and augmentation of the anterior cruciate ligament in cadaver knees. Clin. Orthop. 172: 107–111 (1983)
Benedetto, K. P.: Die Technik der arthroskopischen Kreuzbandplastik. Chirurg 55: 756–759 (1984)
Benedetto, K. P., Glötzer, W.: Die Technik der arthroskopischen Kreuzbandplastik mit dem Ptfe-

Band. Pp. 226–230 In: Hofer, H. (ed.): Fortschritte in der Arthroskopie. Ferdinand Enke – Verlag, Stuttgart, 1985

Boszotta, H., Wendrinsky, R., Sauer, G.: Eine neue Technik zur arthroskopischen Reinsertion und Augmentation des frisch gerissenen vorderen Kreuzbandes. Unfallchirurgie 14: 46–49 (1988)

Ferkel, R. D., Fox, J. M., Wood, D., Del Pizzo, W., Friedman, M. J., Snyder, S. J.: Arthroscopic „second look" at the Gore-Tex ligament. Am. J. Sports Med. 17: 147–152 (1989)

Fox, J. M., Sherman, O. H., Markolf, K.: Arthroscopic anterior cruciate ligament repair: Preliminary results and instrumented testing for anterior stability. Arthroscopy 1: 175–181 (1985)

Fox, J. M.: Arthroscopic insertion of the prothetic Gore-Tex ligament. Pp. 165–179. In: Friedman, M. J., Ferkel, R. D. (eds.): Prosthetic ligament reconstruction of the knee. W. B. Saunders Company, Philadephia, 1988

Fujikawa, K., Iseki, F., Seedhom, B. B.: Arthroscopy after anterior cruciate reconstruction with the Leeds-Keio ligament. J. Bone Joint Surg. (Br.) 71: 566–70 (1989)

Hales, A. L.: Arthroscopically assisted anterior cruciate ligament reconstruction. Aorn. J. 49: 234–255 (1989)

Imbert, J. C.: Acl reconstruction procedure with autogenous graft under arthroscopic control. Pp. 168–169 In: Müller, W., Hackenbruch, W. (eds.): Surgery and Arthroscopy of the knee. Springer, Berlin Heidelberg New York, 1988

Kariya, Y., Kurosawa, H.: Arthroscopically aided anterior cruciate ligament reconstruction using a new drill wire guide. Arthroscopy 5: 227–231 (1989)

Klein, W.: Technik des arthroskopisch-chirurgischen vorderen Kreuzbandersatzes. Pp. 148–153, In: Hofer, H. (ed.): Fortschritte in der Arthroskopie. Ferdinand Enke – Verlag, Stuttgart, 1985

Matthews, L. S., Soffer, S. R.: Pitfalls in the use of interference screws for anterior cruciate ligament reconstruction: brief report. Arthroscopy 5: 225–226 (1989)

Matthews, L. S., Martin, D. F., Wolock, B. S.: Accurate tunnel placement using drill guides in knee ligament reconstruction. Orthop. Rev. 19: 822–824 (1990)

Rehm, K. E.: Die geschlossene Kreuzbandplastik. Unfallchir. 7: 55–59 (1981)

Rehm, K. E., Schultheis, K. H.: Technik des endoskopischen Kreuzbandersatzes. Pp. 231–237 In: Hofer, H. (ed.): Fortschritte in der Arthroskopie. Ferdinand Enke – Verlag, Stuttgart, 1985

Rosenberg, T. D., Paulos, L. E., Parker, R. D.: Allograft anterior cruciate ligament reconstruction: an arthroscopically guided technique. Pp. 193–201. In: Friedman, M. J., Ferkel, R. D. (eds.): Prosthetic ligament reconstruction of the knee. W. B. Saunders Company, Philadephia, 1988

Rusch, R. M., Nelson, E. F., Noel, D.: Integraft™ anterior cruciate ligament reconstruction: arthroscopic technique. Pp. 59–64 In: Friedman, M. J., Ferkel, R. D. (eds.): Prosthetic ligament reconstruction of the knee. W. B. Saunders Company, Philadephia, 1988

Schmid, A., Schmid, F., Tiling, T.: Arthroskopische Versorgung der frischen vorderen Kreuzbandruptur. Entwicklung einer neuen OP-Technik und eines neuen Nahtmaterials. Arthroskopie 1: 83–89 (1988)

Shino, K., Inoue, M., Nakamura, H., Hamada, M., Ono, K.: Arthroscopic follow-up of anterior cruciate ligament reconstruction using allogeneic tendon. Arthroscopy 5: 165–171 (1989)

Springer, S. I.: Anterior cruciate ligament substitution: endoscopic technique. Pp. 213–220 In: Parisien, J. S. (ed.): Arthroscopic surgery. McGraw-Hill Book Company, New York, 1988

Springer, S. I.: Technique, complications and results of arthroscopic anterior cruciate ligament reconstructions with bioprothetic ligaments. Pp. 243–245 In: Müller, W., Hackenbruch, W. (eds.): Surgery and Arthroscopy of the knee. Springer, Berlin Heidelberg New York, 1988

Stadler, J., Steenblock, U., Holzach, P., Matter, P.: Arthroskopische Ersatzoperation des vorderen Kreuzbandes. Pp. 238–241 In: Hofer, H. (ed.): Fortschritte in der Arthroskopie. Ferdinand Enke – Verlag, Stuttgart, 1985

Strümper, R., Hertel, E.: Arthroskopische Naht des vorderen Kreuzbandes. Eine neue Technik und ein neues Instrumentarium. Arthroskopie 1: 78–82 (1988)

Whipple, T. L.: Arthroscopic anterior cruciate ligament reconstruction with Procol xenograft bioprothesis. Pp. 112–117. In: Friedman, M. J., Ferkel, R. D. (eds.): Prosthetic ligament reconstruction of the knee. W. B. Saunders Company, Philadephia, 1988

Wuschech, K., Kundiger, R., Heller, G., Wuschech, C.: Die Technik der arthroskopischen vorderen Kreuzbandplastik mit dem Kohlenstoffband. Zbl. Chir. 111: 409–413 (1986)

Yasuda, K., Tomiyama, Y., Ohkoshi, Y., Kaneda, K.: Arthroscopic observations of autogeneic quadriceps and patellar tendon grafts after anterior cruciate ligament reconstruction of the knee. Clin. Orthop. 246: 217–224 (1989)

Yasuda K., Aoki Y., Tomiyama Y., Ohkoshi Y., Kaneda K.: Maturation of autogenous tendon grafts in anterior cruciate ligament reconstruction of the human knee--an arthroscopic study. Nippon. Seikeigeka Gakkai Zasshi 63: 59–66 (1989)

17.6.10 Synovectomy

Aritomi, H., Yamamoto, M.: A method of arthroscopic surgery: Clinical evaluation of synovectomy with the electric resector scope and removal of loose bodies in the knee joint. Orthop. Clin. North Am. 10: 565–584 (1989)

Arnold, W. J., Kalunian, K.: Arthroscopic synovectomy by rheumatologists: time for a new look. Arthritis. Rheum. 32: 109–111 (1989)

Beguin, J., Locker, B., Vielpeau, C., Souquieres G.:

Pigmented villonodular synovitis of the knee: results from 13 cases. Arthroscopy. 5: 62–64 (1989)
BITTAR, E. S.: Arthroscopic knee synovectomy. Pp. 688 – 689 In: MÜLLER, W., HACKENBRUCH, W. (eds.): Surgery and Arthroscopy of the knee. Springer, Berlin Heidelberg New York, 1988
COHEN, S., JONES, R.: An evaluation of the efficiency of arthroscopic synovectomy of the knee in rheumatoid arthritis: 12–24 month results. J. Rheumatol. 14: 452–455 (1987)
COMBE, B., KRAUSE, E., SANY, J.: Treatment of chronic knee synovitis with arthroscopic synovectomy after failure of intraarticular injection of radionuclide. Arthritis Rheum. 32: 10–14 (1989)
DORFMANN, H., DE BIE, B., BONVARLET, J. P., BOYER, T.: Arthroscopic treatment of synovial chondromatosis of the knee. Arthroscopy 5: 48–51 (1989)
GUAYDIER SOUQUIERES, C., BEGUIN, J., OLLIVIER, D., LOYAU, G.: Knee arthroscopy after yttrium or osmic acid injection. Arthroscopy 5: 70–5 (1989)
HIGHGENBOTEN, C.: Arthroscopic synovectomy. Clin. Orthop. North Am. 13: 399–405 (1982)
HIGHGENBOTEN, C.: Arthroscopic synovectomy. Arthroscopy 1: 190–193 (1985)
HIGHGENBOTEN, C.: Synovial disease. Pp. 147–154 In: PARISIEN, J.S. (ed.): Arthroscopic surgery. McGraw-Hill Book Company, New York, 1988
KLEIN, K. S., ALAND, C. M., KIM, H. C., EISELE, J., SAIDI, P.: Long term follow-up of arthroscopic synovectomy for chronic hemophilic synovitis. Arthroscopy 3: 231–236 (1987)
KLEIN, W.: Die arthroskopische Synovektomie beim künstlichen Kniegelenk. Fallbericht. Arthroskopie 1: 148–152 (1988)
LOCKER, B., BEGUIN, J., VIELPEAU, C., LOYAU, G.: Pigmented villonodular synovitis of the knee: advantages of arthroscopy. Pp. 661 – 665 In: MÜLLER, W., HACKENBRUCH, W. (eds.): Surgery and Arthroscopy of the knee. Springer, Berlin Heidelberg New York, 1988
MATSUI, N., TANEDA, Y., OHTA, H., ITOH, T., TSUBOGUCHI, S.: Arthroscopic versus open synovectomy in the rheumatoid knee. Int. Orthop. 13: 17–20 (1989)
MORALDO, M., SCHLEBERGER, R., HEDTMANN, A.: Synovectomy applied to inflammatory rheumatic diseases of the knee unter arthroscopic control. Pp. 690 – 694 In: MÜLLER, W., HACKENBRUCH, W. (eds.): Surgery and Arthroscopy of the knee. Springer, Berlin Heidelberg New York, 1988
SHIBATA, T., SHIRAOKA, K., TAKUBO, N.: Comparison between arthroscopic and open synovectomy for the knee in rheumatoid arthritis. Arch. Orthop. Trauma. Surg. 105: 257–262 (1986)
WIEDEL, J. D.: Arthroscopic synovectomy for chronic hemophilic synovitis of the knee. Arthroscopy 1: 205–209 (1985)

17.6.11
Fracture of the tibial head

CASPARI, R. B.: Arthroscopy and the management of fractures of the tibial plateau. Pp. 197–200 In: SHAHRIAREE, H. (ed.): O'Connor's textbook of arthroscopic surgery. J. B. Lippincott Company, Philadelphia, 1984
CASPARI, R. B., HUTTON, P. M., WHIPPLE, T. L., MEYERS, J. F.: The role of arthroscopy in the management of tibial plateau fractures. Arthoscopy 1: 76 (1985)
HOLZACH, P., MATTER, P.: Arthroskopie und Osteosynthese von Tibiaplateaufrakturen. Arthroskopie 1: 74–77 (1988)
JENNINGS, J. C.: Arthroscopic management of tibial plateau fractures. Arthroscopy 1: 160 (1985)

17.6.12
Patellar dislocation – lateral release

AGLIETTI, P., PISANESCHI, A., BUZZI, R., GAUDENZI, A., ALLEGRA, M.: Arthroscopic lateral release for patellar pain or instability. Arthroscopy 5: 176–183 (1989)
BRAY, R. C., ROTH, J. H., JACOBSEN, R. P.: Arthroscopic lateral release for anterior knee pain: a study comparing patients who are claiming worker's compensation with those who are not. Arthroscopy 3: 237–247 (1987)
DANDY, D. J., GRIFFITHS, D.: Lateral release for recurrent dislocation of the patella. J. Bone Joint Surg. (Br.) 71: 121–125 (1989)
DZIOBA, R. B., STROKON, A., MULBRY, L.: Diagnostic arthroscopy and longitudinal open lateral relaese: A safe and effective treatment for „chondromalacia patellae". Arthroscopy 1: 131–135 (1985)
DZIOBA, R. B.: Diagnostic arthroscopy and longitudinal open lateral release. A four year follow-up study to determine predictors of surgical outcome. Am. J. Sports Med. 18: 343–348 (1990)
FARID, F.: Indikation und Technik der arthroskopischen Patella-Realignment- Operation (Fesselung) nach Johnson mit Hilfe von neu entwickeltem Instrumentarium. Orthop. Praxis 24: 162–167 (1988)
HENRY, J. H., GOLETZ, T. H., WILLIAMSON, B.: Lateral retinacular release in patellofemoral subluxation. Indications, results and comparison to open patellofemoral reconstruction. Am. J. Sports Med. 14: 121–129 (1986)
HERTEL, P., VERSCHL, J.: Arthroskopie bei der akuten Patellaluxation. Arthroskopie 1: 68–73 (1988)
HUGHSTON, J. C., DEESE, M.: Medial subluxation of the patella as a complication of lateral retinacular release. Am. J. Sports Med. 16: 383–388 (1988)
LANKENNER, P. A., MICHELI, L., CLANCY, R., GERBINO, P. G.: Arthroscopic percutaneous lateral patellar retinacular release. Am. J. Sports Med. 14: 267–269 (1986)
MCGINTY, J. B., MCCARTHY, J. C.: Endoscopical lateral retinacular release of the subluxating or dislocating patella. Clin. Orthop. 167: 9–17 (1982)

METCALF, R. W.: An arthroscopic method for lateral release of the subluxating or dislocating patella. Clin. Orthop. 167: 9–18 (1982)

MILLER, R., BARTLETT, J.: Recurrent dislocation of the patella treated by arthroscopic lateral release. J. Bone Joint Surg. (Br.) 71: 159 (1989)

SCHLEBERGER, R., MORALDO, M., PEISELER, U.: Die Behandlung der chronischen, therapieresistenten Chondropathia patellae durch die arthroskopisch kontrollierte laterale Kapselspaltung. Orthop. Praxis 24: 160–161 (1988)

SCHONHOLTZ, G. J., ZAHN, M. G., MAGEE, C. M.: Lateral retinacular release of the patella. Arthroscopy 3: 269–272 (1987)

SHERMAN, O. H., FOX, J. M., SPERLING, H., DEL PIZZO, W., FRIEDMANN, M. J., SNYDER, S. J., FERKEL, R. D.: Patellar instability: treatment by arthroscopic electrosurgical lateral release. Arthroscopy 3: 152–160 (1987)

SIMPSON, L. A., BARRETT, J. P.: Factors associated with poor results following arthroscopic subcutaneous lateral release. Clin. Orthop. 186: 165–171 (1984)

VERNACE, J. V., ROTHMAN, R. H., BOOTH, R. E., BALDERSTON, R. A.: Arthroscopic management of the patellar clunk syndrome following posterior stabilized total knee arthroplasty. J. Arthroplasty. 4: 179–82 (1989)

WASILEWSKI, S. A., PURNELL, M. B., COHEN, S.: Rehabilitation after arthroscopic lateral retinacular release. Orthop. Rev. 18: 1011–1018 (1989)

YERYS, P.: A technique for lateral retinacular release. Arthroscopy 1: 233- 236 (1985)

17.7 Komplikationen

ANDERSON, A. F., ALFREY, D., LIPSCOMB, A. B.: Acute pulmonary edema, an unusual complication following arthroscopy: a report of three cases. Arthroscopy 6: 235–7 (1990)

BACHNER, E. J., PARKER, R. D., ZAAS, R. D.: Resection of the patellar ligament: a complication of arthroscopic synovectomy. Arthroscopy 5: 76–78 (1989)

BECK, D. E., ROBISON, J. G., HALLETT, J. W.: Popliteal artery pseudoaneurysm following arthroscopy. J. Trauma 26: 87–89 (1986)

BERNHANG, A. M.: Clostridium pyoarthrosis following arthroscopy. Arthroscopy 3: 56–58 (1987)

BLASIER, R. B., CIULLO, J. V.: Rupture of the quadriceps tendon after arthroscopic lateral release. Arthroscopy 2: 262–263 (1986)

BUNKER, T. D., THOMAS, E.: Ruptured semimembranosus bursa: a complication of arthroscopy. Injury 15: 182 (1984)

CARLSEN, A.: A broken telescope: A complication of arthroscopy. Arthroscopy 2: 182–183 (1986)

CHRISTOPHER, G. W., JURIK, J. A., JANECKI, C. J., HAAKE, P. W., RILEY, G. J., CHESSIN, L. N.: Meningococcal arthritis, bacteremia and osteomyelitis following arthroscopy. Report of a case. Clin. Orthop. 171: 127–130 (1982)

COLLINS, J. J.: Knee-joint arthroscopy--early complications. Med. J. Aust. 150: 702–706 (1989)

DELEE, J. C.: Complications of arthroscopy and arthroscopic surgery: Results of a national survey. Arthroscopy 1: 214–220 (1985)

DICK, W., GLINZ, W., HENCHE, H. R., RUCKSTUHL, J., WRUHS, O., ZOLLINGER, H.: Komplikationen der Arthroskopie. Eine Analyse von 3714 Fällen. Arch. Orthop. Trauma. Surg. 92: 69–73 (1978)

DUNN, P. M., POST, R. H., JONES, S. R.: Thromboembolic complications of knee arthroscopy. Western J. Med. 140: 291 (1984)

FARBER, B. F., BROOME, C. V., HOPKINS, C. C.: Fulminant hospital acquired toxic shock syndrome. Am. J. Med. 77: 331–332 (1984)

FIDDAN, N. J., PORRIER, H.: The morbidity of arthroscopy of the knee. J. Bone Joint Surg. (Br.) 63: 630 (1981)

FOX, J. M., MESSINEO, B. L.: Vascular complications. Pp. 107–124. In: SPRAGUE, N. F. (ed.) Complications in arthroscopy. Raven Press, New York 1989

GAMBARDELLA, R. A., TIBONE, J. E.: Knife blade in the knee joint: A complication of arthroscopic surgery. A case report. Am. J. Sports Med. 11: 267–268 (1983)

GROSS, M. L., FINERMAN, G. A. M.: Thromboembolic complications. p 21–26. In: SPRAGUE, N. F. (ed.) Complications in arthroscopy. Raven, New York, 1989

GRÜNWALD, J., KIESER, C.: Zwei tödliche Luftembolien während Akut- Arthroskopie im gasförmigen Medium. Arthroskopie 1: 90–93 (1988)

GRÜNWALD, J.: Fatal air embolism during arthroscopy. J. Bone Joint Surg. (Br.) 72: 929 (1990)

HABEGGER, R., SIEBENMANN R., KIESER C.: Lethal air embolism during arthroscopy. A case report. J. Bone Joint Surg. (Br.) 71: 314–316 (1989)

HADIED, A. M.: An unusual complication of arthroscopy: A fistula between the knee and the prepatellar bursa. Case report. J. Bone Joint Surg. (Am.) 66: 624 (1984)

HARNER, C. D., FU F. H., MASON G. C., WISSINGER H. A., RABIN B. S.: Cidex-induced synovitis. Am-J. Sports Med. 17: 96–102 (1989)

HENDERSON, C. E., HOPSON, C. N.: Pneumoscrotum as a complication of arthroscopy. J. Bone Joint Surg. (Am.) 64: 1238–1240 (1982)

JACKSON, R. W.: Septic and aseptic synovitis. p. 11–20. In: SPRAGUE, N. F. (ed.) Complications in arthroscopy. Raven, New York, 1989

JEFFRIES, J. T., GAINOR, B. J., ALLEN, W. C., CIKRIT, D.: Injury to the popliteal artery as a complication of arthroscopic surgery. J. Bone Joint Surg. (Am.) 69: 783–785 (1987)

JURIST, K. A., GREENE, P. W., SHIRHODA, A.: Peroneal nerve disfunction as a complication of lateral meniscus repair: a case report and anatomic dissection. Arthroscopy. 5: 141–147 (1989)

KATZ, M. M., HUNGERFORD, D. S.: Reflex sympathetic dystrophy affecting the knee. J. Bone Joint Surg. (Br.) 69: 797–803 (1987)

KETTERL, R., BECKURTS T., KOVACS J., STUBINGER B., HIPP R., CLAUDI B.: Gas-gangrene following arthroscopic surgery. Arthroscopy. 5: 79–83 (1989)

KOHL, J. M.: Anesthesia complications. Pp. 27–52. In: SPRAGUE, N. F. (ed.) Complications in arthroscopy. Raven, New York, 1989

KOORNNEEF, M. L., VAN HOUTE, D. P. F., OLSTHOORN, P. G. M., FIDLER, M. W.: Hepatitis B antigen in joint irrigation fluid. J. Bone Joint Surg. (Br.) 69: 662–663 (1987)

LAIS, E., HERTEL, P., GEORGOULIS, A.: Cartilaginous lesions following medial arthroscopic meniscectomy. S. 77–79 In: TRICKEY, E. L., HERTEL, P. (eds.): Surgery and arthroscopy of the knee. Springer, Berlin Heidelberg New York, 1986

LINDENBAUM, B. L.: Complications of knee joint arthroscopy. Clin. Orthop. 160: 158 (1981)

LOEW, M.: Sudecksche Dystrophie nach Arthroskopie des Kniegelenkes – eine Fallbeschreibung. Aktuel. Traumatol. 18: 157–159 (1988)

LOTMANN, D. B.: Pneumoperitoneum and acidosis during arthroscopy with CO_2. Arthroscopy 3: 185–186 (1987)

MANNING, M. P., MARSHALL, J. H.: Aneurysm after arthroscopy. J. Bone Joint Surg. (Br.) 69: 151 (1987)

MCGINTY, J. B.: Complications of arthroscopy and arthroscopic surgery. Pp. 221–228 In: PARISIEN, J. S. (ed.): Arthroscopic surgery. McGraw-Hill Book Company, New York, 1988

MCGINTY, J. B.: Ligament, bone, and nerve complications. p 87–106. In: SPRAGUE, N. F. (ed.) Complications in arthroscopy. Raven, New York, 1989

METCALF, R. W.: Instrumented related complications. Pp. 75–86. In: SPRAGUE, N. F. (ed.) Complications in arthroscopy. Raven, New York, 1989

NOYES, F. R., SPIEVACK, E. S.: Extra-articular fluid dissection in tissue during arthroscopy. Am. J. Sports Med. 10: 346 (1982)

PEEK, R. D., HAYNES, D. W.: Compartment syndrome as a complication of arthroscopy: A case report and a study of interstitial pressures. Am. J. Sports Med. 12: 464–468 (1984)

POEHLING, G. G., KOMAN, L. A., POLLOCK, F. E.: Reflex sympathetic dystrophy of the knee. Pp. 53–74. In: SPRAGUE, N. F. (ed.) Complications in arthroscopy. Raven, New York, 1989

ROBERTS, T. S., DREZ, D., BANTA C. J.: Complications of the anterior cruciate ligament reconstruction. pp, 169–178. In: SPRAGUE, N. F. (ed.) Complications in arthroscopy. Raven, New York, 1989

ROSENBERG, T. D., KOLOWICH, P. A.: Complications of the lateral retinacular release. Pp. 145–156. In: SPRAGUE, N. F. (ed.) Complications in arthroscopy. Raven, New York, 1989

SHERMAN, O. H., FOX, J. M., SNYDER, S. J., DEL PIZZO, W., FRIEDMAN, M. J., FERKEL, R. D., LAWELY, M. J.: Arthroscopy „no problem surgery". An analysis of complications in 2640 cases. J. Bone Joint Surg. (Am.) 68: 256–265 (1986)

SHUPACK, R. C., SHUSTER, H., FUNCH, R. S.: Airway emergency in a patient during CO_2 arthroscopy. Anesthesiology 60: 171 (1984)

SMALL, N. C.: Complications in arthroscopy: the knee and other joints. Arthroscopy 2: 253–258 (1986)

SMALL, N. C.: Complications in arthroscopic surgery performed by experienced arthroscopists. Arthroscopy 4: 215–221 (1989)

Small, N. C.: Overview of arthroscopic surgery complications. p,. 1–10. In: SPRAGUE, N. F. (ed.) Complications in arthroscopy. Raven, New York, 1989

SPRAGUE, N. F.: Minor and soft tissue complications. Pp. 125–144. In: SPRAGUE, N. F. (ed.) Complications in arthroscopy. Raven, New York, 1989

STONE, R. G., SPRAGUE, N. F.: Complications of arthroscopic menical repair. Pp. 157–168. In: SPRAGUE, N. F. (ed.) Complications in arthroscopy. Raven, New York, 1989

STRINGER, M. D., STEADMAN, C. A., HEDGES, A. R., THOMAS, E. M., MORLEY, T. R., KAKKAR, V. V.: Deep vein thrombosis after elective knee surgery. An incidence study in 312 patients. J. Bone Joint Surg. (Br.) 71: 492–7 (1989)

TOYE, B.: Staphylococcus epidermidis septic arthritis post arthroscopy. Clin. Exp. Rheumatol. 5: 165–166 (1987)

WALKER, R. M., DILLINGHAM, M.: Thrombophlebitis following arthroscopic surgery of the knee. Contemp. Orthop. 6: 29–33 (1983)

WALTHER, H., TURBA, M., AIGNER, K. R.: Splenic rupture following arthroscopy. Unfallchirurgie 16: 210–212 (1990)

17.8 Documentation

BROWN, C. H.: Producing still images in arthroscopy. Arthroscopy 5: 87–92 (1989)

EICHHORN, J., STROBEL, M.: Dokumentation und Therapiekontrolle. In: CHASSAING, V., PARIER, J.: Arthroskopie des Kniegelenkes, Diagnostik und operative Therapie. Deutscher Ärzte – Verlag, Cologne, 1988

JOHNSON, L. L.: A rationale for systematized record keeping and improved documentation. Arthroscopy 3: 258–264 (1987)

KLEIN, W.: Praxisgerechte Dokumentation arthroskopischer Eingriffe am Kniegelenk mit grafischer Darstellung und MS-Dos Software. (personal communication) (1989)

Subject Index

MIX
Papier aus verantwortungsvollen Quellen
Paper from responsible sources
FSC® C105338

If you have any concerns about our products,
you can contact us on
ProductSafety@springernature.com

In case Publisher is established outside the EU,
the EU authorized representative is:
Springer Nature Customer Service Center GmbH
Europaplatz 3, 69115 Heidelberg, Germany

Printed by Libri Plureos GmbH
in Hamburg, Germany